ADVANCES IN CIRRHOSIS, HYPERAMMONEMIA, AND HEPATIC ENCEPHALOPATHY

ADVANCES IN EXPERIMENTAL MEDICINE AND BIOLOGY

Recent Volumes in this Series

Volume 411
OXYGEN TRANSPORT TO TISSUE XVIII
Edited by Edwin M. Nemoto and Joseph C. LaManna

Volume 412
MECHANISMS IN THE PATHOGENESIS OF ENTERIC DISEASES
Edited by Prem S. Paul, David H. Francis, and David A. Benfield

Volume 413
OPTICAL IMAGING OF BRAIN FUNCTION AND METABOLISM 2: Physiological Basis and Comparison to Other Functional Neuroimaging Methods
Edited by Arno Villringer and Ulrich Dirnagl

Volume 414
ENZYMOLOGY AND MOLECULAR BIOLOGY OF CARBONYL METABOLISM 6
Edited by Henry Weiner, Ronald Lindahl, David W. Crabb, and T. Geoffrey Flynn

Volume 415
FOOD PROTEINS AND LIPIDS
Edited by Srinivasan Damodaran

Volume 416
PLATELET-ACTIVATING FACTOR AND RELATED LIPID MEDIATORS 2: Roles in Health and Disease
Edited by Santosh Nigam, Gert Kunkel, and Stephen M. Prescott

Volume 417
DENDRITIC CELLS IN FUNDAMENTAL AND CLINICAL IMMUNOLOGY, Volume 3
Edited by Paola Ricciardi-Castagnoli

Volume 418
STREPTOCOCCI AND THE HOST
Edited by Thea Horaud, Anne Bouvet, Roland Leclercq, Henri de Monclos, and Michel Sicard

Volume 419
ADP-RIBOSYLATION IN ANIMAL TISSUES: Structure, Function, and Biology of Mono (ADP-ribosyl) Transferases and Related Enzymes
Edited by Friedrich Haag and Friedrich Koch-Nolte

Volume 420
ADVANCES IN CIRRHOSIS, HYPERAMMONEMIA, AND HEPATIC ENCEPHALOPATHY
Edited by Vicente Felipo and Santiago Grisolía

ADVANCES IN CIRRHOSIS, HYPERAMMONEMIA, AND HEPATIC ENCEPHALOPATHY

Edited by

Vicente Felipo and
Santiago Grisolía
Instituto de Investigaciones Citologicas de la F. V. I. B.
Valencia, Spain

SPRINGER SCIENCE+BUSINESS MEDIA, LLC

Library of Congress Cataloging-in-Publication Data

Advances in cirrhosis, hyperammonemia, and hepatic encephalopathy / edited by Vicente Felipo and Santiago Grisolia.
p. cm. -- (Advances in experimental medicine and biology ; v. 420)
"Proceedings of the International Symposium on Cirrhosis, Hyperammonemia, and Hepatic Encephalopathy, held December 2-4, 1996, in Valencia, Spain"--T.p. verso.
Includes bibliographical references and index.
ISBN 978-0-306-45598-8 ISBN 978-1-4615-5945-0 (eBook)
DOI 10.1007/978-1-4615-5945-0
1. Hepatic encephalopathy--Congresses. 2. Ammonia--Toxicology--Congresses. 3. Liver--Cirrhosis--Complications--Congresses.
I. Grisolía, Santiago, 1923- . II. International Symposium on Cirrhosis, Hyperammonemia, and Hepatic Encephalopathy (1996 : Valencia, Spain) III. Series.
[DNLM: 1. Liver Cirrhosis--congresses. 2. Ammonia--metabolism--congresses. 3. Ammonia--pharmacokinetics--congresses. 4. Urea--metabolism--congresses. 5. Hepatic Encephalopathy--congresses.
W1 AD559 v.420 1997 / WI 725 A244 1997]
RC848.H4A375 1997
616.3'62--dc21
DNLM/DLC
for Library of Congress 97-4391
CIP

Proceedings of the International Symposium on Cirrhosis, Hyperammonemia, and Hepatic Encephalopathy, held December 2 – 4, 1996, in Valencia, Spain

ISBN 978-0-306-45598-8

http://www.plenum.com

10 9 8 7 6 5 4 3 2 1

PREFACE

This volume contains the papers presented at the International Symposium on "Cirrhosis, Hyperammonemia and Hepatic Encephalopathy," held in Valencia, Spain, December 2nd–4th, 1996.

Liver cirrhosis is one of the main causes of death in occidental countries. There are other hepatic dysfunctions such as fulminant hepatic failure, Reye's syndrome, or congenital deficiencies of urea cycle enzymes which can also lead to hepatic encephalopathy, coma and death. However, the molecular bases of the pathogenesis of hepatic encephalopathy remain unclear.

One of the consequences of hepatic failure is the reduced ability to detoxify ammonia by incorporating it into urea. This leads to increased blood ammonia levels. Hyperammonemia is considered one of the main factors responsible for the mediation of hepatic encephalopathy and classical clinical treatments are directed towards reducing blood ammonia levels.

Altered neurotransmission is an essential step in the pathogenesis of hepatic encephalopathy. The first part of the book is devoted to the discussion of the recent advances in the understanding of the alterations of different neurotransmitter systems in hepatic encephalopathy.

The alterations of tryptophan metabolism and neurotransmission in hepatic encephalopathy and the implications for the clinical use of neuropsychoactive drugs are reviewed.

The alterations in glutamate transport and neurotransmission in hepatic encephalopathy due to acute liver failure are also reviewed.The role of NMDA receptors in the molecular mechanism of acute ammonia toxicity is discussed as well as its modulation by metabotropic glutamate receptors and muscarinic receptors.

The possible role of some endogenous indole derivatives, affecting neurotransmission, in the pathogenesis of hepatic encephalopathy is also discussed.

The effects of ammonia on GABAergic neurotransmission and the contribution of alterations in this neurotransmitter system to the pathogenesis of hepatic encephalopathy are discussed.

The role of astrocytes and of the alterations in peripheral benzodiazepine receptors and neurosteroids in hepatic encephalopathy are reviewed.

In the following chapter there is a detailed discussion of the possible utility of ornithine aminotransferase as a therapeutic target in hyperammonemias.

To clarify the mechanisms involved in hyperammonemia and hepatic encephalopathy suitable animal models are required. Sparse-fur mice are congenitally deficient in ornithine trancarbamylase and are, therefore, a suitable model of hyperammonemia, resembling human congenital deficiencies in the enzyme. The main characteristics of the model as well as the alterations in neurotransmitter systems are reviewed.

Another mutant mouse showing autosomal recessive juvenile visceral steatosis presents symptoms very similar to those of Reye's syndrome, including hyperammonemia, fatty liver, hypoglycemia and growth retardation. The mechanisms of abnormal gene expression causing hyperammonemia in these mice as well as the reversion by carnitine treatment are discussed.

The differences between the encephalopathy caused by ammonia in rats with portal systemic shunting and in normal rats and the possible implications are also discussed.

The use of noninvasive techniques for diagnosis and study of human illnesses is very convenient. The application of in vivo magnetic resonance spectroscopy in the study of hyperammonemia and hepatic encephalopathy and the new findings provided by this technology are reviewed.

Acute liver failure is usually associated with cell swelling and increased intracraneal pressure. The recently discovered intracellular signalling mechanisms which link the osmotic water shift across the plasma membrane to changes in cell function are reviewed in detail.

The interplay between ammonia metabolism and detoxification, and the regulation of acid-base balance is also presented.

It is well known that liver cirrhosis is associated with abnormalities of carbohydrate metabolism, alteration of insulin levels and insulin resistance. The current knowledge about the mechanisms involved in these alterations is reviewed.

There is increasing evidence that Alzheimer's disease is associated with increased brain ammonia. The possible contribution of ammonia to the deletereous effects of Alzheimer's disease is discussed.

Finally, by this moment, the more efficient treatment for hepatic failure is in many cases liver transplantation. However, the number of donors is insufficient. This problem is very important in the pediatric population. One possibility to solve this problem is to transplant liver grafts from living related donors. The results of the use of this technique are presented in the last chapter of the book.

The book provides therefore an update of the knowledge about certain crucial aspects of the causes and mechanisms of hyperammonemia and hepatic encephalopathy.

We would like to express our gratitude to all participants for their written contributions and for their enlightened and fruitful discussion.

We also acknowledge with deep gratitude, the financial support of the Ministerio de Sanidad y Consumo, Ministerio de Educación y Ciencia, Consellerías de Sanidad y Educación de la Generalitat Valenciana and Sigma-Tau Laboratories. We also thank the Fundación Valenciana de Estudios Avanzados, which provided both the facilities for organizing the Symposium and for the sessions.

Vicente Felipo
Santiago Grisolía

CONTENTS

BRAIN TRYPTOPHAN PERTURBATION IN HEPATIC ENCEPHALOPATHY: IMPLICATIONS FOR EFFECTS BY NEUROPSYCHOACTIVE DRUGS IN CLINICAL PRACTICE

Finn Bengtsson, Peter B.F. Bergqvist and Gustav Apelqvist

Department of Clinical Pharmacology, Lund University Hospital
S-221 85 Lund, SWEDEN

INTRODUCTION

The neuropsychiatric disorder resulting from hepatocerebral dysfunction

The syndromes encountered within the term metabolic encephalopathy may be defined as "any metabolic disease that disrupts normal cerebral function" (Conn and Bircher, 1988). In the case of liver dysfunction, the terms hepatic encephalopathy (HE) or portal-systemic encephalopthy (PSE) are frequently used. In the human and clinical situation, these HE/PSE disorders are recognized as acute, chronic or, most commonly, acute-on-chronic events. The central nervous system (CNS) processes accompanying the patient suffering from HE/PSE probably include a mixture of reversible as well as irreversible changes of neuronal function (Victor *et al.* 1965; Victor 1974, 1979; see also Conn and Lieberthal, 1979). Thus, clinical HE/PSE, which almost inexclusively have included previous or even ongoing exposure to e.g. liver affecting agents, like those related to a variety of acute or chronic infectious or immunological processes, as well as intake of liver toxins such as ethanol. Since the chronic abuse of alcohol is not an uncommon major cause for a subsequently appearing liver cirrhosis, in turn related to the etiology chronic PSE in many clinical cases by blood vessel collateral development bypassing the liver parenchyma, it should be kept in mind that this type of abuse will most certainly exert effects of its own on the CNS in patients with chronic PSE involving aspects of acute, chronic as well as acute-on-chronic CNS effects of ethanol concomitantly to the encephalopathy component provided by the "isolated" PSE per se. Of course, in the clinical setting the isolated effects on the brain of chronic PSE is almost impossible to purify in scientific terms whereas, however, this pure type of chronic PSE may be identified in experimental in vivo models available such as most prominently evidenced by the advent of the surgically induced end-to-side portacaval shunt (PCS) in the rat (Lee and Fisher, 1961).

In contrast to a multitude of usually mixed neuronal and glial (and frequently also endothelial; notably the blood-brain barrier) morphology or structurally defined lesions of the brain parenchyma that may display a reversible or irreversible rostral-caudal progression of CNS symptomatology (as also an indicator of changes in severity within such conditions), the metabolic encephalopathies are usually referred to a group of disorders that exhibit fluctuating CNS-symptoms sometimes rapidly altering also in location of brain region of engagement, indicating a continuous change on the level at which the brain functions are disturbed. In the clinical situation of HE/PSE this is also true, but differently to the idealised PSE situation in the chronic PCS rat, the former situation will comprise a progressive disorder whereas the latter seems to be rather non-progressive and completely without morphological changes in the brain except those typically engaging astrocytes in an hyperammonemic state (i.e. the so called Alzheimer type-II astrocytosis; see e.g. Bengtsson *et al.*, 1988a).

Despite immense research efforts to clarify the pathological mechanisms involved, the more precise pathogenesis of PSE is still mainly unknown, also that which refers to the involvement of brain tryptophan (TRP)/serotonin (5-hydroxytryptophan; 5-HT) (for recent reviews, Conn and Bircher, 1988; Bengtsson *et al.*, 1989b; Butterworth, 1992b, 1993, 1994; Rao *et al.*, 1992; Mousseau and Butterworth, 1994b; Bengtsson and Bergqvist, 1996). As mentioned above, rats subjected to a permanent PCS do display that some amino acids transport systems across the blood-brain barrier are specifically affected (James *et al.*, 1978, 1979; Mans *et al.*, 1982) but otherwise no major structural or functional alterations of the blood-brain barrier in chronic PSE have been reported (Sarna *et al.*, 1977; Crinquette *et al.*, 1982). The energy state of the CNS has been suspected to be influenced in severe PSE (Bessman and Bessman, 1955; Schenker and Mendelson, 1964) but it seems more likely that this change in the cerebral energy state is the result rather than the cause of the coma associated with more severe forms of PSE. This indicates that a reduced neuronal activity in the brain in PSE may result in a decreased energy need and, consequently, reduced glucose consumption (Hindfelt *et al.*, 1977).

Neuropsychiatric symptomatology in HE/PSE. The importance of the notion above concerning the PCS rat versus the human conditions encountering chronic PSE in relation to the neuropsychiatric symptomatology are thus, at least, two-fold: Firstly, differently to the human situation of HE/PSE the chronic PCS rat most likely displays the manifold of CNS-derived behavioral abnormalities reproducibly evidenced (see e.g. Bengtsson *et al.*, 1985, 1986; Theander *et al.*, 1996; Apelqvist *et al.*, 1996a) primarily based on a more or less purely neurotransmission-related disturbance involving dynamic neuronal dysfunction rather than including also a structural neuronal damage. Secondly, the great variety of CNS-effects as has been evidenced to accompany the chronic PCS rat (for overviews, see e.g. Bengtsson *et al.*, 1989; Mans *et al.*, 1990; Butterworth 1994) are most likely all of them of some relevance to the clinical condition of chronic HE/PSE. However, the further features adding to the complexity for the CNS-symptoms as seen in clinical picture of HE/PSE may not necessarily adhere to the PCS rat behavioral abnormality. A spectrum of some of the more commen neuropsychiatric symptoms displayed in clinical HE/PSE of different severity (HE/PSE grade 0-4) are shown in Table 1.

Table 1. Spectrum of disordered mental state in portal-systemic encephalopathy (modified from reference Conn and Lieberthal, 1979)

Grade of HE/PSE	State of Consciousness	Intellectual Function	Personality-Behavior
0 (Normal)	- No abnormality	- No abnormality	- No abnormality
1 (Mild impairment)	- Hyperinsomnia	- Subtly impaired computations	- Euphoria or depression
	- Inversed sleep pattern	- Shortened attention span	- Irritability
2 (Moderate impairm.)	- Slow responses	- Loss of time	- Overt personality change
	- Minimal disorientation	- Impaired computations	- Anxiety or apathy
	- Lethargy	- Amnesia for past events	- Schizotypic behaviors
3 (Severe impairm.)	- Somnolence	- Loss of place	- Paranoia or anger
	- Confusion	- Inability to compute	- Rage
4 (Coma)	- Stupor	- Loss of self	- None
	- Unconscious	- No intellect	

Neurotransmission failure in HE/PSE

A substantial body of evidence suggests PSE to be associated with disturbances in different neurotransmitter systems in the brain. For example, perturbations have been demonstrated in the cholinergic system (Rao *et al.*, 1994a) as well as in the glutamatergic (Butterworth, 1992a; Rao *et al.*, 1992), GABA-ergic (Basile *et al.*, 1991), and other amino acidergic systems (Bucci *et al.*, 1980; Rao *et al.*, 1995; for overview, Conn and Lieberthal, 1979; Conn and Bircher, 1988; Butterworth, 1994, 1996; Mousseau and Butterworth,

1994b). In 1971, Fischer and Baldessarini proposed the fascinating so-called "false neurotransmitter" hypothesis to explain the pathogenesis of HE/PSE (Fischer and Baldessarini, 1971). According to this hypothesis there is a reduction in the ratio of branched-chain amino acids (BCAAs) to aromatic amino acids (AAAs) in liver failure (Smith *et al.*, 1978). This phenomenon can partly be explained by the fact that the BCAAs are not broken down in the liver unlike the other amino acids and, thus, the normal clearance for other amino acids than BCAAs is diminished in liver dysfunction states (Soeters and de Boer, 1984). In a coupled exchange with glutamine (GLN) across the blood-brain barrier a competitive influx of AAA and BCAAs into the brain is likely to exist (James *et al.*, 1976, 1978, 1979; Pardridge, 1977). This means that if brain levels of GLN is increased resulting from an elevated brain concentration of ammonia, and blood levels of BCAAs are decreased, relative to the AAAs, more AAAs will be transported into the brain in a condition of liver failure. The AAAs are in turn precursors of the monoaminergic neurotransmitters dopamine (DA), noradrenaline (NA), and 5-HT. It could therefore be anticipated that an increase in the concentrations of AAAs in the brain may affect the metabolism and perhaps also the release and function of these monoamine neurotransmitters. According to the false neurotransmitter hypothesis, despite an increase in the brain levels of phenylalanine (PHE) and tyrosine (TYR), a net depletion of DA and NA can occur during liver failure due to the excessive formation of false (or weak) neurotransmitters such as octopamine from the same amino acid substrates (Fischer and Baldessarini, 1971, 1976; Baldessarini and Fischer, 1978). In turn, in the chronic situation these false neurotransmitters may accumulate in the brain and a CNS-neurotransmission failure in the catecholaminergic systems could follow due both to an excess of the false neurotransmitters and to a deficit of DA and NA. However, data on the true existence of brain DA alterations in PSE *in vivo* are still contradictory. Thus reports of either an increase (Simert *et al.*, 1978), a decrease (Faraj *et al.*, 1981) or no change (Bengtsson *et al.*, 1985; Bergeron *et al.*, 1995) of the DA metabolism in the brain have been presented. A decrease in DA receptor density has been demonstrated in the globus pallidus from patients who died in hepatic coma possibly suggesting an increased rather than a decreased synaptic DA activity prevailing in liver failure and HE/PSE, at least in this brain region (Mousseau *et al.*, 1993). Furthermore, infusions of octopamine directly into the rat brain produced no mental disturbances (Zieve and Olsen, 1977) and clinical trials with BCAAs and dopaminergic drugs (L-DOPA and bromocriptine) are ineffective in improving the PSE (Maddrey and Weber, 1975; Uribe *et al.*, 1979). In human autopsy study on patients dying with PSE, brain octopamine levels were shown to be decreased, whereas NA and DA levels were increased (Cuilleret *et al.*, 1980).

Serotonergic neurotransmission in HE/PSE. Now, what may be of so critical concern to, for example, the scrutiny on e.g. brain TRP/5-HT perturbations associated with HE/PSE in relation to the conceptual analysis as presented above when comparing the PCS rat model with the clinical condition comprising HE/PSE? Well, the possibilities to study brain TRP pathology in HE/PSE *in vivo* in much closer detail is available by access to the PCS rat model and modern techniques such as e.g. in vivo brain microdialysis (Bergqvist *et al.*, 1995c). However, the results hereof may not describe the real extracerebral and CNS-related tryptophan disturbance as it eventually will appear in the HE/PSE seen in patients. Intriguingly, for example, it has been clearly shown that intake of ethanol itself both acutely and chronically will affect the brain TRP and 5-HT homeostasis (Badawy *et al.* 1989). Thus, whereas the PCS rat model will define a basic TRP and 5-HT disturbance of relevance to the clinical condition of HE/PSE there may in fact be further factors contributing to the importance of the ultimate TRP and/or 5-HT dysfunction that may prevail in the clinical condition. Hence, the disturbance seen in the PCS rat may thus be considered as possibly a minimum of impact of entities such as the found brain TRP/5-HT disturbance to that which will eventually come into play in the clinical setting. The bottom line for this recollection is therefore in the present context that the caution suggested in the text below for a to vividly and uncontrolled utility of TRP/5-HT neuroactive compounds in clinical situations where HE/PSE may be of concern is very adequate as of today. This warning is thus not only based on e.g. pharmacokinetic problems inherited by the many novel neuroactive compounds acting on for example the monoaminergic systems in the brain when an intercurrent liver dysfunction is at hand (for overview, see Hale, 1993, see also Morgan and McLean, 1995), but also that yet very poorly defined direct pharmacodynamic effects on the brain TRP/5-HT and/or other monoaminergic systems may be present in a clinical HE/PSE situation that in the worst case could work in concert to provoke dangerous or even fatal outcomes to patients in these situations if the mechanisms are not adequately understood.

In essence, on the grounds described above a deeper analysis of the brain TRP/5-HT involvement in HE/PSE as mirrored trough a scrutiny on e.g. the in vivo PCS rat model seems highly justified also in the clinical perspective of modern drug utility today. It seems warranted, however, to begin this survey by relating some basic outlines for the present understanding on essential factors relevant to TRP as well as brain 5-HT of particular interest to HE/PSE.

TRYPTOPHAN METABOLISM

There are two major metabolic fates of dietary TRP: it may be metabolized either 1) by way of the oxidative pathway (the kynurenine pathway; see below) or 2) by way of 5-hydroxyindole synthesis leading to the neurotransmitter 5-HT (the 5-HT pathway; see below). The oxidative pathway is the major route of TRP metabolism. Under normal conditions, 99% of the TRP metabolism in the body is by way of oxidative metabolism. There are some additional minor metabolic pathways that TRP might enter. For example, the metabolism of TRP can lead to the formation of tryptamine and ß-carbolines.

Importantly, the effect of altered L-TRP availability in the brain with regard to the release of neuronal 5-HT seems to critically depend on the ambient conditions prevailing in the 5-HT system at the time when the L-TRP availability is altered (Young and Teff, 1989). To this end, several papers have reported lack of changes in 5-HT release following L-TRP administration (Elks *et al.*, 1979; Wolf and Kuhn, 1986; De Simoni *et al.*, 1987; Sleight *et al.*, 1988; Sharp *et al.*, 1992; Thorré *et al.*, 1996) probably reflecting a generally low potential to alter 5-HT release and function by L-TRP augmentation under normal conditions. For example, Sharp and colleagues have demonstrated that elevation of brain L-TRP availability increases neuronal 5-HT release in hippocampus only under conditions when an already increased serotonergic neuronal activity is at hand (Sharp *et al.*, 1992). It has also been shown that exogenous systemic administration of L-TRP induces a much more pronounced increase in brain extracellular 5-HT levels in food-deprived or exercised rats than in ad lib fed rats or rats at rest, respectively (Schwartz *et al.*, 1990; Meeusen *et al.*, 1995). Furthermore, studies have shown that certain behavioral changes thought to be mediated by 5-HT do not occur following L-TRP administration unless accompanied by a simultaneous MAO inhibition (Grahame-Smith, 1971). Based on findings like these it has been proposed that any increase in 5-HT biosynthesis is accompanied by a subsequent increase in 5-hydroxyindole metabolism which degrades the additionally produced 5-HT before it is released (Grahame-Smith, 1974). It is important to recall, however, that several studies indeed have reported that L-TRP augmentation may also increase the neuronal 5-HT release in the brain (Ternaux *et al.*, 1976; Suter and Collard, 1983; Carboni *et al.*, 1989; Schaechter and Wurtman, 1990; Sarna *et al.*, 1991; Westerink and De Vries, 1991). It should therefore be kept in mind that these various reports refer to different methodology applied including for example varying doses or dose regimens for the L-TRP supplementation, etc. More detailed study protocols addressing this topic are thus still clearly warranted to uncover the relation between 5-HT biosynthesis and 5-HT release.

It should be clearly noted that issues like blood-brain extraction of L-TRP, plasma-free versus bound L-TRP (for further discussion, see e.g. Salerno *et al.*, 1984), as well as brain L-TRP toxicity in general have been investigated rather extensively in HE/PSE. In relation to the latter, already in 1956 it was shown that L-TRP could be a cerebrotoxic amino acid when administered to rats (Gullino *et al.*, 1956). Increased plasma levels of L-TRP have thereafter also frequently been reported accompany animals (Curzon *et al.*, 1973; James *et al.*, 1978; Smith *et al.*, 1978) and humans (Hirayama, 1971; Fischer *et al.*, 1974; Knell *et al.*, 1974; Young *et al.*, 1975; Cascino *et al.*, 1982) with liver insufficiency. Increased brain tissue concentrations of L-TRP were early on observed in PCS rats (Baldessarini and Fischer, 1973; Curzon *et al.*, 1975; Cummings *et al.*, 1976a; Jellinger and Riederer, 1977; Bloxam and Curzon, 1978; Tricklebank *et al.*, 1978; James *et al.*, 1979; Mans *et al.*, 1979, 1982, 1984, 1990; Bucci *et al.*, 1980; Jessy *et al.*, 1990; Bengtsson *et al.*, 1991) as well as in the cerebrospinal fluid of patients with varying types of hepatocerebral dysfunction (Young *et al.*, 1975; Ono *et al.*, 1978; Hutson *et al.*, 1979; Cascino *et al.*, 1982; Rössle *et al.*, 1984) and in postmortem brain tissue from patients dying of HE (Jellinger *et al.*, 1978; Bergeron *et al.*, 1989a). Long-term oral feeding with L-TRP to PCS rats was demonstrated to negatively affect the behavior as well as the brain histology of these animals (Bucci *et al.*, 1982). Studies like these above make a strong case for profound changes in the disposition of L-TRP to occur in the brain in HE/PSE that ultimately may exert a major toxic effect in these situations.

Quinolinic acid

L-TRP may also degrade to yield many potentially active metabolites other than 5-HT (such as e.g. those belonging to the group of kynurenines) and it is therefore not excluded that certain effects seen following perturbations in the L-TRP handling could be attributed to such metabolite activity. Kynurenic acid (KYNA) was recognized as a TRP metabolite in canine urine already in 1904 (Ellinger, 1904). However, it was not until in the mid 1940's that the kynurenine pathway was recognized as a major route for the conversion of TRP to nicotinamide (Beadle *et al.*, 1947). In 1964, another kynurenine metabolite, quinolinic acid (QUIN; pyridine-2,3-dicarboxylic acid), was accepted as an intermediate in this oxidative pathway (Gholson *et al.*, 1964). Interest in the kynurenine pathway was long centred around its importance as a source of NAD and NADP (Stone, 1993). This situation prevailed until it was discovered that QUIN and KYNA had pronounced effects of neuronal activity, showing activity at excitatory amino acid (EAA) receptors on neurons in the CNS (Stone and Perkins, 1981; Perkins and Stone, 1982, 1983a, 1983b). Interestingly, already some years prior to the reports by Perkins and Stone, Lapin had reported marked convulsing activity of QUIN and KYNA when injected directly into the brain of rodents (Lapin, 1978, 1981), but the significance of these observations did initially remain unattended (Stone, 1993). In parallel with the substantial increase in the interest in the role of excitatory amino acid receptors in neurotransmission, both under normal conditions but also under pathophysiological conditions such as excitotoxicity and neurodegeneration, there has been an accompanying expansion of interest in the analysis and understanding of functions of the kynurenine pathway in the CNS (Stone, 1993). The interest for perturbations in the excitatory neurotransmission as a possible pathogenic event in HE/PSE has been indicated during the later part of the 1980's (Moroni *et al.*, 1986a,b; Peterson *et al.*, 1990).

QUIN is an endogenous competitive agonist of the *N*-methyl-D-aspartate (NMDA) subclass of EAA receptors (McLennan, 1983; Perkins and Stone, 1983a) mediating neuronal membrane calcium ion transients and thereby excitatory neurotransmission in the brain. Under normal circumstances, QUIN concentrations in brain tissue are in the nanoM range. In general around microM concentrations of QUIN are excitotoxic, but some studies have, however, reported excitotoxicity exerted by QUIN to certain neuronal cell types *in vitro* only in reasonably hyper-physiological concentrations (Whetsell and Schwarcz, 1989). QUIN has been suggested to be involved in the pathogenesis of several neurologic diseases such as Huntington's disease, temporal lobe epilepsy, glutaric aciduria, the neuropathology frequently associated with AIDS, as well as in HE/PSE (for overview, see Freese *et al.*, 1990). Neurotoxicity induced by QUIN occurs preferentially in the neocortex, striatum, and hippocampus (Perkins and Stone, 1983a, 1983b), regions in the brain particularly affected by the CNS disorders mentioned above. Important in this context is the recollection that this specific type of neurotoxicity is by no means any trademark for e.g. HE/PSE. Nevertheless, Moroni and colleagues reported increased QUIN levels in the cerebral neocortex and cerebellum but in no other brain regions of PCS rats and, moreover, following a coma-inducing NH_4Ac challenge to these PCS rats an about 50% increase in the neocortical brain QUIN levels in this the acute hyperammonemic state could also be evidenced (Moroni *et al.*, 1986a). Increased QUIN concentrations were also found in the cerebrospinal fluid from patients suffering from HE as well as postmortem in the frontal neocortex from patients dying in hepatic coma reported by the same investigators (Moroni *et al.*, 1986b). These observations led to the hypothesis that increased L-TRP availability in the brain may subsequently increase brain QUIN levels in HE and that QUIN could contribute to the neurological alterations observed in HE/PSE (Moroni *et al.*, 1986a,b). A hypothesis for that of increased brain levels of EAA ligands in HE was further supported by the down-regulation of NMDA receptor binding sites in the brain as demonstrated in the PCS rat (Peterson *et al.*, 1990). Furthermore, in children with congenital hyperammonemia increased cerebrospinal fluid levels of QUIN were recently also demonstrated to prevail (Batshaw *et al.*, 1993). In a rat model of this hyperammonemia syndrome, however, no changes of cerebrospinal fluid QUIN levels were found (Robinson *et al.*, 1992a).

Conversely, in a series of most recent experiments, though, elevated brain parenchymal as well as extracellular QUIN levels have been critically questioned to exist either in chronic or acute PSE as shown in the PCS rat (Bergqvist *et al.*, 1995b; 1996a). Moreover, the challenge with ammonia did not display an increment in brain QUIN levels that correlated with the neurological deterioration accompanying these PCS rats (Bergqvist *et al.*, 1995b). In addition, elevated brain QUIN levels were demonstrated only in patients dying in acute but not chronic liver failure (Basile *et al.*, 1995). The elevated brain QUIN levels in the patients succumbed in acute HE did, however, not correlate with the severity of the neurological impairments of the patients at time of death (Basile *et al.*, 1995). Experimental chronic HE/PSE, such as in the PCS rat, will be accompanied by glial rather than neuronal degeneration (Bengtsson *et al.*, 1988a) which in turn would speak against at least traditional neuronal excitotoxicity to exist in this situation, although patients dying from HE/PSE may exhibit indications of also neuronal degeneration (Victor *et al.*, 1965; see also discussion above). Furthermore, in PSE an overall depressed neuronal activity that includes a general EEG slowing appears (Conn and Lieberthal, 1979) which is opposite to that expected on the traditional basis of excitotoxicity (for overview, see Stone 1993). These finding are all important caveats for the possible involvement of QUIN in the pathogenesis of HE/PSE. In summary, therefore, although it is likely that perturbations in the brain EEAs are accompanying HE (Moroni *et al.*, 1986b; Butterworth, 1992a, 1996), for almost a decade the suspicion of QUIN as a potential major pathogenetic factor in HE/PSE was not refuted by other independent researchers than the excellent group around professor Moroni. This was probably mainly due to methodological difficulties in establishing reliable and reproducible assays for determinations of QUIN levels in the brain, and now also in the brain dialysate (Bergqvist *et al.*, 1995b). However, by the advent of new methods to overcome these vital methodological difficulties a possible false indication of an endogenous neurotoxin to be involved in the pathogenesis of HE can now be settled. Accordingly, although seemingly negative as an overall result, the detailed recent studies (Basile 1995; Bergqvist *et al.*, 1995b; 1996a) clearly suggests QUIN <u>not</u> to be closely related to the pathogenesis of, at least, chronic HE/PSE perhaps providing e.g. textbooks as of today to omit elaborating further in great length on the brain QUIN story as a causative factor for this condition.

Tryptamine

A minor portion of ingested L-TRP is not metabolized by way of the kynurenine pathway or the 5-HT pathway but converted into various trace compounds (e.g. indoles other than 5-hydroxyindoles, skatoles, ß-carbolines, etc) among which tryptamine seems to be of possible specific importance due to its potential biological activities. Tryptamine is an endogenous neuroactive L-TRP metabolite with a number of behavioral, physiological, as well as pharmacological effects already known (for comprehensive overview, see Mousseau, 1993). The biosynthesis of tryptamine occurs by decarboxylation of L-TRP via the action of the abundant and unspecific enzyme L-amino acid decarboxylase (AAD). The major route of metabolism of tryptamine is a subsequent enzymatic inactivation by MAO resulting in the formation of an unstable aldehyde that is rapidly converted into indole-3-acetic acid (IAA). Although tryptamine is rapidly metabolized and exists only in minute amounts in brain tissue, its rapid biosynthesis allows for quantities which are comparable to those reported for 5-HT and DA (Wu and Boulton, 1987). While some evidence exist that tryptamine may be acting as a neurotransmitter in the brain, it is generally believed that the major role for tryptamine is modulatory for the neurotransmission, in particular the serotonergic, in the brain. Distinct species-dependent bindings sites for tryptamine have been characterized (Mousseau and Butterworth, 1994a; see also Mousseau, 1993). In the rat, these binding sites are heterogeneously distributed with the highest densities in the striatum, neocortex, and hippocampus (Cascio and Kellar, 1983). Tryptamine has been shown to interact with the 5-HT, DA, and ACh systems in the brain (Ennis *et al.*, 1981; Ennis and Cox, 1982), exert thermoregulatory effects (Dooley and Quock, 1976), affect neuronal firing in the brain (Aghajanian and Haigler, 1975), etc (Mousseau, 1993). Disturbances in the biosynthesis and/or metabolism of tryptamine have been suggested as possible factors in the pathogenesis of various psychiatric disorders such as depression, Parkinson's disease, schizophrenia, and Tourette's syndrome (Mousseau, 1993). Direct evidence for the involvement of tryptamine in the etiology of such diseases is, however, relatively poor but future work on these issues are clearly warranted. Tryptamine metabolism has also been shown to be much more responsive than serotonin metabolism to changes in the ambient L-TRP availability (Young *et al.*, 1980). Using IAA levels as index of brain tryptamine turnover, it has been observed that patients with hepatic coma have significantly higher brain tryptamine turnover when compared with cirrhotic patients not in coma (Young and Lal, 1980; see also Mousseau, 1993). Furthermore, the grade of coma was proportional to IAA levels in cerebrospinal fluid in these patients. Consistent with these findings, decreases in [^{3}H]-tryptamine binding site density in postmortem brain tissue from patients who died in hepatic coma have recently also been reported (Mousseau *et al.*, 1994). The possible involvement of tryptamine in the pathogenesis of various neuropsychiatric conditions, including chronic HE/PSE, should be studied further.

Melatonin

In the pineal gland, a large portion of 5-HT is metabolized into the hormone *N*-acetyl-5-methoxytryptamine (more frequently referred to as melatonin; for review see Arendt, 1988). Noradrenergic sympathetic nerves, originating from the superior cervical ganglia, innervate the pineal gland and stimulate the pineal biosynthesis of melatonin. It is generally assumed that the *N*-acetylation of 5-HT is the rate-limiting step in melatonin formation (Klein and Weller, 1970). The activity of this enzyme shows a diurnal variation in the pineal gland that corresponds to the variation in melatonin levels in the brain and the circulation through the light-dark cycle (Deguchi, 1975). In the rat for example, as much as a 60-fold increase in the activity of serotonin *N*-acetyltransferase has been demonstrated during the hours of darkness. The biosynthesis and secretion of melatonin is greatest during the hours of darkness and a 3-fold increase in the level of circulating melatonin from the minimum level during daytime to the peak at night has been demonstrated (Wetterberg *et al.*, 1976; Arendt, 1988).

The exact physiological and behavioral effects of melatonin are still unclear. Perhaps the strongest case can be made in reproduction, particularly in seasonally breeding animals (Arendt, 1995). The rhythmic secretion of melatonin and its control by light and adrenergic neurons have proved to be of particular interest in psychiatric studies (Arendt, 1988). For example, a disturbed melatonin function has been implicated in depression (Wetterberg *et al.*, 1982), mania (Lewy *et al.*, 1978), schizophrenia (Ferrier *et al.*, 1982) etc (for review, Reppert and Weaver, 1995). Melatonin has also been implicated in normal physiological processes such as aging (Sandyk, 1990). It has even been claimed that melatonin can reverse aging (Pierpaoli and Regelson, 1994). This assertion is, however, speculative and not scientifically founded since it is based on a debated study performed in mice (for further discussion, Reppert and Weaver, 1995). Biosynthesis of melatonin has also been found to exist in the retina and the hormone is believed to have several important regulatory functions in the mammalian retina (Krause and Dubocovich, 1990; Cahill and Besharse, 1995). Perturbations in the melatonin metabolism have also recently been described both in PCS rats (Zee *et al.*, 1991) and in patients with cirrhosis of the liver (Steindl *et al.*, 1995a). Such changes in melatonin metabolism have been suggested to be involved in the disruption of diurnal rhythms frequently observed both in PCS rats (Beaubernard *et al.*, 1977; Steindl *et al.*, 1995b) as well as in HE patients (Bergonzi *et al.*, 1978). Sound therapeutic applications of melatonin have been developed around its circadian effects (Arendt, 1995). Melatonin administered orally to humans has been used successfully to treat symptomes of jet lag as well as for some more problematic and chronic circadian-based sleep disorders (James *et al.*, 1990; Garfinkel *et al.*, 1995). An essential critical feature to keep in mind for the possible circadian effect exerted by melatonin is the time of its administration during the day, since melatonin can only alter circadian rhythms during a restricted portion of the circadian cycle (Arendt, 1995). However, since circadian rhythm disturbances are most likely to be a central feature accompanying chronic PSE (e.g. Apelqvist *et al.*, 1996a), further scrutiny on the melatonin involvement in neuropsychiatric syndromes like this are clearly warranted in the future.

BRAIN SEROTONIN IN HE/PSE

In a historic perspective, the first hypotheses dealing with the possible involvement of serotonergic disturbances in the brain in HE/PSE suggested either that an excess of indoleamines to reach the CNS were recruited from the gut or that, in fact, a decrease in the formation and possibly also the release of 5-HT in the brain was prevailing in this condition (Conn and Lieberthal, 1979). Later, though, most studies performed in this field have suggested unaltered or increased brain 5-HT and/or in combination with other brain L-TRP perturbations to be most likely associated with HE/PSE (for recent overviews, see e.g. Bengtsson, 1992; Bengtsson and Bergqvist , 1996).

Brain 5-HT biosynthesis and metabolism

5-HT is synthesized from L-TRP by a two step reaction: hydroxylation of L-TRP catalyzed by an enzymatic process involving TPH producing 5-hydroxytryptophan (5-HTP), immediately followed by decarboxylation of 5-HTP catalyzed by unspecific AAD resulting in 5-HT. The enzyme AAD is found in both serotonergic and catecholaminergic neurons where it converts 5-HTP to 5-HT and L-DOPA to dopamine (DA), respectively (Sourkes, 1977). Thus, if 5-HTP is administered it can be converted to 5-HT in other cells than the serotonergic ones (Melamed *et al.*, 1980; Gartside *et al.*, 1992). However, substantial doses of 5-HTP are demanded in order to detect any 5-HT formation within non-serotonergic neurons (Fuxe *et al.*, 1971). AAD is present in the brain in far greater amounts than is TPH (Ichiyama *et al.*, 1968) and, hence, only trace amounts of 5-HTP can be found in brain tissue (Tappaz and Pujol, 1980). This suggests that 5-HTP can be decarboxylated almost as readily as it is formed. This also supports the hypothesis that the TRP hydroxylation is the rate-limiting step in the 5-HT formation (Carlsson and Lindqvist, 1978). TPH seems to be restricted to cells that normally synthesize 5-HT as it is best located near the raphe nuclei, the tectum, the hypothalamus, the septum, the pons medulla, and the spinal cord (areas all rich in 5-HT; Meek and Lofstrandh, 1976; Hamon *et al.*, 1979). The K_m of TPH for L-TRP is about 50 microM but the normal physiological L-TRP concentration *in vivo* in brain tissue is only about 20 microM. Hence, the enzyme is approximately only half-saturated with its substrate (Fernstrom and Wurtman, 1971; Costa and Meek, 1974; Young and Sourkes, 1977; Carlsson and Lindqvist, 1978; Curzon, 1986). As a consequence, the rate of TRP hydroxylation in the brain would fluctuate with the concentration of the precursor amino acid according to first-order kinetics (Neckers *et al.*, 1977; Hamon *et al.*, 1979). Indeed, central as well as peripheral administrations of L-TRP have been shown to induce large increases in the concentrations of 5-HT and/or the main 5-HT metabolite 5-hydroxyindole-3-acetic acid (5-HIAA) in the brain *in vivo* (Aschcroft *et al.*, 1965; Eccleston *et al.*, 1965, 1970; Fernstrom and Wurtman, 1971; Grahame-Smith, 1971; Knott and Curzon, 1974; Curzon and Marsden, 1975; Marsden and Curzon, 1976; Curzon *et al.*, 1978; Elks *et al.*, 1979; Hamon *et al.*, 1979; Gibson *et al.*, 1982; Johnston and Moore, 1983; Tracqui *et al.*, 1983; Hutson *et al.*, 1985; Lookingland *et al.*, 1986; Wolf and Kuhn, 1986; De Simoni *et al.*, 1987; Carboni *et al.*, 1989; Schwartz *et al.*, 1990; Bengtsson *et al.*, 1991; Sarna *et al.*, 1991). However, the impact of increased brain L-TRP availability in terms of 5-HT function, i.e. neuronal 5-HT release, is still subjected to discussion (Curzon, 1986; Bengtsson, 1992; Bengtsson and Bergqvist, 1996).

In addition to L-TRP, molecular oxygen and the reduced cofactor tetrahydrobiopterin (BH_4) are both required for TRP hydroxylation *in vivo* (Friedman *et al.*, 1972; Fukushima and Nixon, 1980). BH_4 is of endogenous origin in the brain and can be synthesized via two distinct pathways; a *de novo* synthetic pathway using the nucleotide GTP as precursor and a salvage pathway which uses the compounds sepiapterin and/or 7,8-dihydrobiopterin. The enzyme GTP-cyclohydrolase I (GTPCHI) catalyzes the first and rate-limiting step in the *de novo* synthetic pathway of BH_4 (Nichol *et al.*, 1985). The GTPCHI activity has been shown to be inhibited by reduced pterins in a negative feed-back manner (Schoedon *et al.*, 1987) but the GTPCHI activity can also be induced by compounds like interferon-gamma and bacterial lipopolysaccharide (Werner *et al.*, 1989; Werner-Felmayer *et al.*, 1993). The oxidized L-TRP hydroxylation reaction product, quinonoid dihydrobiopterin, is inactive and regenerated into the reduced and active BH_4 by the action of the NADH-dependent enzyme quinonoid dihydropteridine reductase. The TPH activity can also be altered by means other than substrate availability. Besides L-TRP, TPH requires molecular oxygen and BH_4 for TRP hydroxylation *in vivo* (Friedman *et al.*, 1972; Fukushima and Nixon, 1980). The K_m of TPH for BH_4 is estimated to be about 30 microM (Friedman *et al.*, 1972) and the level of BH_4 in rat brain is about 1 microM, although it may reach levels up to 10 microM in monoamine-containing neurons (Levine *et al.*, 1979). Therefore, the activity of TPH under physiological *in vivo* conditions seems to depend largely on the BH_4 concentration (Lovenberg *et al.*, 1967; Knapp and Mandell, 1984; Miwa *et al.*, 1985; Nagatsu, 1985; Sawada *et al.*, 1986; Levine *et al.*, 1987) and the availability of BH_4 in the brain has therefore also been suggested to be one possible regulatory mechanism of brain 5-HT biosynthesis *in vivo* (Bengtsson *et al.*, 1991).

A way of altering the brain 5-HT biosynthesis is by changing the activity of the rate-limiting enzyme TPH *per se*. This can be achieved by several ways. As electrical stimulation of serotonergic nuclei likely induces a Ca^{2+}-dependent increase in the biosynthesis of 5-HT in the nerve terminals, it seems as if TPH activity and 5-HT biosynthesis also may be modulated by depolarization of the neurons (Shields and Eccleston, 1972; Elks *et al.*, 1979). It is therefore not unlikely that the increased 5-HT biosynthesis at least in part results also from alterations in the kinetic properties of TPH, perhaps due to a Ca^{2+}-dependent phosphorylation of the enzyme in response to increased neuronal activity. Short-term requirements for increases in the biosynthesis of 5-HT can thus probably be effectively met by processes that change the kinetic properties of TPH without necessitating the biosynthesis of more TPH molecules. By contrast, situations requiring long-term increases in the biosynthesis of 5-HT result in *de novo* biosynthesis of TPH protein (Frazer and Hensler, 1994). TPH is normally unsaturated with its substrate (Fernstrom and Wurtman, 1971; Costa and Meek, 1974; Young and Sourkes, 1977; Carlsson and Lindqvist, 1978; Curzon, 1986; Bengtsson *et al.*, 1991), and, consequently, modifying levels of L-TRP in the brain can rapidly influence the saturation of the enzyme with substrate and, thus, the rate at which L-TRP is converted into 5-HT. However, in some cases, e.g. following treatment with the antidepressant clomipramine, despite decreased brain L-TRP levels the brain TPH activity has been shown to be unaltered (Neckers *et al.*, 1977). The possible involvement of BH_4 in enhancing the brain 5-HT synthesis in chronic HE/PSE has recently been challenged, but the results hereof so far are still unequivocal on this point (Bergqvist *et al.*, 1995b). In L-TRP challenged PCS rats the extracellular TRP levels in the neocortex during brain microdialysis were found to reach a peak value within a similar time frame as the L-TRP challenged sham rats (Bergqvist *et al.*, 1996b). This value for the PCS rats, however, remained constant throughout the repeated L-TRP challenge of lower additional doses administered in the experiment for the first time in the literature displaying these effects in PCS rats (Bergqvist *et al.*, 1996b). This different time-course may be explained by the fact that PCS rats already prior to the L-TRP challenge exhibit an elevated brain extracellular TRP level possibly due to an impaired liver TRP metabolism. The ability to metabolize TRP has for example been demonstrated to be reduced in cirrhotic patients (Rössle *et al.*, 1986). Accordingly, following a superimposed L-TRP load to PCS rats the plasma TRP levels might substantially increase and the transport of TRP from the blood to the CNS may hence be saturated (for further discussion, Salerno *et al.*, 1984). Although the plasma TRP levels are further increased following the L-TRP challenges the transport of TRP into the brain might be kept at a constant level and the brain extracellular TRP levels do therefore not increase any further in the L-TRP challenged PCS rats.

5-HT in the nerve terminal can be subjected to metabolism either prior to release or after it has been recaptured into the presynaptic nerve terminal (or glia cell) by the reuptake mechanism. Some data indicate that newly synthesized 5-HT is preferentially released by the neurons (Elks *et al.*, 1979; Lookingland *et al.*, 1986; Pei *et al.*, 1989) but this preference is still under discussion (Reinhardt and Wurtman, 1977; Whittaker and Roed, 1982; Curzon, 1986). Although 5-HT is usually protected from metabolism because of its localization in storage vesicles and that the metabolizing enzymes are present mainly outside of these structures, 5-HT can be very rapidly degraded mainly as a result of the activity of the enzyme monoamine oxidase (MAO) to yield 5-hydroxyindoleacetaldehyde (5-HIAL), which in turn is a very reactive aldehyde, and the majority of 5-HIAL is rapidly oxidized to the biologically inert metabolite 5-HIAA by aldehyde dehydrogenase.

Since early studies, like one with dogs bearing a PCS given L-TRP in combination with an irreversible and non-selective MAO-inhibitors (Ogihara *et al.*, 1967), were reported to result in a non-ammonia related encephalopathy it was suggested that the amine metabolites of L-TRP, 5-HT and tryptamine, to be likely to be responsible for the encephalopathy rather than L-TRP itself. Indeed, the increased brain tissue turnover of 5-HT in PSE is, for example, supported by the increased brain 5-HT levels seen after complete MAO-inhibition (Bengtsson *et al.*, 1987a) and by increased brain MAO activities demonstrated to be prevailing both in PCS rats (Rokicki *et al.*, 1989) and in postmortem human brain tissue from cirrhotic patients with HE (Rao *et al.*, 1993). Earlier studies also verified the high 5-HT and/or 5-HIAA brain concentrations and/or 5-HIAA/5-HT ratios and/or the enhanced turnover of 5-hydroxyindoles to be prevailing in almost all conditions of hepatocerebral dysfunction (Tyce *et al.*, 1967; Baldessarini and Fischer, 1973; Knell *et al.*, 1974; Knott and Curzon, 1974; Curzon *et al.*, 1975; Reichle and Reichle, 1975; Young *et al.*, 1975; Cummings *et al.*, 1976a, 1976b; Jellinger and Riederer, 1977; Bloxam and Curzon, 1978; Jellinger *et al.*, 1978; Smith *et al.*, 1978; Tricklebank *et al.*, 1978; Bucci *et al.*, 1980; Mans *et al.*, 1984, 1987; Bengtsson *et al.*, 1985, 1986, 1987a, 1987b, 1988a, 1988b, 1991; Bugge *et al.*, 1986, 1989b; Mans and Hawkins, 1986; Bergeron *et al.*, 1989b, 1990; for reviews, Bengtsson *et al.*, 1989b; Bergeron *et al.*, 1991; Bengtsson, 1992; Bengtsson and Bergqvist, 1996). In fact, though, such studies have generally suggested brain L-TRP and 5-HIAA levels to be markedly increased while the 5-HT concentrations increments as such were usually much less pronounced. Thus, elevations in brain 5-HT did not appear to correlate well with hepatocerebral dysfunction unless ratios of L-TRP/5-HT/5-HIAA (usually 5-HIAA/5-HT) were calculated and used as indicator of brain 5-HT turnover. However, measurements of absolute levels of L-TRP and L-TRP metabolites always have the disadvantage of imaging static events from which the dynamics of the system cannot be inferred. In addition, wholebrain analyses of these compounds probably also frequently can obscure important regional variations, especially so since it has been shown that TPH activities under normal conditions vary substantially in different parts of the brain (Baumgarten *et al.*, 1973). Moreover, the normal day-night rhythm variations for brain L-TRP and L-TRP metabolites has to be taken into account when doing experiments, especially so in PSE research where there are reasons to believe that the normal circadian pattern may be disturbed in this condition (Bergeron *et al.*, 1991; Apelqvist *et al.*, 1996a).

A minor portion of 5-HIAL is not oxidized into 5-HIAA but reduced by the enzymes alcohol dehydrogenase or aldehyde reductase resulting in the formation of the 5-hydroxyindole derived alcohol 5-hydroxytryptophol (5-HTOL; Davis *et al.*, 1966; Bulat *et al.*, 1970; Diggory *et al.*, 1979; Cheifetz and Warsh, 1980). 5-HTOL can induce sleep in mice and chicks (Feldstein *et al.*, 1970; Taborsky, 1971) and displays certain electrophysiological effects in rabbit brain (Sabelli and Giardina, 1970). 5-HTOL may also interfere with the action of 5-HT on 5-HT binding sites in the brain and thereby elicit cerebroarterial contractions (Fu *et al.*, 1980). Under normal conditions, brain 5-HTOL occurs scarsely compared with 5-HIAA (pmolar versus mmolar concentrations). However, when changes in the brain redox potential occur (measured e.g. as brain NADH-to-NAD^+ratio), the 5-HTOL/5-HIAA ratio can be shifted (Beck *et al.*, 1986). The 5-HTOL/5-HIAA ratio can also be altered by administration of drugs that affect the 5-HT system such as MAOIs (such as pargyline), 5-HT neurotoxins (such as 5,7-dihydroxytryptamine), and probenecid (Beck *et al.*, 1987) or by alcohol dehydrogenase inhibitors such as disulfiram (Beck *et al.*, 1995). In addition, L-TRP administration has been shown to cause an increase in the 5-HTOL content in the rat pineal gland (Young and Anderson, 1982). The increased brain tissue turnover of 5-HT prevailing in PSE is further supported by a recent preliminar study showing increased brain tissue levels of 5-HTOL to be accompanying PCS rats (Bergqvist *et al.*, 1996d).

Brain 5-HT storage and release

As for catecholeamines, 5-HT is stored primarily in vesicles within the nerve terminals. There is still an unsettled discussion of a possible existence for (at least) two different neuronal pools of 5-HT in the brain (Grahame-Smith, 1971, 1973, 1974; Shields and Eccleston, 1973; Curzon and Marsden, 1975; Schaub and Meyers, 1975; Mennini *et al.*, 1981; Morot-Gaudry *et al.*, 1981; Tamir *et al.*, 1982; Kleven *et al.*, 1983; Kuhn *et al.*, 1985; Wolf and Kuhn, 1986; Bengtsson *et al.*, 1989b). According to this hypothesis, the serotonergic nerve terminals contain one small functionally active and readily releasable pool of 5-HT and one larger but functionally inactive, and thus non-releasable, 5-HT storage pool (Grahame-Smith, 1973). The functionally active pool of 5-HT is believed to be stored in regular presynaptic vesicles and participating in serotonergic neurotransmission while the function of the non-releasable pool is more obscure. It has been suggested that the non-releasable pool of 5-HT might serve as a buffer-like compartment. Hence, if the neuronal biosynthesis of 5-HT is in excess of that required to fulfill the functional needs of the brain, in order to avoid a 5-HT induced hyperactivity the surplus 5-HT might be taken up and stored by the non-releasable pool. The "buffered" 5-HT might subsequently either be subjected to intraneuronal metabolism or, if the demand of the nerve terminal for releasable 5-HT increases, be restored into the functional pool. This latter capability may be of great significance to e.g. conditions of diseases where a primary disturbance in the CNS 5-HT systems can be involved. Furthermore, it is also believed that the two pools share the same metabolic pathways in the nerve cell. This means that a measured overall 5-HT turnover may not reflect the metabolism of the functionally active compartment but instead mirror the sum of both the active and the inactive 5-HT pool in the nerve cell. The uptake of 5-HT into synaptic vesicles is an active process fueled by ATP. Certain drugs, such as reserpine, interfere with this uptake process and causes a leakage of the 5-HT stored in vesicles out into the preterminal cytoplasm where the 5-HT is then degraded by MAO (Shore and Giachetti, 1978). The tissue level of 5-HT after e.g. reserpine administration thus drops (Brodie *et al.*, 1955) and the preterminal exocytotic 5-HT release is therefore also subsequently affected (Heslop and Curzon, 1994). Interestingly, despite a reduction in brain 5-HT content, prior reserpine treatment does not block the behavioral effects (e.g. the 5-HT behavioral syndrome) induced by the application of certain 5-HT releasing drugs such as amphetamine and its derivative pCA (Kuhn *et al.*, 1985; Adell *et al.*, 1989; Heslop and Curzon, 1994). This phenomenon has been suggested to result from a release of 5-HT by a reserpine-insensitive (i.e. extravesicular) cytosolic pool of the transmitter (Kuhn *et al.*, 1985; Adell *et al.*, 1989). It should also be emphasized that there are substantial regional differences among serotonergic neurons in the brain in the response to reserpine (Long *et al.*, 1983).

Brain 5-HT release in acute and subacute HE. Acute HE condition is possibly associated with a profound decrease of the 5-HT release in the neocortex (Bergqvist *et al.*, 1995c). In the dialysate samples from these acutely and severely encephalopathic rats significantly elevated 5-HIAA concentrations were observed. On the other hand, subacute HE and thus less overtly CNS-affected condition resulted in significant elevations of the dialysate 5-HIAA content but the extracellular 5-HT level did not appear to change *per se* as compared to normal control rats. These data may indicate that a large metabolic increase in intraneuronal 5-HT biosynthesis (Bengtsson *et al.*, 1988a) do <u>not</u> necessarily have to correlate with, or result in, an increase in neuronal release of 5-HT in the brain as previously suggested from the observations of increases in the CNS tissue 5-HT metabolism in experimental HE (Cummings *et al.*, 1976a, 1976b; Mans and Hawkins, 1986; for further detailed discussion, see e.g Bengtsson *et al.*, 1989b). In fact, even a relative decrease in serotonergic tone in the CNS in some severe conditions of HE may be at hand at least in the neocortex as evidenced from the data obtained in the present investigation. Moreover, though, also in some condition of severe and acute HE, notably in complete ischemia of the liver but <u>not</u> in partial (i.e. only main hepatic artery ligation) or in total hepatectomy of the rat, the brain 5-HT turnover has been shown to be decreased rather than increased (for further discussion, see Bengtsson *et al.*, 1989).

Brain 5-HT release in steady-state chronic PSE. No significant differences between sham and PCS rats with regard to the basal extracellular neocortical 5-HT concentrations were obtained in any of the many separate recent experiments comprising such data (Bergqvist *et al.*, 1995c; 1996a-d; 1997a-c). The 5-HIAA levels were, however, almost obligately elevated in the PCS group as compared to the sham-operated group of animals. Accordingly, it can be envisaged that under the current experimental conditions, albeit an increased brain intraneuronal 5-HT metabolism is clearly prevailing (for reviews, Bengtsson *et al.*, 1989b; Bergeron *et al.*, 1991; Bengtsson, 1992), neuronal release of the transmitter 5-HT and thereby possibly also 5-HT function is probably not altered in the brain in conditions of chronic steady-state PSE. These findings thus speak <u>against</u> a functional overactivity in the monoaminergic systems in the CNS as a direct cause for, at least, chronic PSE. An alternative explanation to the present finding may be that neuronal 5-HT release is indeed altered in the resting state of experimental PSE, but that this is compensated for by an enhanced reuptake of 5-HT hence, maintaining the extracellular 5-HT at a more or less constant level. Partially based on this assumption, the last trial applying an SSRI (Bergqvist *et al.*, 1997c) was performed. However, the 5-HT-enhancing effect of local extracellular neocortical administration of the potent SSRI citalopram was equally pronounced in the PCS as it was in control rats indicating that the neocortical 5-HT reuptake is similarly effective in both chronic PSE as under normal conditions. It may thus be suggested that the the previously reported unchanged brain 5-HT output (Bergqvist *et al.*, 1995c, 1996b-c, 1997a-b) accompanying PCS in the rat, despite the profoundly increased brain 5-HT turnover in this condition, is probably not due to an increased 5-HT reuptake mechanism in the brain being exerted by these animals. The lack of major changes in the brain extracellular 5-HT levels seen in sham-operated control rats of the present study in the immediate period following systemic L-TRP administration (Bergqvist *et al.*, 1996b) is in agreement with observations reported from other authors (Elks *et al.*, 1979; Wolf and Kuhn, 1986; De Simoni *et al.*, 1987; Sleight *et al.*, 1988; Sharp *et al.*, 1992; Thorré *et al.*, 1996). Furthermore, the lack of changes in neocortical extracellular 5-HT levels in the PCS rats is probably reflecting a generally low potential to alter brain neuronal 5-HT release (and 5-HT function) by L-TRP augmentation not only under normal conditions but during chronic PSE as well. The hypothesis of the existence for two different pools of 5-HT in the brain may offer some help for explanation. Without demonstrable changes in extracellular 5-HT levels in either PCS or control rats following even multiple L-TRP administrations could indicate that the amount of 5-HT in a releasable pool of this transmitter is sufficient to meet the demand for a normal serotonergic neurotransmission and the L-TRP-induced increase in 5-HT biosynthesis may therefore speculatively be "functionally buffered" by primary being solely metabolized in a non-releasable (or "less"-releasable; see below) compartment/pool of 5-HT. Following the L-TRP augmentation procedure, the 5-HIAA levels tended to be increased but to a different degree in both sham and PCS rats possibly indicating that an increased intraneuronal 5-HT metabolism in response to this treatment had been evolving. The present findings thus further emphasize the importance of distinguishing between brain 5-HT metabolism and brain 5-HT release which in turn may alter differently under normal conditions compared with that appearing during a state of CNS-disease.

Additional factors of relevance for brain 5-HT release

The nerve terminal release of 5-HT is dependent on the firing rate of the serotonergic soma in the raphe nuclei located in the midbrain (Héry and Ternaux, 1981). Numerous studies have revealed that procedures that increased the raphe firing rate also increase the 5-HT release in terminal regions, whereas the opposite effect is observed when raphe firing rate decreases. This means that drugs or other manipulations that change the firing rate of the serotonergic soma in the raphe nuclei can modify the release of 5-HT in terminal regions as well (Aghajanian, 1978; Frazer and Hensler, 1994; Matos *et al.*, 1996). For example, electrical stimulation of the DRN *in vivo* has been shown to cause a frequency-dependent rapid rise in the 5-HT output from the rat hippocampus (Sharp *et al.*, 1989). With regard to drugs that may change the firing rate of 5-HT neurons, important targets for such drugs are the somatodendritic autoreceptors, which are of the 5-HT_{1A} subclass. Hence, activation of these receptors by e.g. administration of 5-HT_{1A} receptor agonists such as 8-hydroxy-2-(di-n-propylamino)-tetralin (8-OH-DPAT) into the DRN slows the rate of firing of serotonergic soma (De Montigny *et al.*, 1984) and decreases in the release of 5-HT in serotonergic terminal regions thereby follow (Hutson *et al.*, 1989; Sharp *et al.*, 1989; Sharp and Hjorth, 1990; Hjorth and Sharp, 1991). Analogously, inhibition of these somatodendritic autoreceptors, by drugs such as pindolol and WAY-100635, causes an increased firing rate of the 5-HT neurons and, subsequently, an enhanced 5-HT release in the serotonergic projection areas in the brain can be observed (Artigas, 1993; Fornal *et al.*, 1996; Hjorth, 1996; for review, Artigas *et al.*, 1996; Gardier *et al.*, 1996). The firing rate of the serotonergic soma in the raphe nuclei is also under the influence of afferent neurons that innervate this brain region. In addition, a number of different (depending on brain region) receptors such as those for NA (a_2; Gobbi *et al.*, 1990; Tao and Hjorth, 1992; Numazawa *et al.*, 1995), DA (Ferré and Artigas, 1993), glutamate (GLU; Whitton *et al.*, 1992; Ohta *et al.*, 1994; Tao and Auerbach, 1996), GABA (Kalén *et al.*, 1989), opioids (Matos *et al.*, 1992; Yoshioka *et al.*, 1993) etc, innervate the serotonergic neurons (for overview, Chesselet, 1984). Administration of ligands affecting these receptors or altering the release of these other neurotransmitters may under certain circumstances accordingly provide yet other ways of regulating the brain 5-HT release that may be of importance. Depending on the species, serotonergic presynaptic autoreceptors in terminal fields appear to be either the 5-HT_{1B} (in the rat) or 5-HT_{1D} (in the man) subclass (Hoyer *et al.* 1994). These presynaptic autoreceptors exert upon activation a negative feedback on the preterminal vesicular 5-HT release (Chesselet, 1984; Engel *et al.*, 1986; El Mansari and Blier, 1996). Administration of agonists for these presynaptic autoreceptors into areas receiving serotonergic innervation have accordingly been shown to decrease the terminal vesicular release of 5-HT in such projection areas (Hjorth and Tao, 1991). The amount of 5-HT released (as well as many other neurotransmitters) is classically viewed upon as proportional to the degree of rise in intracellular Ca^{2+} (although a minor portion of the 5-HT release is probably Ca^{2+}-independent). The 5-HT release can thus in principle also be altered by changing the intracellular Ca^{2+}concentrations. An obvious way of establishing a change in the intracellular Ca^{2+} concentration is to change the level of Ca^{2+} on the outside, i.e. in the extracellular space. By increasing or decreasing the extracellular Ca^{2+} concentrations, a significant change in the 5-HT release has been demonstrated (Westerink *et al.*, 1987; Kalén *et al.*, 1988; Auerbach *et al.*, 1989; Carboni *et al.*, 1989; Carboni and Di Chiara, 1989; Adell *et al.*, 1993; Taylor and Basmann, 1995; see also Di Chiara, 1990). The brain 5-HT release can, analogously, be manipulated by changing the extracellular K^+ concentration (Westerink *et al.*, 1987; Kalén *et al.*, 1988; Carboni and Di Chiara, 1989; Adell *et al.*, 1993; Taylor and Basmann, 1995). Another unspecific way of manipulating the brain 5-HT release is by applying certain types of drugs. Besides the effects exerted by e.g. reserpine (as mentioned above), drugs like amphetamine enter the preterminal neuron and displace 5-HT from its vesicles into the cytosol, where this 5-HT is either metabolized by MAO or escapes by a carrier-mediated diffusion into the synaptic cleft to act on 5-HT receptors.

Brain 5-HT release and ammonia. In conditions of liver failure, these pathways for ammonia detoxification are impaired and overwhelmed by the gut-derived ammonia load. In addition, the presence of portal-systemic shunts allows the ammonia to bypass the liver unmetabolized into the systemic circulation. The resulting high plasma ammonia concentration leads to increased ammonia diffusion into the brain and it has been suggested that the PSE may be primarily (or basically) induced in this way (Lockwood *et al.*, 1979; Butterworth *et al.*, 1987). In the brain there is no urea cycle available and the most important ammonia utilizing and thus detoxifying pathway is the GLN synthesis reaction. GLN levels in autopsied brain samples from cirrhotic patients or from patients with FHF dying in hepatic coma have been demonstrated to be increased 2- to 5-fold, suggesting profound exposure to ammonia having been a prevailing condition before death (Lavoie *et al.*, 1987). The enzyme responsible for ammonia detoxification in brain (i.e. glutamine synthetase) has an almost exclusively astrocytic localization (Norenberg, 1987). This glial localization for detoxification of ammonia may provide an explanation for why the histopathological picture of PSE is one of astrocytic, rather than neuronal damage. Furthermore, a clear brain regional difference in the capacity for removal of ammonia has been demonstrated in PCS rats (Butterworth *et al.*, 1988). Such regional differences might provide an explanation why some brain areas are more affected than others in PSE (Mans *et al.*, 1987). Ammonia exerts a deleterious effect on brain function by both direct and indirect mechanisms (Schenker *et al.*, 1967; Butterworth *et al.*, 1987; Jessy *et al.*, 1990; for comprehensive and excellent overview on this topic, see Szerb and Butterworth, 1992). Millimolar levels of ammonium ions, equivalent to those levels observed in postmortem brain tissue in hepatic coma patients (Lockwood *et al.*, 1979) may affect normal neurotransmission in the brain. For example, the ammonium ion behaves electrophysiologically very much like K^+ and because of this resemblance, ammonium ions can depolarize the resting membrane potential of a nerve cell probably by reducing the intracellular K^+ concentration (Gallego and Lorente de No, 1947). Such a decrease in the resting potential of a neuron may be responsible for an impaired effectivness of the extrusion of Cl^- from nerve cells, thus possibly explaining the well-known postsynaptic inhibition that has been shown to be exerted by ammonia (Raabe, 1987). In this context, it should be noted that membrane potential of astrocytes has been demonstrated to be significantly more depolarized in the brain of PCS rats as compared to sham-operated controls (-72 ± 5 mV versus -81 ± 6 mV, $p<0.001$; Swain *et al.*, 1991). Whether the resting potental of the nerve cells also are increased in conditions of experimental PSE has, at least to my knowledge, not been investigated. Furthermore, ammonia has been shown to suppress excitatory neurotransmission e.g. by preventing the excitatory amino acid GLU to act on its postsynaptic receptors resulting in a decrease in excitatory postsynaptic potentials of the nerve cell (Raabe, 1987).

Importantly for the present discussion of HE/PSE is that ammonia is a compound that also has been shown to cause a release of 5-HT (and DA) from rat brain synaptosomes *in vitro* (Erecinska *et al.*, 1987). The mechanism of such a 5-HT releasing effect of e.g. amphetamine and ammonia may be related to the so called "weak base model" of DA release (Sulzer and Rayport, 1990; Sulzer *et al.*, 1992, 1993). According to this model, weak bases such as amphetamine and ammonium ions may reduce synaptic vesicular pH gradients by alkalinization of the vesicles resulting in impaired uptake and storage of DA into cytoplasmatic vesicles leading to increased cytoplasmic DA levels (Sulzer and Rayport, 1990; Sulzer *et al.*, 1992, 1993). Elevated cytoplasmatic DA concentrations in this way may then in turn promote a reverse carrier-transport of DA out from the neurons into the extracellular compartment. Indeed, microdialysis experiment with the addition of ammonium chloride (NH_4Cl) in the dialysate fluid entering into the brain has been shown to cause substantially increases in neuronal DA release (Sulzer *et al.*, 1992). Whether this model is valid also for the neuronal 5-HT output has recently been addressed in a study on PCS rats (Bergqvist *et al.*, 1996c). It was thus demonstrated that increased extracellular neocortical levels of 5-HT *in vivo* were present following NH_4Ac administration to PCS rats (Bergqvist et al. 1996c). This finding is thereby also consistent with previous *in vitro* results suggesting an ammonia-induced increase in 5-HT output from rat brain synaptosomal preparations to exist (Erecinska *et al.*, 1987). Moreover, a single dose of NH_4Ac was here shown induce a reversible coma in PCS rats during a period when also the neuronal 5-HT release was transiently increased in the brain closely paralleling the presence of coma in these rats (Bergqvist et al. 1996c). Based on these novel *in vivo* data obtained from using the PCS rat it seems highly warranted to investigate also the release pattern of the important monoamine 5-HT after administration of longer periods of lower doses of ammonia, since it from the presently available data can be speculated that such an increase in the neocortical 5-HT release may, in fact, be involved in the development of coma in this model of acutely deteriorating PSE. Mechanisms like this could thereby also be implicated in conditions of latent PSE resulting from other ammoniagenic clinical situations such as gastrointestinal bleeding and protein loading in cirrhotic patients and closely has to be studied further in the future. Moreover, if an exogenous load of ammonia in this way may not only affect the neurological status but also the brain 5-HT output, perhaps the use of modern potent CNS 5-HT-acting drugs should be avoided in conditions of hyperammonemia in general until further notice about the more detailed effects on the brain serotonergic systems by such compounds have been outlined. Notably, hyperammonemic conditions in clinical practice comprise a mulitude of common situations besides liver failure and inborn error of metabolism like e.g. cancer and starvation, several infectious and immunological diseases, uremia and other renal disorders, etc. At present, therefore, at least a stress for caution and increased measures in pharmacovigilance is called for when novel e.g. 5-HT-acting drugs are utilized concomitantly with clinical conditions where perturbations in the handling of ammonia may be at hand.

Brain 5-HT release during a KCl challenge in chronic HE/PSE. Increasing the extracellular K^+ concentration has been considered a well-established technique to evaluate the depolarization-dependency of neurotransmitter release (Westerink *et al.*, 1987; Di Chiara, 1990). A clearcut increase in the sensitivity to a depolarzing KCl challenge with regard to neuronal 5-HT output has recently been shown to prevail in PCS as compared to control rats (Bergqvist et al. 1997a). This finding suggests that, despite the unaltered neocortical 5-HT release in experimental PSE in the resting state, there may very well be a larger amount than normal of the transmitter available for release upon depolarization from serotonin-containing nerve terminals of the neocortex in PCS rats *in vivo*. Alternatively, the difference in 5-HT output between PCS and sham following the KCl depolarization may result from changes in the resting membrane potentials of nerve cells in the brain between the two groups possibly due to an increased ammonia level in the brain of the PCS rats. Given the fact that the resting membrane potential of astrocytes in the brain from PCS rats have been found to be more depolarized than those from sham-operated controls (Swain *et al.*, 1991), it seems tempting to speculate that maybe the membrane potential of neurons in the brains of PCS rats are more depolarized than those in the brains of sham-operated rats and therefore more sensitive to a depolarizing KCl challenge? This hypothesis clearly has to be further studied e.g. by *in vivo* electrophysiological measurements of the membrane potentials of neurons in the brain of PCS and sham-operated controls. The depolarizing KCl pulse proved to release 5-HT from the nerve terminals in both a Ca^{2+}-dependent as well as Ca^{2+}-independent way in the present study (Bergqvist *et al.*, 1997a). The lack of differences in the KCl evoked 5-HT release between PCS and sham-operated rats in Ca^{2+}-free medium, however, possibly indicates that the mechanism responsible for the higher 5-HT response to the K^+ pulses in the PCS rats may be Ca^{2+}-dependent. In turn, this may suggest that the enhanced 5-HT response to KCl in the PCS rats is primarily exocytotic in nature. The underlying mechanism for such a feature could possibly be that the 5-HT granula in the PCS rats contain more 5-HT than do those of sham-operated controls, and/or that a larger number of 5-HT containing granula is released from the nerve terminals of PCS rats in response to same degree of depolarizing stimulus (in this case by introducing high extracellular K^+ levels *in vivo*). Alternatively, the Ca^{2+} uptake of the neurons in the PCS rats may be more effective than in sham-operated controls, thus explaining the increased sensitivity to depolarization evoked 5-HT release in PCS rats. These very speculative suggestions for how an increasing neuronal 5-HT output may be brought about in experimental chronic PSE under depolarization-provoked conditions have to be more closely investigated in future work before any firm or conclusive statement can be made. Using only a single high KCl concentration as in the present study (Bergqvist *et al.*, 1997a) the fact still remains that some mechanism responsible for the different response to such a depolarizing KCl challenge between PCS and sham-operated rats has to be further classified since it may also have a certain bearing on perhaps other depolarizing affecting situations possibly appearing in the PSE condition that that produced by KCl. Situations like these may include other electrolyte/body fluid imbalances, diuretic or other drug treatment instituted and/or simply the fact that the PSE condition could worsen to a more severe neurologic status where possibly brain edema development is a contributing membrane depolarizing factor. Speaking against these latter events, however, may be the observations also made in the present study that neither acute HE nor subacute HE/PSE seemed to be accompanied by any major increments in monoaminergic release in the neocortex of the brain (Bergqvist *et al.*, 1995c). In essence, therefore, this issue has to be further investigated not only in the chronic but preferably also in acute conditions of HEPSE. The KCl evoked 5-HT release was found to be TTX-insensitive in both the PCS rats and the sham-operated controls (Bergqvist *et al.*, 1997a). The neocortical 5-HT output was, however, still clearly higher in the PCS rats compared with sham as the result of being subjected to a similar KCl perfusion in the presence of TTX. TTX is a frequently used inhibitor of the voltage-sensitive Na^+ channels on the nerve cell membrane and, hence, serves as a depolarization blocking agent. The fact that both in experimental chronic PSE and in controls did indeed release 5-HT occur in the presence of TTX is, however, probably not due to a depolarization-independent release of the transmitter but rather to that of a K^+ induced direct depolarization of the nerve cell membranes independently of the blocking of the Na^+ channels. In parallel with the TTX results, in the presence of citalopram (Bergqvist et al. 1997c), the depolarizing KCl challenge produced a higher elevation of extracellular 5-HT in the neocortex of PCS when citalopram was administered as compared to control rats. The difference between PCS and sham-operated rats in the 5-HT response both with regard to amplitude and duration to the KCl challenge was more pronounced in the former group, most likelyprimarily due to the fact that a 5-HT reuptake inhibitor such as citalopram now also had been introduced in a concentration-equal fashion into the perfusion medium. This finding thus supports the hypothesis that the 5-HT granula in the PCS rats may very well contain more 5-HT than do those of sham-operated controls, and/or that a larger number of 5-HT containing granula is released from the nerve terminals of PCS rats in response to depolarizing stimulus. Differences in the 5-HT content of granulae from PCS rats and sham-operated controls may be investigated in the future by the use of sophisticated available histological techniques such as electronmicroscopy.

Brain 5-HT releasing effects of pCA and dFEN in chronic HE/PSE. The brain 5-HT release induced by local pCA or dFEN perfusion appeared equally pronounced when exposed to controls but in the PCS rats, however, the 5-HT release response to the pCA perfusion challenge was significantly more pronounced as compared to the 5-HT response in the sham rats, whereas the 5-HT effect of dFEN perfusion in the PCS rats remained at the same level as in sham controls (Bergqvist et al. 1997b). The apparent discrepancy between the results obtained by pCA and dFEN in the PCS rats may be explained by the somewhat different mechanisms of action of these two drugs. At such low dFEN concentrations as used in the actual paper (Bergqvist *et al.*, 1997b), the drug is likely to enter the serotonergic nerve terminals through the reuptake carrier and whereby the release of vesicular 5-HT is elicited and, hence, probably mainly via a Ca^{2+}dependent exocytotic-like mechanism (Bonanno *et al.*, 1994; de Parada *et al.*, 1995). On the other hand, the pCA in the presently used concentration probably release both vesicular as well as, in particular, extravesicular 5-HT from the nerve terminals in Ca^{2+}-dependent plus Ca^{2+}-independent ways, respectively (Kuhn *et al.*, 1985; Adell *et al.*, 1989; Wichems *et al.*, 1995). Accordingly, the more pronounced elevation of the brain 5-HT release in the PCS rats relative to controls after the given pCA perfusion challenge may be explained by assuming that the serotonergic nerve terminals in the PCS brain contains more extravesicular 5-HT than the nerve terminals in the brain of the sham-operated controls. Such an excess, and possibly extravesicularly located, neuronal 5-HT in the PCS rat brains is congruent with the previously demonstrated elevated brain 5-HT biosynthesis shown to be localized intraneuronally in this type of rats (Bengtsson *et al.*, 1988a). The finding that dFEN administration induced a similar 5-HT response in the PCS and sham-operated rats appears to be at variance with a previous suggestion (see above) that a Ca^{2+}-dependent mechanism may likely be responsible for the higher 5-HT response to a depolarizing KCl challenge in PCS rats as compared to controls. It should be recalled in this context that since dFEN probably enters the nerve terminals via the reuptake carriers and, the ultimate effects observed following dFEN perfusion is possibly unlikely to be that of induction of 5-HT release but rather that of inhibition of the 5-HT reuptake. This observation that the 5-HT output did not clearly differ between PCS and sham rats following the dFEN administration could thus be in accordance with the similar brain 5-HT output seen in PCS and sham-operated rats following local perfusion of the reuptake inhibitor citalopram (see below; Bergqvist *et al.*, 1997c) of the present thesis work. Based on such results obtained here recently (Bergqvist *et al.*, 1997a-b) it seems reasonable to be concluded 1) that the extravesicular amount of 5-HT is larger in the brains of the PCS rats and that this amount of 5-HT may possibly be in the form of a stationary that may be available also for release under certain pathophysiological and/or pharmacological conditions (in this case evidenced by pCA administration in experimental PSE), and 2) that the vesicular 5-HT release may be enhanced as well in PCS rats as compared to sham-operated controls when a depolarizing stimulus is used (in this case high KCl level). The reason why the presently used KCl challenge resulted in increases in the brain 5-HT release in PCS rats relative to sham animals but dFEN failed to induce any difference in 5-HT output between the two groups may be related to the possibility that maybe also different vesicular stores of 5-HT are available for release from the nerve terminal when depolarization- and pharmacology-induced 5-HT release are at hand. This discrepancy could also be explained by the speculative idea forwarded above that if the neurons in the brain in e.g. the hyperammonemic state of the PCS rats are in fact more depolarized the ambient transmembranal voltage upholds in the normal condition whereby dFEN administration will exert no effect on 5-HT release in the presence of such electrophysiological changes whereas following KCl perfusion a differently graded depolarization-release effect may come into play. Moreover, in vivo such a K+-induced graded depolarization effect between PCS and controls may arise secondary to modulation of afferent input exerted by other neurotransmitters which maybe are, in turn, insensitive to dFEN administration.

Brain 5-HT receptors and termination of 5-HT activity

With regard to brain 5-HT receptors in PSE, two radioligand binding studies in the mid 1980's were unable to demonstrate any major alterations in either the B_{max} or the K_d for the two major types of 5-HT receptors (5-HT_1 and 5-HT_2) best known at that time (Bengtsson *et al.*, 1989a; Bugge *et al.*, 1989a). Some years later, though, the B_{max} values for the 5-HT_{1A} receptor ligand [^{3}H]-8-OH-DPAT and the 5-HT_2 receptor ligand [^{3}H]ketanserin were 26% increased and 21% decreased, respectively, in neocortical tissue homogenates from hyperammonemic sparse-fur mice (Robinson *et al.*, 1992b). This animal model can, however, not simply be referable to the HE/PSE condition. Using the same ligands and ligand concentrations as Robinson *et al.*, Rao and Butterworth (1994b) demonstrated significant decreases in the [^{3}H]-8-OH-DPAT binding in the hippocampus and frontal neocortex in patients dying in HE. Furthermore, in the same study a clearly increased B_{max} value of [^{3}H]ketanserin was demonstrated in hippocampal brain tissue from the same patients (Rao and Butterworth, 1994b). Furthermore, acute ammonia intoxication in rats results in increased 5-HT_{1A} receptor expression (evidenced as increased 5-HT_{1A} receptor mRNA) in the hippocampus (Alexander *et al.*, 1995). In the light of these seemingly discrepant findings on brain 5-HT receptor changes associated with the HE/PSE condition we recently performed an autoradiographic study and screened for possible alterations in brain 5-HT_{1A}, 5-HT_{1B}, and 5-HT_{2A} receptors in PCS rats (Apelqvist *et al.*, 1996b). The results revealed a general decrease in the 5-HT_{1A} receptor binding density in most serotonergic projection areas of the brain including the frontal neocortex. Interestingly, there were no changes in the 5-HT_{1A} receptor density observed in the raphe nuclei in this screening study. A general decrease in the 5-HT_{1B} receptor binding site density was however observed, most prominently displayed in the olfactory tubercle, the midbrain, and in the frontal neocortex. Essentially, no changes could be seen in the binding site density of the 5-HT_{2A} receptor (Apelqvist *et al.*, 1996b).

Termination of 5-HT activity and reuptake inhibition. The predominant mechanism for the termination of a neurotransmitting compound effect, such as that for 5-HT, is by the removal of the released transmitter via an active transport into presynaptic neurons or into surrounding glial cells through specific membrane-bound transport proteins (Descarries and Beaudet, 1983; Kimelberg, 1988; Adell *et al.*, 1991; for review, Borowsky and Hoffman, 1995). Back inside the nerve terminal, the 5-HT can be reused in storage granules or subjected to metabolism but in the glia cells, however, no other fate for the 5-HT taken up other than inactivation by metabolism seems likely (Kimelberg, 1988). Pharmacological studies have suggested that distinct reuptake transporters exist for each of the monoaminergic and amino acid neurotransmitters, respectively. The monoaminergic transporters have been of particular interest because they are sites of action for most of the clinically utilized thymoleptic (more commonly refrerred to as antidepressants) drugs today. The 5-HT reuptake system is an active, temperature sensitive, and Na^+- and Cl^--dependent process, that is saturable and of high affinity for 5-HT with a K_m value of around 10^{-7} M.

Since the early 1980's, selective serotonin reuptake inhibitors (SSRIs) have been available as pharmacological agents (i.e. as antidepressants) which effectively promote serotonergic neurotransmission. Fluoxetine was one of the the first compound reported to exert such properties *in vitro* (Wong *et al.*, 1974). Paradoxically, administration of racemic fluoxetine decreases biosynthesis and turnover of 5-HT in the brain (Fuller and Wong, 1990). Consistent with its apparent effect on biosynthesis and turnover of brain 5-HT, fluoxetine has been shown to lower the firing rate of serotonergic soma in the raphe nuclei (Clemens *et al.*, 1977). Other SSRIs (e.g. indalpine) produced similar decreases in activity of 5-HT neurons in the raphe area (Blier *et al.*, 1984). These findings may be explained by an SSRI-induced increased autoinhibition by activation of the somatodendritic 5-HT_{1A} receptors by non-reuptaken 5-HT also at the serotonergic soma (see *5-HT receptors* above). By using *in vivo* microdialysis it has been demonstrated that whereas single administration of an SSRI produces a large increase in extracellular 5-HT levels in the raphe region, the extracellular 5-HT concentrations in terminal areas are, by comparison, only moderately affected (Adell and Artigas, 1991; Bel and Artigas, 1992). Chronic treatment with SSRIs in rats have been shown to restore normal firing rate of 5-HT neurons suggesting a desensitization of the autoreceptors to occur and may be one possible explanation for the delay in onset of antidepressive action of the SSRIs (Blier *et al.*, 1984). Recent studies show that co-administration of 5-HT_{1A} receptor antagonists, such as (*S*)-UH-301, pindolol, or WAY 100635, concomitantly with an SSRI will result in significantly higher extracellular 5-HT levels in the serotonergic terminal areas than following administration of the SSRI alone (Hjorth, 1993, 1996; Artigas *et al.*, 1996; Dreshfield *et al.*, 1996; Hjorth and Auerbach, 1996; for review, see Gardier *et al.*, 1996).

Administration of citalopram in experimental chronic HE/PSE. Activation of somatodendritic 5-HT_{1A} autoreceptors located in the midbrain raphe nuclei have been evidenced to decrease the 5-HT neuronal firing rate (Aghajanian, 1987), and thereby also release of the transmitter in e.g. the neocortical forebrain structures. When the nerve terminal 5-HT reuptake sites at this location are already blocked by a preceeding local neocortical application of citalopram by reversed dialysis (like in the present study; VIII), systemic administration of citalopram has previously been shown to result in a decrease of the 5-HT output in terminal areas like the neocortex and hippocampus (Hjorth and Auerbach, 1994; Auerbach *et al.*, 1995). This latter phenomenon is likely brought about by the activation of 5-HT_{1A} autoreceptors due to the citalopram-induced elevated extracellular 5-HT also found in the raphe region where this increment in 5-HT will act on such somatodendritic 5-HT_{1A} receptors to subsequently decrease the neocortical 5-HT output. Interestingly, using this experimental set up we observed that such combined effect of local and systemic citalopram administrationpreviously known to decrease the neuronal 5-HT output in the neocortex, was now found significantly more pronounced in the rats with liver insufficiency than in controls. (Bergqvist *et al.*, 1997c) This could then suggest a) that the reuptake machinery in the raphe region is more sensitive to inhibition by this SSRI in PCS rats and/or b) that the 5-HT_{1A}-mediated inhibition of the serotonergic neuronal activity is more effectively exerted by this drug in PCS versus normal rats. Up to date, no studies have been conducted in order to investigate possible differences in raphe 5-HT reuptake mechanisms in experimental PSE. Partly due to indications for affected drug metabolism of citalopram when given systemically to PCS rats (Bergqvist *et al.*, 1997c), a slightly higher than normal concentration of citalopram (as evidenced in the brain parenchymal determinations of this SSRI in the midbrain) may in the present study be suggested as the main reason for also a more pronounced such 5-HT effect exerted in the raphe region of PCS rats secondary to the simply more concentration effective reupotake inhibitor here. However, the possibility for a more outspoken ability in itself in PCS rats than normally seen of peripheral citalopram administration to decrease the brain 5-HT output has to be further investigated in liver insufficiency, since the presently observed difference in citalopram concentrations in the brain in PCS versus controls clearly could be considered of likely minor relevance in absolute terms compared to the high potency for an SSRI-effect by this drug at any of the high levels obtained. It is relevant in this context that, in an autoradiographic study from our group, no changes in 5-HT_{1A} receptor density were detected in the dorsal raphe of PCS rats (Apelqvist *et al.*, 1996b). However, the latter referred study is as of yet only preliminary and do thus not allow us to exclude possible differences between the normal and PSE condition in, for example, 5-HT_{1A} receptor affinities for 5-HT or in the efficiency of post-receptor transduction mechanisms to be present (Apelqvist *et al.*, 1996b).

IMPLICATIONS FOR THE CLINICAL USE OF SSRIs IN LIVER FAILURE

The state-of-the-art, as presented above for brain TRP/5-HT in HE/PSE, may be summed up in a few general conceptual terms of relevance for the present use of novel neuropsychoactive drugs in clinical practice today. It is thus common knowledge that patients with liver insufficiency most often display altered pharmacokinetics for SSRIs as well as for other CNS serotonin-active agents and, in fact, most CNS-active compounds in general (Holm *et al.*, 1986; Doogan and Caillard, 1988; Schenker *et al.*, 1988; Krastev *et al.*, 1989; Royer *et al.*, 1989; DeVane *et al.*, 1990; Stoeckel *et al.*, 1990; Dahlhoff *et al.*, 1991; Goodnick, 1991; Ferry *et al.*, 1994; Orlando *et al.*, 1995; Sonne, 1996). However, for unclear reasons it has been forwarded that such clinical pharmacokinetic aberrations observed with the novel serotonin-active agents that frequently accompany conditions of liver failure are probably of only minor practical concern in giving and even dosing of these drugs to patients with any type of liver disease (Holm *et al.*, 1988; for overviews, Hale, 1993; DeVane, 1994). The basis for this type of blunt statement seems to be relying primarily on one secondary published open-labeled study of the SSRI fluvoxamine conducted without adequate kinetic control (Holm *et al.*, 1988). In this latter study the main motive for establishment of this conclusion was based on the observation that no overt worsening of the PSE was seen in a few patients with chronic liver disease when exposed to this SSRI for as short time as only two weeks (Holm *et al.*, 1988). It is clear, though, as evidenced by the results obtained by us (Bergqvist *et al.*, 1997c), and with regard solely to the pharmacodynamic complexity exerted by serotonin-active drugs in PCS rats, caution appears warranted to raise against uncontrolled and widespread use of e.g. SSRIs today in subjects having affected liver function. The main reason for this warning has a bearing on improvement of drug safety in general for such modern potent psychoactive medications that are introduced in the "decade of the brain" i.e. just prior to entering into the third millenium. Importantly, though, the recent study by us (Bergqvist *et al.*, 1997c) did not encompass complete investigations of the pharmacokinetics of citalopram in experimental PSE. It was, however, observed that in addition to the differences between PCS and sham-operated rats in pharmacodynamic responses to citalopram, also the kinetic behavior of this compound displayed major alterations likely to be associated with experimental chronic PSE. In agreement with results obtained from patients with liver disease (Baumann and Larsen, 1995), the serum levels of citalopram in PCS rats were found to be about two-fold compared to controls following only a single subcutaneous dose administred. This is not a surprising finding since citalopram is primarily metabolized by enzymes in the cytochrome P_{450} system (Baumann and Larsen, 1995), enzymes that to a major quantitative part are localized to the liver and in conditions of liver impairment this metabolism is likely to be compromised (George *et al.,* 1995) and the clearance of citalopram may thus be decreased. Certainly, therefore, it is not unlikely that pharmacodynamic and pharmacokinetic factors for citalopram, and probably also other SSRIs or similar agents in general, are concomitantly altered in conditions of liver impairment with or without PSE. Hence, the net effect of such changes in pharmacodynamics and pharmacokinetics in such conditions of pending encephalopathy if working in concert may eventually be truely hazardous. In order to minimize the risk for demonstrated but erronously denoted "paradoxical" drug reactions appearing in clinical practice and to enhance drug safety in patients with liver impairment administered novel potent 5-HT-psychoactive compounds a better delineation of the potential combined dynamic and kinetic effects exerted of such compounds (including e.g. their metabolitesand, in the case of racemates, their selective enantiomere effects) should be considered a high priority demand today. From the incomplete kinetic citalopram and metabolite data obtained in our study (Bergqvist *et al.,* 1997c) it could be seen that the racemic serum levels of the parent compound but not the main quantitative metabolite, desmethylcitalopram, were altered in experimental chronic PSE compared to controls. The reason for this is clearly that after, still only a single, subcutaneous injection the delayed maximum concentration (C_{max}) and longer elimination half-life ($t_{1/2}$) of desmethylcitalopram in blood serum will in this situation present itself as artefactually low desmethylcitalopram concentrations to what would be obtained if this metabolite were to be determined in serum at a later time point or after repeated dosing of the drug were investigated. Nevertheless, by the present observation of higher than normal serum citalopram concentrations accompanying the PCS rat after a single systemic challenge this should call for further scrutiny on pharmacokinetic parameters including kinetics also for the main metabolites upon repeated dosing and put in perspective of the pharmacodynamic effects possibly exerted by all these compounds when this condition is prevailing. The precise interpretation of the brain tissue levels of citalopram as obtained in this investigation (Bergqvist *et al.,* 1997c) is rather complicated. The reason for this is, of course, that the impact of both local as well as systemic administration effects intermingle here. The rational for this procedure in the present study was to obtain similar citalopram levels in the functional extracellular neocortical compartment in order to compare concentration-equal effects exerted by this compound on the output of 5-HT in PCS rats versus sham-operated controls. This prerequisite criterion was also met in the present experiment (as evidenced by the similar dialysis level of drug and main metabolite), and by the findings from brain parenchyma levels of citalopram it is suggested 1) that the comparably higher levels of citalopram in brain tissue versus dialysate probably result from a net contribution of citalopram to the tissue by the subsequent systemic dose given of the drug, and 2) that the higher levels of citalopram found in the tissue of neocortex and even more pronounced elevation in mesencephalon (raphe region) of PCS versus control rats most likely signify that the contribution to the brain of systemically administered citalopram to liver insufficiency with or without PSE probably is greater than normal if the same dose is given. Interpretation on the otherwise important serum-to-brain ratio of citalopram in has no meaningful purpose in the present study due to the clinically abnormal mixed fashion of local and systemic administration of the drug herein. However, these observations clearly warrant further detailed pharmacokinetic investigations to be conducted in conditions of compromised liver function if drugs like this are to be used more readily in broader groups of patients suffering also from such concurrent somatic disorders like those that may alter the metabolism of the drug.

REFERENCES

Adell, A. and Artigas, F., 1991, Differential effects of clomipramine given locally or systemically on extracellular5-hydroxytryptamine in raphe nuclei and frontal cortex. An in vivo brain microdialysis study. *Naunyn-Schmiedeberg's Arch. Pharmacol.* 343: 237-244.

Adell, A., Carceller, A., and Artigas, F., 1991, Regional distribution of extracellular 5-hydroxytryptamine and5-hydroxyindoleacetic acid in the brain of freely moving rats. *J. Neurochem.* 56: 709-712.

Adell, A., Sarna, GS., Hutson, PH., and Curzon, G., 1989, An in vivo dialysis and behavioural study of the release of 5-HT by p-chloroamphetamine in reserpine-treated rats. *Br. J. Pharmac.* 97: 206-212.

Adell, A., Carceller, A., and Artigas, F., 1993, In vivo brain dialysis study of the somatodendritic release of serotonin in the raphe nuclei of the rat: effects of 8-hydroxy-2-(di-n-propylamino)tetralin. *J. Neurochem.* 60: 1673-1681.

Aghajanian, G.K. and Haigler, H.J., 1975, Hallucinogenic indoleamines: preferential action upon presynaptic serotonin receptors. *Psychopharmacol. Comm.* 1: 619-629.

Aghajanian, G.K., 1978, Feedback regulation of central monoaminergic neurons: evidence from single cell recording studies. In (Youdim MBH, Lovenberg W, Sharman DF, and Lagnado JR, eds), Essays in Neurochemistry and Neuropharmacology. New York, John Wiley & Sons. pp. 1-32.

Alexander, J.J., Banerjee, P., Dawson, G., and Tonsgard, J.H., 1995, Hyperammonemia increases serotonin1A receptor expression in both rat hippocampus and a transfected hippocampal cell line, HN2-5. *J. Neurosci. Res.* 41: 105-110.

Apelqvist, G., Hindfelt, B., Andersson, G., and Bengtsson, F., 1996a, Diurnal and gender effects by chronic portacaval shunting in rats on spontaneous locomotor and rearing activities in an open-field. *Submitted.*

Apelqvist, G., Bergqvist, P.B.F., Larsson, B., Bugge, M., and Bengtsson, F., 1996b, Regional brain serotonin receptor changes in chronic experimental hepatic encephalopathy. *Submitted.*

Arendt, J., 1988, Melatonin. *Clin. Endocrinol.* 29: 205-229.

Arendt, J., 1995, Melatonin and the Mammalian Brain. London, Chapman and Hill.

Artigas, F., 1993, 5-HT_{1A} receptor antagonists in combination therapy. 5-HT and antidepressants: new views from microdialysis studies. *Trends Pharmacol. Sci.* 14: 262.

Aschcroft, G.W., Eccleston, D., and Crawford, T.B.B., 1965, 5-Hydroxyindole metabolism in rat brain. A study of intermediate metabolism using the technique of tryptophan loading-I. Methods. *J. Neurochem.* 12: 483-492.

Auerbach, S.B., Minzenberg, M.J., and Wilkinson, L.O., 1989, Extracellular serotonin and 5-hydroxyindoleacetic acid in hypothalamus of the unanesthetized rat measured by in vivo microdialysis coupled to high-performance liquid chromatography with electrochemical detection: dialysate serotonin reflects neuronal release. *Brain Res.* 499: 281-290.

Auerbach, S.B., Lundberg, J.F., and Hjorth, S., 1995, Differential inhibition of serotonin release by 5-HT and NA reuptake blockers after systemic administration. *Neuropharmacology* 34: 89-96.

Badawy, A.A-B., Morgan, C.J., Lane, J., Dhaliwal, K., and Bradley, DM., 1989, Liver tryptophan pyrrolase. A major determinant of the lower brain 5-hydroxytryptamine concentration in alcohol-preferring C57BL mice. *Biochem. J.* 264: 597-599.

Baldessarini, R.J. and Fischer, J.E., 1973, Serotonin metabolism in rat brain after surgical diversion of the portal venous circulation. *Nature New Biol.* 245: 25-27.

Baldessarini, R.J. and Fischer, J.E., 1978, Trace amines and alternative neurotransmitters in the central nervous system. *Biochem. Pharmacol.* 27: 621-626.

Basile, A.S., Jones, E.A., and Skolnick, P., 1991, The pathogenesis and treatment of hepatic encephalopathy: evidence for the involvement of benzodiazepine receptor ligands. *Pharmacol. Rev.* 43: 28-71.

Basile, A.S., Saito, K., Al-Mardini, H., Record, C.O., Hughes, R.D., Harrison, P., Williams R, Li Y, and Heyes MP ., 1995, The relationship between plasma and brain quinolinic acid levels and the severity of hepatic encephalopathy. *Gastroenterology* 108: 818-823.

Batshaw, M.L., Robinson, M.B., Hyland, K., Djali, S., and Heyes, M.P., 1993, Quinolinic acid in children with congenital hyperammonemia. Ann. Neurol. 34: 676-681.

Baumann, P. and Larsen, P., 1995, The pharmacokinetics of citalopram. Rev. Contemp. Pharmacother. 6: 287-295.

Baumgarten, H.G., Victor, S.J., and Lovenberg, W., 1973, Effect of intraventricular injection of 5,7-dihydroxytryptamine on regional tryptophan hydroxylase of rat brain. *J. Neurochem.* 21: 251-253.

Beadle, G.W., Mitchell, H.K., and Nyc, J.F., 1947, Kynurenine as an intermediate in the formation of nicotinic acid from tryptophane by Neurospora. *Proc. Natl. Acad. Sci.* 33: 155-158.

Beaubernard, C., Salomon, F., Grange, D., Thangapregassam, M.J., and Bismuth, J., 1977, Experimental hepaticencephalopathy. Changes of the level of wakefulness in the rat with portacaval shunt. *Biomedicine* 27: 169-171.

Beck, O., Eriksson, C.J.P., Kiinamaa, K., and Lundman, A., 1986, 5-hydroxyindoleacetic acid and 5-Hydroxytryptophol levels in rat brain: effects of ethanol, pyrazole, cyanamide and disulfiram treatment. *Drug and Alcohol Dependence* 16: 303-308.

Beck, O., Lundman, A., and Jonsson, G., 1987, 5-Hydroxytryptophol and 5-hydroxyindoleacetic acid levels in rat brain: effects of various drugs affecting serotonergic transmitter mechanisms. *J. Neural Transm.* 69: 287-298.

Beck, O., Helander, A., Carlsson, S., and Borg, S., 1995, Changes in serotonin metabolism during treatment with the aldehyde dehydrogenase inhibitors disulfiram and cyanamide. *Pharmacol. Toxicol.* 77: 323-326.

Bel, N. and Artigas, F., 1992, Fluvoxamine preferentially increases extracellular 5-hydroxytryptamine in the raphe nuclei: an in vivo microdialysis study. *Eur. J. Pharmacol.* 229: 101-103.

Bengtsson, F., Gage, F.H., Jeppsson, B., Nobin, A., and Rosengren, E., 1985, Brain monoamine metabolism and behavior in portacaval-shunted rats. Exp. Neurol. 90: 21-35.

Bengtsson, F., Nobin, A., Falck, B., Gage, F.H., and Jeppsson, B., 1986, Portacaval shunt in the rat: selective alterations in behavior and brain serotonin. Pharmacol. Biochem. Behav. 24: 1611-1616.

Bengtsson, F., Bugge, M., Hansson, L., Fyge, K., Jeppsson, B., and Nobin, A., 1987a, Serotonin metabolism in the central nervous system following sepsis or portacaval shunt in the rat. J. Surg. Res. 43: 420-429.

Bengtsson, F., Bugge, M., Vagianos, C., Jeppsson, B., and Nobin, A., 1987b, Brain serotonin metabolism and behavior in rats with carbon tetrachloride-induced liver cirrhosis. *Res. Exp. Med.* 187: 429-438.

Bengtsson, F., Bugge, M., Brun, A., Falck, B., Henriksson, K.G., and Nobin, A., 1988a, The impact of time after portacaval shunt in the rat on behavior, brain serotonin, and brain and muscle histology. *J. Neurolog. Sci.* 83: 109-122.

Bengtsson, F., Nobin, A., Falck, B., Gage, F.H., and Jeppsson, B., 1988b, Effect of oral branched chain amino acids on behavior and brain serotonin metabolism in portacaval shunted rats. *World J. Surg.* 12: 246-254.

Bengtsson, F., Bugge, M., Hall, H., and Nobin, A., 1989a, Brain 5-HT_1 and 5-HT_2 binding sites following portacaval shunt in the rat. *Res. Exp. Med.* 189: 249-256.

Bengtsson, F., Bugge, M., and Nobin, A., 1989b, Hepatocerebral dysfunction and brain serotonin. In (Butterworth RF and Pomier Layrargues G, eds), *Hepatic Encephalopathy: Pathophysiology and Treatment.* Clifton, NJ, The Humana Press, Inc. pp. 355-385.

Bengtsson, F., Bugge, M., Johansen, K.H., and Butterworth, R.F., 1991, Brain tryptophan hydroxylation in the portacaval shunted rat: a hypothesis for the regulation of serotonin turnover in vivo. *J. Neurochem.* 56: 1069-1074.

Bengtsson, F., 1992, Neurotransmission failure in hepatic encephalopathy involving the combined action of different brain tryptophan-related pathology: a speculative synthesis. In (Ishiguro I, Kido R, Nagatsu T, Nagamura Y, and Ohta Y, eds), *Advances in Tryptophan Research 1992.* Toyoake, Japan, Fujita Health University Press. pp. 303-308.

Bengtsson, F. and Bergqvist, P.B.F., 1996, Neuropsychiatric implications of brain tryptophan: Perturbations appearing in hepatic encephalopathy. In (Filippini GA, Costa CVL, and Bertazzo A, eds), Recent Advances in Tryptophan Research. New York, NY, Plenum Publ. Corp. pp. 387-395.

Bergeron, M., Pomier Layrargues, G., and Butterworth, RF., 1989a, Aromatic and branched-chain amino acids in autopsied brain tissue from cirrhotic patients with hepatic encephalopathy. *Metab. Brain Dis.* 4: 169-176.

Bergeron, M., Reader, T.A., Pomier Layrargues, G., and Butterworth, R.F., 1989b, Monoamines and metabolites in autopsied brain tissue from cirrhotic patients with hepatic encephalopathy. *Neurochem. Res.* 14: 853-859.

Bergeron, M., Swain, M.S., Reader, T.A., Grondin, L., and Butterworth, R.F., 1990, Effect of ammonia on brain serotonin metabolism in relation to function in the portacaval shunted rat. *J. Neurochem.* 55: 222-229.

Bergeron, M., Reader, T.A., and Butterworth. RF., 1991, Early changes of serotonin turnover in brain following portacaval anastomosis: Relation to altered sleep patterns and diurnal rhythms. In (Bengtsson F, Jeppsson B, Almdal T, and Vilstrup H, eds), Progress in Hepatic Encephalopathy and Metabolic Nitrogen Exchange. Boca Raton, FL, CRC Press, Inc. pp. 219-232.

Bergeron, M., Swain, M.S., Reader, T.A., and Butterworth, R.F., 1995, Regional alterations of dopamine and its metabolites in rat brain following portacaval anastomosis. *Neurochem. Res.* 20: 79-86.

Bergonzi, P., Bianco, A., Mazza, A., and Mennuni, G., 1978, Night sleep organization in patients with severe hepatic failure. Its modifications after L-DOPA treatment. *Eur. Neurol.* 17: 271-275.

Bergqvist, P.B.F., Werner, E.R., Apelqvist, G., Bugge, M., Wachter, H., and Bengtsson, F., 1995a, Brain biopterin metabolism in chronic experimental hepatic encephalopathy. *Metab. Brain Dis.* 10: 143-157.

Bergqvist, P.B.F., Heyes, M.P., Bugge, M., and Bengtsson, F., 1995b, Brain quinolinic acid in chronic experimental hepatic encephalopathy: Effects of an exogenous ammonium acetate challenge. *J. Neurochem.* 65: 2235-2240.

Bergqvist, P.B.F., Vogels, B.A.P.M., Bosman, D.K., Maas, M.A.W., Hjorth, S., Chamuleau, R.A.F.M., and Bengtsson, F., 1995c, Neocortical dialysate monoamines of rats after acute, subacute, and chronic liver shunt. *J. Neurochem.* 64: 1238-1244.

Bergqvist, P.B.F., Heyes, M.P., Apelqvist, G., Butterworth, R.F., and Bengtsson, F., 1996a, Brain extracellular quinolinic acid in chronic experimental hepatic encephalopathy as assessed by in vivo microdialysis: Acute effects of L-tryptophan. *Neuropsychopharmacology,* 15: 382-389.

Bergqvist, P.B.F., Hjorth, S., Apelqvist, G., and Bengtsson, F., 1996b, Acute effects of L-tryptophan on brain extracellular 5-HT and 5-HIAA in chronic experimental portal-systemic encephalopathy. *Metab. Brain Dis.,* 11: 269-278.

Bergqvist, P.B.F., Hjorth, S., Audet, R., Apelqvist, G., Bengtsson, F., and Butterworth, R.F., 1996c, Ammonium acetate challenge in experimental hepatic encephalopathy induces a transient increase of brain 5-HT release in vivo. *Eur. Neuropsychopharmacology, In press.*

Bergqvist, PBF, Some, M, Apelqvist, G, Helander, A, and Bengtsson, F., 1996d, Elevated brain 5-hydroxytryptophol levels in chronic experimental portal-systemic encephalopathy. *Submitted.*

Bergqvist, P.B.F., Hjorth, S., Apelqvist, G., and Bengtsson, F., 1997a, Potassium-evoked neuronal serotonin release in experimental portal-systemic encephalopathy. *Submitted.*

Bergqvist, P.B.F., Hjorth, S., Wikell, C., Apelqvist, G., and Bengtsson, F., 1997b, p-Chloroamphetamine- and d-fenfluramine induced brain serotonin release in experimental portal-systemic encephalopathy. *Submitted.*

Bergqvist, P.B.F., Wikell, C., Hjorth, S., Apelqvist, G., and Bengtsson, F., 1997c, Citalopram and release of brain serotonin in experimental portal-systemic encephalopathy: Implications for the clinical use of selective serotonin reuptake inhibitors in liver insufficiency. *Submitted.*

Bessman, S.P. and Bessman, A.N., 1955, The cerebral and peripheral uptake of ammonia in liver disease with an hypothesis for the mechanism of hepatic coma. *J. Clin. Invest.* 34: 622-628.

Blier, P., de Montigny, C., and Tardif, D., 1984, Effects of the two antidepressant drugs mianserin and indalpine on the serotonergic system: single-cell studies in the rat. *Psychopharmacology* 84: 242-249.

Bloxam, D.L. and Curzon, G., 1978, A study of proposed determinants of brain tryptophan concentration in rat after portocaval anastomosis or sham operation. *J. Neurochem.* 31: 1255-1263.

Bonanno, G., Fassio, A., Severi, P., Ruelle, A., and Raiteri, M., 1994, Fenfluramine releases serotonin from human brain nerve endings by a dual mechanism. *J. Neurochem.* 63: 1163-1166.

Borowsky, B. and Hoffman, B.J., 1995, Neurotransmitter transporters: molecular biology, function, and regulation. *Int. Rev. Neurobiol.* 38: 139-199.

Brodie, B.B., Pletscher, A., and Shore, PA., 1955, Evidence that serotonin has a role in brain function. *Science* 122: 968.

Bucci, L., Cardelli, M., Chiavarelli, R., Massotti, M., and Morisi, G., 1980, Behavioral, electroencephalographic, and biochemical changes in porta-cava shunted rats. *Intern. J. Neuroscience* 10: 129-134.

Bucci, L., Ioppolo, A., Chiavarelli, R., and Bigotti, A., 1982, The central-nervous-system toxicity of long-term oral administration of L-tryptophan to porto-caval-shunted rats. *Br. J. exp. Path.* 63: 235-241.

Bugge, M., Bengtsson, F., Nobin, A., Holmin, T., Jeppsson, B., Hultberg, B., Falck, B., and Herlin, P., 1986, Amino acids and indoleamines in the brain after infusion of branched-chain amino acids to rats with liver ischemia. *J. Parent. Ent. Nutr.* 10: 474-478.

Bugge, M., Bengtsson, F., Nobin, A., Hall, H., Wedel, I., Jeppsson, B., and Herlin, P., 1989a, Serotonin receptors in the brain following total hepatoectomy in rats treated with branched-chain amino acids. *J. Parent. Ent. Nutr.* 13: 235-239.

Bugge, M., Bengtsson, F., Nobin, A., Jeppsson, B., Hultberg, B., Jonung, T., and Herlin, P., 1989b, The effect of ammonia infusion on brain monoamine metabolism in portacaval-shunted rats. *Res. Exp. Med.* 189: 101-111.

Bulat, M., Iskric, S., Stancic, L., Kveder, S., and Zivkovic, B., 1970, The formation of 5-hydroxytryptophol from exogenous 5-hydroxytryptamine in cat spinal cord in vivo. *J. Pharm. Pharmacol.* 22: 67-68.

Butterworth, R.F., Giguère, J.F., Michaud, J., Lovoie, J., and Layrargues, G.P., 1987, Ammonia: key factor in the pathogenesis of hepatic encephalopathy. *Neurochem. Pathol.* 6: 1-12.

Butterworth, R.F., Girard, G., and Giguère, J-F., 1988, Regional differences in the capacity for ammonia removal by brain following portocaval anastomosis. *J. Neurochem.* 51: 486-490.

Butterworth, R.F., 1992a, Evidence that hepatic encephalopthy results from a defect of glutamatergic synaptic regulation. *Mol. Neuropharmacol.* 2: 229-232.

Butterworth, R.F., 1992b, Pathogenesis and treatment of portal-systemic encephalopathy: An update. *Dig. Dis. Sci.* 37: 321-327.

Butterworth, R.F., 1993, Portal-systemic encephalopathy: A disorder of neuron-astrocytic metabolic trafficking. *Dev. Neurosci.* 15: 313-319.

Butterworth, R.F., 1994, Hepatic encephalopathy. In (Arias IM, Boyer JL, Fausto N, Jakoby WB, Schachter DA, and Shafritz DA, eds), *The Liver: Biology and Pathology.* New York, N.Y., Raven Press, Ltd., pp. 1193-1208.

Butterworth, R.F., 1996, Neuroactive amino acids in hepatic encephalopathy. *Metab. Brain Dis.* 11: 165-173.

Cahill, G.M. and Besharse, J.C., 1995, Circadian rhythmicity in vertebrate retinas: regulation by a photoreceptor oscillator. *Prog. Ret. Eye Res.* 14: 267-291.

Carboni, E., Cadoni, C., Tanda, G.L., and Di Chiara, G., 1989, Calcium-dependent, tetrodotoxin-sensitive stimulation of cortical serotonin release after a tryptophan load. *J. Neurochem.* 53: 976-978.

Carboni, E. and Di Chiara, G., 1989, Serotonin release estimated by transcortical dialysis in freely-moving rats. *Neuroscience* 32: 637-645.

Carlsson, A. and Lindqvist, M., 1978, Dependence of 5-HT and catecholamine synthesis on concentrations of precursor amino-acids in rat brain. *Naunyn-Schmiedeberg's Arch. Pharmacol.* 303: 157-164.

Cascino, A., Cangiano, C., Fiaccadori, F., Ghinelli, F., Merli, M., Pelosi, G., Riggio, O., Rossi-Fanelli, F., Sacchini, D., Stortoni, M., and Capocaccia, L., 1982, Plasma and cerebrospinal fluid amino acid patterns in hepatic encephalopathy. *Dig. Dis. Sci.* 27: 828-832.

Cascio, C.S., and Kellar, K.J., 1983, Characterization of [^{3}H]tryptamine binding sites in brain. *Eur. J. Pharmacol.* 95: 31-39.

Cheifetz, S. and Warsh, J,J., 1980, Occurence and distribution of 5-hydroxytryptophol in the rat. *J. Neurochem.* 34:1093-1099.

Chesselet, M.-F., 1984, Presynaptic regulation of neurotransmitter release in the brain: facts and hypothesis. *Neuroscience* 12: 347-375.

Clemens, J.A., Sawyer, B.D., and Cerimele, B., 1977, Further evidence that serotonin is a neurotransmitter involved in the control of prolactin secretion. *Endocrinology* 100: 692-698.

Conn, H.O., and Lieberthal, M.M., 1979, *The hepatic coma syndromes and lactulose.* Baltimore, MD, The Williams & Williams Co.

Conn, H.O. and Bircher, J., 1988, *Hepatic Encephalopathy: Management with Lactulose and Related Carbohydrates.* East Lansing, Michigan, Medi-Ed Press.

Costa, E., and Meek, J.L., 1974, Regulation of biosynthesis of catecholamines and serotonin in the CNS. *Ann. Rev. Pharmacol.* 14: 491-511.

Crinquette, J-F., Boschat, M., Rapin, J-R., Delorme, M-L., and Opolon, P., 1982, Early changes in blood-brain barrier permeability after porto-caval shunt and liver ischaemia. *Clin. Physiol.* 2: 241-250.

Crossley, I.R. and Williams, R., 1984, Progress in the treatment of chronic portasystemic encephalopathy. *Gut* 20: 85-98.

Cuilleret, G., Pomier Layrargues, G., Pons, F., Cadilhac, J., and Michel, H., 1980, Changes in brain catecholamine levels in human cirrhotic hepatic encephalopathy. *Gut* 21: 565-569.

Cummings, M.G., Soeters, P.B., James, J.H., Keane, J.M., and Fischer, J.E., 1976a, Regional brain indoleamine metabolism following chronic portacaval anastomosis in the rat. *J. Neurochem.* 27: 501-509.

Cummings, M.G., Soeters, P.B., James, J.H., Keane, J.M., and Fischer, J.E., 1976b, Regional brain study of indoleamine metabolism in the rat in acute hepatic failure. *J. Neurochem.* 27: 741-746.

Curzon, G., Kantamaneni, B.D., Winch, J., Rojas-Bueno, A., Murray-Lyon, I.M., and Williams, R., 1973, Plasma and brain tryptophan changes in experimental acute hepatic failure. *J. Neurochem.* 21: 137-145.

Curzon, G., Kantamaneni, B.D., Fernando, J.C., Woods, M.S., and Cavanagh, J.B., 1975, Effects of chronic porto-caval anastomosis on brain tryptophan, tyrosine and 5-hydroxytryptamine. *J. Neurochem.* 24: 1065-1070.

Curzon, G., and Marsden, C.A., 1975, Metabolism of a tryptophan load in the hypothalamus and other brain regions. *J. Neurochem.* 25: 251-256.

Curzon, G., Fernando, J.C.R., and Marsden, C.A., 1978, 5-Hydroxytryptamine: the effects of impaired synthesis on its metabolism and release in rat. *Br. J. Pharmac.* 63: 627-634.

Curzon, G., 1986, Serotonin neurochemistry revisited: a new look at some old axioms. *Neurochem. Int.* 8: 155-159.

Dalhoff, K., Almdal, T.P., Bjerrum, K., Keiding, S., Mengel, H., and Lund, J., 1991, Pharmacokinetics of paroxetine in patients with cirrhosis. *Eur. J. Clin. Pharmacol.* 41: 351-354.

Davis, V.E., Cashaw, J.L., Huff, J.A., and Brown, H., 1966, Identification of 5-hydroxytryptophol as a serotonin metabolite in man. *Proc. Soc. Exp. Biol. Med.* 122: 890-893.
de Montigny, C., Blier, P., and Chaput, Y., 1984, Electrophysiologically-identified serotonin receptors in the rat CNS. Effect of antidepressant treatment. *Neuropharmacology* 23: 1511-1520.
de Parada, M.P., Parada, M.A., Pothos, E., and Hoebel, B.G., 1995, d-Fenfluramine, but not d-norfenfluramine, uses calcium to increase extracellular serotonin. *Life Sci.* 56: 415-420.
De Simoni, M.G., Sokola, A., Fodritto, F., Dal Toso, G., and Algeri, S., 1987, Functional meaning of tryptophan-induced increase of 5-HT metabolism as clarified by in vivo voltammetry. *Brain Res.* 411: 89-94.
Deguchi, T., 1975, Ontogenesis of a biological clock for serotonin:acetyl coenzyme A *N*-acetyltransferase in pineal gland of rat. *Proc. Natl. Acad. Sci.* 72: 2814-2818.
Descarries, L., and Beaudet, A., 1983, The use of radioautography for investigating transmitter-specific neurons. In (Björklund A and Hökfelt T, eds), *Handbook of Chemical Neuroanatomy. Vol 1: Methods in Chemical Neuroanatomy*. Amsterdam, Elsevier, pp. 286-364.
DeVane, C.L., Laizure, S.C., Stewart, J.T., Kolts, B.E., Ryerson, E.G., Miller, R.L., and Lai, A.A., 1990, Disposition of bupropion in healthy volunteers and subjects with alcoholic liver disease. *J. Clin. Psychopharmacol.* 10: 328-332.
DeVane, C.L., 1994, Pharmacokinetics of newer antidepressants: clinical relevance. *Am. J. Med.* 97(suppl 6A): 13S-23S.
Dewhurst, W.G., and McKim, HR., 1980, Pharmacological effects of p-chloroamphetamine with respect to current amine hypotheses of affective disorders. *Neuropsychobiology* 6: 66-71.
Di Chiara, G., 1990, Brain dialysis of neurotransmitters: a commentary. *J. Neurosci. Meth.* 34: 29-34.
Diggory, G.L., Ceasar, P.M., Hazelby, D., and Taylor, K.T., 1979, Endogenous 5-hydroxytryptophol in mouse brain. *J. Neurochem.* 32: 1323-1325.
Doogan, D.P., and Caillard, V., 1988, Sertraline: A new antidepressant. *J. Clin. Psychiat.* 49(8, suppl): 46-51.
Dooley, D.J., and Quock, R.M., 1976, Tryptamine and 5-hydroxytryptamine-induced hypothermia in mice. *J. Pharm. Pharmacol.* 28: 775-776.
Dreshfield, L.J., Wong, D.T., Perry, K.W., and Engleman, E.A., 1996, Enhancement of fluoxetine-dependent increase of extracellular serotonin (5-HT) levels by (-)-pindolol, an antagonist at 5-HT_{1A} receptors. *Neurochem. Res.* 21: 557-562.
Eccleston, D., Aschcroft, G.W., and Crawford, T.B.B., 1965, 5-Hydroxyindole metabolism in rat brain. A study of intermediate metabolism using the technique of tryptophan loading-II. Applications and drug studies. *J. Neurochem.* 12: 493-503.
Eccleston, D., Aschcroft, G.W., Crawford, T.B.B., Stanton, J.B., Wood, D., and McTurk, P.H., 1970, Effect of tryptophan administration on 5HIAA in cerebrospinal fluid in man. *J. Neurol. Neurosurg. Psychiat.* 33: 269-272.
El Mansari, M., and Blier, P., 1996, Functional characterization of 5-HT_{1D} autoreceptors on the modulation of 5-HT release in guinea-pig mesencephalic raphe, hippocampus and frontal cortex. *Br. J. Pharmacol.* 118: 681-689.
Elks, M.L., Youngblood, W.W., and Kizer, J.S., 1979, Serotonin synthesis and release in brain slices: independece of tryptophan. *Brain Res.* 172: 471-486.
Ellinger, A., 1904, Die Entstehung der Kynurensäure. Z. *Physiol. Chem.* 43: 325-337.
Engel, G., Göthert, M., Hoyer, D., Schlicker, E., and Hillenbrand, K., 1986, Identity of inhibitory presynaptic 5-hydroxytryptamine (5-HT) autoreceptors in the rat brain cortex with 5-HT_{1B} binding sites. *Naunyn-Schmiedeberg's Arch. Pharmacol.* 332: 1-7.
Ennis, C., Kemp, J.D., and Cox, B., 1981, Characterisation of inhibitory 5-hydroxytryptamine receptors that modulate dopamine release in the striatum. *J. Neurochem.* 36: 1515-1520.
Ennis, C. and Cox, B., 1982, Pharmacological evidence for the existence of two distinct serotonin receptors in rat brain. *Neuropharmacology* 21: 41-44.
Erecinska, M., Pastuszko, A., Wilson, D.F., and Nelson, D., 1987, Ammonia-induced release of neurotransmitters from rat brain synaptosomes: differences between the effects on amines and amino acids. *J. Neurochem.* 49: 1258-1265.
Faraj, B.A., Camp, V.M., Ansley, J.D., Scott, J., Ali, F.M., and Malveaux, E.J., 1981, Evidence for central hypertyraminemia in hepatic encephalopathy. *J. Clin. Invest.* 67: 395-402.
Feldstein, A., Chang, F.H., and Kucharski, J.M., 1970, Tryptophol, 5-hydroxytryptophol and 5-methoxytryptophol induced sleep in mice. *Life Sci.* 9: 323-329.
Fernstrom, J.D., and Wurtman, R.J., 1971, Brain serotonin content: physiological dependence on plasma tryptophan levels. *Science* 173: 149-151.

Ferré, S., and Artigas, F., 1993, Dopamine D_2 receptor-mediated regulation of serotonin extracellular concentration in the dorsal raphe nucleus of freely moving rats. *J. Neurochem.* 61: 772-775.

Ferrier, I.N., Arendt, J., Johnstone, E.C., and Crow, T.J., 1982, Reduced nocturnal melatonin secretion in chronic schizophrenia: relationship to body weight. *Clin. Endocrinol.* 17: 181-187.

Ferry, N., Bernard, N., Cuisinaud, G., Rougier, P., Trepo, C., and Sassard, J., 1994, Influence of hepatic impairment on the pharmacokinetics of nefazodone and two of its metabolites after single and multiple oral doses. *Fundam. Clin. Pharmacol.* 8: 463-473.

Fischer, J.E., and Baldessarini, R.J., 1971, False neurotransmitters and hepatic failure. *The Lancet* ii: 75-79.

Fischer, J.E., Yoshimura, N., Aguirre, A., James, J.H., Cummings, M.G., Abel, R.M., and Deindoerfer, F., 1974, Plasma amino acids in patients with hepatic encephalopathy. Effects of amino acid infusions. *Am. J. Surg.* 127: 40-47.

Fischer, J.E., and Baldessarini, R.J., 1976, Pathogenesis and therapy of hepatic coma. In (Popper H and Schaffner F, eds), *Progress in Liver Diseases*. New York, Grune & Stratton., pp. 363-397.

Fornal, C.A., Metzler, C.W., Gallegos, R.A., Veasey, S.C., McCreary, A.C., and Jacobs, B.L., 1996, WAY-100635, a potent and selective 5-hydroxytryptamine$_{1A}$ antagonist, increases serotonergic neuronal activity in behaving cats: comparison with (*S*)-WAY-100135. *J. Pharmacol. Exp. Ther.* 278: 752-762.

Freese, A., Swartz, K.J., During, M.J., and Martin, J.B., 1990, Kynurenine metabolites of tryptophan: Implications for neurologic diseases. Neurology 40: 691-695.

Friedman, P.A., Kappelman. A.H., and Kaufman. S., 1972, Partial purification and characterization of tryptophan hydroxylase from rabbit hindbrain. *J. Biol. Chem.* 247: 4165-4173.

Fu, L.H.W., Hayashi, S., and Toda, N., 1980, Effects of 5-hydroxytryptophol, a 5-hydroxytryptamine metabolite, on isolated cerebral arteries of the dog. *Br. J. Pharmac.* 68: 17-18.

Fukushima, T., and Nixon, J.C., 1980, Analysis of reduced forms of biopterin in biological tissues and fluids. Anal. Biochem. 102: 176-188.

Fuller, R.W., and Wong, D.T., 1990, Serotonin uptake and serotonin uptake inhibition. N.Y. Acad. Sci. 600: 68-78.

Fuxe, K., Butcher, L.L., and Engel, J., 1971, DL-5-hydroxytryptophan-induced changes in central monoamine neurons after peripheral decarboxylase inhibition. *J. Pharm. Pharmacol.* 23: 420-424.

Gallego, A., and Lorente de No, R., 1947, On the effect of several monovalent ions upon frog nerve. J. Cell. Comp. Physiol. 29: 189-206.

Garfinkel, D., Laudon, M., Nof, D., and Zisapel, N., 1995, Improvement of sleep quality in elderly people by controlled-release melatonin. Lancet 346: 541-544.

Gartside, S.E., Cowen, P.J., and Sharp, T., 1992, Effect of 5-hydroxy-L-tryptophan on the release of 5-HT in rat hypothalamus *in vivo* as measured by microdialysis. *Neuropharmacology* 31: 9-14.

George, J., Murray, M., Byth, K., and Farrell, G.C., 1995, Differential alterations of cytochrome P450 proteins in livers from patients with severe chronic liver disease. *Hepatology* 21: 120-128.

Gholson, R.K., Ueda, I., Ogasawara, N., and Henderson, L.M., 1964, The enzymatic conversion of quinolinate to nicotinic acid mononucleotide in mammalian liver. *J. Biol. Chem.* 239: 1208-1214.

Gibson, C.J., Deikel, S.M., Young, S.N., and Binik, Y.M., 1982, Behavioural and biochemical effects of tryptophan, tyrosine and phenylalanine in mice. Psychopharamacology 76: 118-121.

Gobbi, M., Frittoli, E., and Mennini, T., 1990, The modulation of [^{3}H]noradrenaline and [^{3}H]serotonin release from rat brain synaptosomes is not mediated by the α_{2B}-adrenoceptor subtype. Naunyn-Schmiedeberg's Arch. Pharmacol. 342: 382-386.

Goodnick, P.J., 1991, Pharmacokinetics of second generation antidepressants: fluoxetine. Psychopharmacol. Bull. 27: 503-512.

Grahame-Smith, D.G., 1971, Studies *in vivo* on the relationship between brain tryptophan, brain 5.HT synthesis and hyperactivity in rats treated with a monoamine oxidase inhibitor and L-tryptophan. *J. Neurochem.* 18: 1053-1066.

Grahame-Smith, D.G., 1973, Does the total turnover of brain 5-HT reflect the functional activity of 5-HT in brain. In (Barchas J and Usdin E, eds), *Serotinin and Behavior*. New York, NY, Academic Press., pp. 5-7.

Grahame-Smith, D.G., 1974, How important is the synthesis of brain 5-hydroxytryptamine in the physiological control of its central function? Adv. Biochem. Psychopharmacol. 10: 83-91.

Gullino, P., Winitz, M., Birnbaum, S.M., Cornfield, J., Otey, M.C., and Greenstein, J.P., 1956, Studies on the metabolism of amino acids and related compounds *in vivo*. I. Toxicity of essential amino acids, individually and in mixtures, and the protective effect of L-arginine. Arch. Biochem. Biophys. 64: 319-332.

Hale, A.S., 1993, New antidepressants: use in high-risk patients. J. Clin. Psychiat. 54: 61-70.

Héry, F., and Ternaux, J.P., 1981, Regulation of release processes in central serotoninergic neurons. J. Physiol. (Paris) 77: 287-301.

Heslop, K.E., and Curzon, G., 1994, Depletion and repletion of cortical tissue and dialysate 5-HT after reserpine. *Neuropharmacology* 33: 567-573.

Hindfelt, B., Plum, F., and Duffy, T.E., 1977, Effect of acute ammonia intoxication on cerebral metabolism in rats with portacaval shunts. *J. Clin. Invest.* 59: 386-396.

Hirayama, C., 1971, Thryptophan metabolism in liver disease. Clin. Chim. Acta 32: 191-197.

Hjorth, S., and Sharp, T., 1991, Effect of the 5-HT_{1A} receptor agonist 8-OH-DPAT on the release of 5-HT in dorsal and median raphe-innervated rat brain regions as measured by in vivo microdialysis. *Life Sci.* 48: 1779-1786.

Hjorth, S., and Tao, R., 1991, The putative 5-HT_{1B} receptor agonist CP-93,129 supresses rat hippocampal 5-HT release in vivo: comparison with RU 24969. *Eur. J. Pharmacol.* 209: 249-252.

Hjorth, S., 1993, Serotonin 5-HT_{1A} autoreceptor blockade potentiates the ability of the 5-HT reuptake inhibitor citalopram to increase nerve terminal output of 5-HT in vivo: a microdialysis study. *J. Neurochem.* 60: 776-779.

Hjorth, S., and Auerbach, S.B., 1994, Further evidence for the importance of 5-HT_{1A} autoreceptors in the activation of selective serotonin reuptake inhibitors. *Eur. J. Pharmacol.* 260: 251-255.

Hjorth, S., and Auerbach, S.B., 1996, 5-HT_{1A} autoreceptors and the mode of action of selective serotonin reuptake inhibitors (SSRI). Behav. *Brain Res.* 73: 281-283.

Hjorth, S., 1996, (-)-Pindolol, but not buspirone, potentaites the citalopram-induced rise in extracellular 5-hydroxytryptamine. *Eur. J. Pharmacol.* 303: 183-186.

Holm, E., Uhl, W., and Stamm, S., 1986, Safety of fluvoxamine for patients with chronic liver disease. Adv. Pharmacother. 2: 151-165.

Holm, E., Jacob, S., Kortsik, C., Leweling, H., and Fischer, B., 1988, Failure of selective serotonin re-uptake inhibition to worsen the mental state of patients with subclinical hepatic encephalopathy. In (Soeters PB, Wilson JHP, Meijer A.J, and Holm E, eds), *Advances in Ammonia Metabolism and Hepatic Encephalopathy.* Amsterdam, Elsevier Science Publishers B.V., pp. 474-486.

Hoyer, D., Clarke, D.E., Fozard, J.R., Hartig, P.R., Martin, G.R., Mylecharane, E.J., Saxena, P.R., and Humphrey, P.P.A., 1994, VII. International union of pharmacology classification of receptors for 5-hydroxytryptamine (serotonin). *Pharmacol. Rev.* 46: 157-203.

Hutson, D.G., Ono, J., Dombro, R.S., Levi, J.U., Livingstone, A., and Zeppa, R., 1979, A longitudinal study of tryptophan involvment in hepatic coma. *Am. J. Surg.* 137: 235-239.

Hutson, P.H., Sarna, G.S., Kantamaneni, B.D., and Curzon, G., 1985, Monitoring the effect of a tryptophan load on brain indole metabolism in freely moving rats by simultaneous cerebrospinal fluid sampling and brain dialysis. *J. Neurchem.* 44: 1266-1273.

Hutson, P.H., Sarna, G.S., O'Connell, M.T., and Curzon, G., 1989, Hippocampal 5-HT synthesis and release in vivo is decreased by infusion of 8-OH-DPAT into the nucleus raphe dorsalis. *Neurosci. Lett.* 100: 276-280.

Ichiyama, A., Nakamura, S., Nishizuka, Y., and Hayaishi, O., 1968, Tryptophan-5-hydroxylase in mammalian brain. Adv. Pharmacol. 6A: 5-17.

Jackson, H.C., Hewitt, K.N., Hutchins, L.J., Cheetham, S.C., and Heal, D.J., 1996, Augmentation of antidepressant action of SSRIs by pindolol may not be explained by 5-HT1A receptor antagonism. Soc. Neurosci. Abstr. 22: 1328.

Jacobs, B.L. and Fornal, C.A., 1991, Activity of brain serotonergic neurons in the behaving animal. *Pharmacol. Rev.* 43: 563-578.

James, J.H., Hodgman, J.M., Funovics, J.M., Yoshimura. N., and Fischer, J.E., 1976, Brain tryptophan, plasma free tryptophan and distribution of plasma neutral amino acids. Metabolism 25: 471-476.

James, J.H., Escourrou, J., and Fischer, J.E., 1978, Blood-brain neutral amino acid transport activity is increased after portacaval anastomosis. *Science* 200: 1395-1397.

James, J.H., Ziparo, V., Jeppsson, B., and Fischer, J.E., 1979, Hyperammonemia, plasma aminoacid imbalance, and blood-brain aminoacid transport: a unified theory of portal-systemic encephalopathy. *Lancet* ii: 772-775.

James, S.P., Sack, D.A., Rosenthal, N.E., and Mendelson, W.B., 1990, Melatonin administration in insomnia. *Neuropsychopharmacology* 3: 19-23.

Jellinger, K. and Riederer, P., 1977, Brain monoamines in metabolic (endotoxic) coma. A preliminary biochemical study in human postmortem material. *J. Neural Transm.* 41: 275-286.

Jellinger, K., Riederer, P., Rausch, W.D., and Kothbauer, P., 1978, Brain monoamines in hepatic encephalopathy and other types of metabolic coma. *J. Neural Transm.* Suppl. 14: 103-120.

Jessy, J., Mans, A.M., DeJoseph, M.R., and Hawkins, R.A., 1990, Hyperammonemia causes many of the changes found after portacaval shunting. *Biochem. J.* 272: 311-317.

Johnston, C.A., and Moore, K.E., 1983, Measurement of 5-hydroxytryptamine synthesis and metabolism in selected discrete regions of the rat brain using high performance liquid chromatography and electrochemical detection: pharmacological manipulations. *J. Neural Transm.* 57: 49-63.

Kalén, P., Strecker, R.E., Rosengren, E., and Björklund, A., 1989, Regulation of striatal serotonin release by the lateral habenula-dorsal raphe pathway in the rat as demonstrated by in vivo microdialysis: role of excitatory amino acids and GABA. *Brain Res.* 492: 187-202.

Kimelberg, H.K., 1988, Serotonin uptake into astrocytes and its implications. In (Osborne NN and Hamon M, eds), *Neuronal Serotonin.* John Wiley & Sons, Ltd., pp. 347-365.

Klein, D.C. and Weller, J.L., 1970, Indole metabolism in the pineal gland: a circadian rhythm in N-acetyltransferase. *Science* 169: 1093-1095.

Kleven, M.S., Dwoskin, L.P., and Sparber, S.B., 1983, Pharmacological evidence for the existence of multiple functional pools of brain serotonin: analysis of brain perfusate from conscious rats. *J. Neurochem.* 41: 1143-1149.

Knapp, S., and Mandell, A.J., 1984, TRH influences the pterin cofactor- and time-dependent instabilities of rat raphe tryptophan hydroxylase activity assessed under far-from-equilibrium conditions. *Neurochem. Int.* 6: 801-812.

Knell, A.J., Davidson, A.R., Williams, R., Kantamaneni, B.D., and Curzon, G., 1974, Dopamine and serotonin metabolism in hepatic encephalopathy. *Br. Med. J.* 1: 549-551.

Knott, P.J. and Curzon, G., 1974, Effect of increased rat brain tryptophan on 5-hydroxytryptamine and 5-hydroxyindolyl acetic acid in the hypothalamus and other brain regions. *J. Neurochem.* 22: 1065-1071.

Krastev, Z., Terziivanov, D., Vlahov, V, Maleev, A., Greb, W.H., Eckl, K.M., Dierdorf H-D., and Wolf D., 1989, The pharmacokinetics of paroxetine in patients with liver cirrhosis. Acta Psychiatr. Scand. 80(suppl 350): 91-92.

Krause, D.N., and Dubocovich, M.L., 1990, Regulatory sites in the melatonin system of mammals. *Trends Neurosci.* 13: 464-470.

Kuhn, D.M., Wolf, W.A., and Youdim, M.B.H., 1985, 5-Hydroxytryptamine release *in vivo* from a cytoplasmic pool: studies on the 5-HT behavioural syndrome in reserpinized rats. *Br. J. Pharmac.* 84: 121-129.

Lapin, I.P., 1978, Stimulant and convulsive effects of kynurenines injected into brain ventricles in mice. *J. Neural Transm.* 42: 37-43.

Lapin, I.P., 1981, Kynurenines and seizures. *Epilepsia* 22: 257-265.

Lavoie, J., Giguère, J.F., Layrargues, G.P., and Butterworth, R.F., 1987, Amino acid changes in autopsied brain tissue from cirrhotic patients with hepatic encephalopathy. *J. Neurochem.* 49: 692-697.

Lee, S.H. and Fisher, B., 1961, Portacaval shunt in the rat. Surgery 50: 668-672.

Levine, R.A., Kuhn, D.M., and Lovenberg, W., 1979, The regional distribution of hydroxylase cofactor in rat brain. *J. Neurochem.* 32: 1575-1578.

Levine, R.A., Zoephel, G.P., Niederwieser, A., and Curtius, H-C., 1987, Entrance of tetrahydrobiopterin derivates in brain after peripheral administration: effect on biogenic amine metabolism. *J. Pharmacol. Exp. Ther.* 242: 514-522.

Lewy, A.J., Wehr, TA., Gold, P.W, and Goodwin, F.K., 1978, Plasma melatonin in manic-depressive illness. In (Usdin E, Kopin IJ, and Barechas J, eds), *Catecholamines: Basic and Clinical Frontiers.* Oxford, Pergamon., pp. 1173-1175.

Lockwood, A.H., McDonald, J.M., Reiman, R.E., Gelbard, A.S., Laughlin, J.S., Duffy, T.E., and Plum, F., 1979, The dynamics of ammonia metabolism in man. Effects of liver disease and hyperammonemia. *J. Clin. Invest.* 63: 449-460.

Long, J.B., Youngblood, WY, and Kizer, J.S., 1983, Regional differences in the response of serotonergic neurons in rat CNS to drugs. *Eur. J. Pharmacol.* 88: 89-97.

Lookingland, K.J., Shannon, N.J., Chapin, D.S., and Moore, K.E., 1986, Exogenous tryptophan increases synthesis, storage, and intraneuronal metabolism of 5-hydroxytryptamine in the rat hypothalamus. *J. Neurochem.* 47: 205-212.

Lovenberg, W., Jequier, E., and Sjoerdsma, A., 1967, Tryptophan hydroxylation: measurement in pineal gland, brainstem, and carcinoid tumor. *Science* 155: 217-219.

Maddrey, W.C., and Weber F.L.Jr., 1975, Chronic hepatic encephalopathy. Symposium on Diseases of the Liver, pp. 937-944.

Mans, A.M., Saunders, S.J., Kirsch, R.E., and Biebuyck, J.F., 1979, Correlation of plasma and brain amino acid and putative neurotransmitter alterations during acute hepatic coma in the rat. *J. Neurochem.* 32: 285-292.

Mans, A.M., Biebuyck, J.F., Shelly, K., and Hawkins, R.A., 1982, Regional blood-brain barrier permeability to amino acids after portacal anastomosis. *J. Neurochem.* 38: 705-717.

Mans, A.M., Biebuyck, J.F., Davis, D.W, and Hawkins, R.A., 1984, Portacaval anastomosis: brain and plasma metabolite abnormalities and the effect of nutritional therapy. *J. Neurochem.* 43: 697-705.

Mans, A.M. and Hawkins, R.A., 1986, Brain monoamines after portacaval anastomosis. *Metab. Brain Dis.* 1: 45-52.

Mans, A.M., Consevage, M.W., DeJoseph, M.R., and Hawkins, R.A., 1987, Regional brain monoamines and their metabolites after portacaval shunting. *Metab. Brain Dis.* 2: 183-193.

Mans, A.M., DeJoseph, M.R., Davis, D.W, Viña, J.R., and Hawkins, R.A., 1990, Early establishment of cerebral dysfunction after portacaval shunting. *Am. J. Physiol.* 259: E104-E110.

Marsden, C.A., and Curzon, G., 1976, Studies on the behavioural effects of tryptophan and *p*-chlorophenylalanine. *Neuropharmacology* 15: 165-171.

Martin, G.R. and Humphrey, P.P.A., 1994, Receptors for 5-hydroxytryptamine: current perspectives on classification and nomenclature. *Neuropharmacology* 33: 261-273.

Masson, P., and Berger, L., 1923, Sur un nouveau mode de sécrétion interne: La neurocrinie. C. R. Acad. Sci. (Paris) 176: 1748-1750.

Matos, F.F., Rollema, H., Brown, J.L., and Basbaum, A.I., 1992, Do opioids evoke the release of serotonin in the spinal cord? An in vivo microdialysis study of the regulation of extracellular serotonin in the rat. *Pain* 48: 439-447.

Matos, F.F., Urban, C., and Yocca, F.D., 1996, Serotonin (5-HT) release in the dorsal raphé and ventral hippocampus: raphé control somatodendrtitic and terminal 5-HT release. *J. Neural Transm.* 103: 173-190.

McLennan, H., 1983, Receptors for the excitatory amino acids in the mammalian central nervous system. *Prog. Neurobiology.* 20: 251-271.

Meek, J.L. and Lofstrandh, S., 1976, Tryptophan hydroxylase in discrete brain nuclei: comparison of activity in vitro and in vivo. *Eur. J. Pharmacol.* 37: 377-380.

Meeusen, R., Thorré, K., Sarre, S., De Meirleir, K., Ebinger, G., and Michotte, Y., 1995, The effect of exercise and L-tryptophan administration on extracellular serotonin metabolism in rat hippocampus. *Soc. Neurosci.* (Abstr.) 21: 1691.

Melamed, E., Hefti, F., and Wurtman, R.J., 1980, L-3,4-Dihydroxyphenylalanine and L-5-hydroxytryptophan decarboxylase activities in rat striatum: effect of selective destruction of dopaminergic or serotoninergic input. *J. Neurochem.* 34: 1753-1756.

Mennini, T, Borroni, E., Samanin, R., and Garattini, S., 1981, Evidence of the existence of two different intraneuronal pools from which pharmacological agents can release serotonin. *Neurochem. Int.* 3: 289-294.

Miwa, S., Watanabe, Y, and Hayaishi, O., 1985, 6*R*-L-Erythro-5,6,7,8-tetrahydrobiopterin as a regulator of dopamine and serotonin biosynthesis in the rat brain. *Arch. Biochem. Biophys.* 239: 234-241.

Morgan, D.J., and McLean, A.J., 1995, Clinical pharmacokinetik and pharmacodynamic considerations in patients with liver disease. *Clin. Pharmacokinet.* 29: 370-391.

Moroni, F., Lombardi, G., Carlà, V, Pellegrini, D., Carassale, G.L., and Cortesini, C., 1986a, Content of quinolinic acid and of other tryptophan metabolites increases in brain regions of rats used as experimental models of hepatic encephalopathy. *J. Neurochem.* 46: 869-874.

Moroni, F., Lombardi, G., Carlà, V, Lal, S., Etienne, P., and Nair, N.P.V., 1986b, Increase in the content of quinolinic acid in cerebrospinal fluid and frontal cortex of patients with hepatic failure. *J. Neurochem.* 47: 1667-1671.

Morot-Gaudry, Y, Bourgoin, S., and Hamon, M., 1981, Kinetic characteristics of newly synthesized ^{3}H-5-HT in the brain of control and reserpinized mice. Evidence for the heterogeneous distribution of 5-HT in serotoninergic neurons. *Naunyn-Schmiedeberg's Arch. Pharmacol.* 316: 311-316.

Mousseau, D.D., 1993, Tryptamine: a metabolite of tryptophan implicated in various neuropsychiatric disorders. *Metab. Brain Dis.* 8: 1-44.

Mousseau, D.D., Perney, P., Pomier Layrargues, G., and Butterworth, R.F., 1993, Selective loss of palladial dopamine D_2 receptor density in hepatic encephalopathy. *Neurosci. Lett.* 162: 192-196.

Mousseau, D.D., and Butterworth, R.F., 1994a, The [^{3}H]tryptamine receptor in human brain: kinetics, distribution, and pharmacologi profile. *J. Neurochem.* 63: 1052-1059.

Mousseau, D.D., and Butterworth, R.F., 1994b, Current theories on the pathogenesis of hepatic encephalopathy. *Exp. Biol. Med.* 206: 329-344.

Mousseau, D.D., Pomier Layrargues, G., and Butterworth, R.F., 1994, Region-selective decreases in densities of [^{3}H]tryptamine binding sites in autopsied brain tissue from cirrhotic patients with hepatic encephalopathy. *J. Neurochem.* 62: 621-625.

Nagatsu, T., 1985, Biopterin cofactor and monoamine-synthesizing monooxygenases. In, (Osborne NN, ed), *Selected Topics in Neurochemistry.* Pergammon., pp. 325-340.

Neckers, L.M., Biggio, G., Moja, E., and Meek, J.L., 1977, Modulation of brain tryptophan hydroxylase activity by braintryptophan content. *J. Pharamcol. Exp. Ther.* 201: 110-116.

Nichol, C.A., Smith, G.K., and Duch, D.S., 1985, Biosynthesis and metabolism of tetrahydrobiopterin and molybdopterin. *Ann. Rev. Biochem.* 54: 729-764.

Norenberg, M.D., 1987, The role of astrocytes in hepatic encephalopathy. *Neurochem. Pathol.* 6: 13-33.

Numazawa, R., Yoshioka, M., Matsumoto, M., Togashi, H., Kemmotsu, O., and Saito, H., 1995, Pharmacological characterization of α_2-adrenoceptor regulated serotonin release in the hippocampus. *Neurosci. Lett.* 192: 161-164.

Ogihara, K., Lowenstein, L.M., and Nakao, K., 1967, Abnormal indole metabolism in hepatic coma. In (Vandenbroucke J, De Groote J, and Standaert LO, eds), *Liver Research. Tijdschrift voor Gastroenterologie.* Antwerpen, pp. 56-67.

Ohta, K., Fukuuchi, Y, Shimazu, K., Komatsumoto, S., Ichijo, M., Araki, N., and Shibata, M., 1994, Presynaptic glutamate receptors facilitate release of norepinephrine and 5-hydroxytryptamine as well as dopamine in the normal and ischemic striatum. *J. Auto Nerv. Syst.* 49: S195-S202.

Ono, J., Hutson, D.G., Dombro, R.S., Levi, J.U, Livingstone, A, and Zeppa, R., 1978, Tryptophan and hepatic coma. *Gastroenterology* 74: 196-200.

Orlando, R., Benvenuti, C., Mazzo, M., and Palatini, P., 1995, The pharmacokinetics of teniloxazine in healthy subjects and patients with hepatic cirrhosis. *Br. J. clin. Pharmac.* 39: 445-448.

Palacios, J.M., Waeber, C., Hoyer, D., and Mengod, G., 1990, Distribution of serotonin receptors. *Ann. N.Y. Acad. Sci.* 600: 36-52.

Pardridge, WM., 1977, Kinetics of competetive inhibition of neutral amino acid transport across the blood-brain barrier. *J. Neurochem.* 28: 103-108.

Perkins, M.N., and Stone, TW., 1982, An iontophoretic investigation of the actions of convulsant kynurenines and their interaction with the endogenous excitant quinolinic acid. *Brain Res.* 247: 184-187.

Perkins, M.N., and Stone, TW., 1983a, Pharmacology and regional variations of quinolinic acid-evoked excitations in the rat central nervous system. *J. Pharmacol. Exp. Ther.* 226: 551-557.

Perkins, M.N., and Stone, TW., 1983b, Quinolinic acid: regional variations in neuronal sensitivity. *Brain Res.* 259: 172-176.

Perry, K.W., and Fuller, R.W., 1993, Extracellular 5-hydroxytryptamine concentration in rat hypothalamus after administration of fluoxetine plus L-5-hydroxytryptophan. *J. Pharm. Pharmacol.* 45: 759-761.

Peterson, C., Giguere, J.F., Cotman, C.W, and Butterworth, R.F., 1990, Selective loss of *N*-methyl-D-aspartate-sensitive L-[^{3}H]glutamate binding sites in rat brain following portacaval anastomosis. *J. Neurochem.* 55: 386-390.

Pierpaoli, W., and Regelson, W., 1994, Pineal control of aging: Effect of melatonin and pieal grafting on aging mice. *Proc. Natl. Acad. Sci.* 91: 787-791.

Raabe, W., 1987, Synaptic transmission in ammonia intoxication. *Neurochem. Pathol.* 6: 145-166.

Rao, V.L.R., Murthy, Ch.R.K., and Butterworth, R.F., 1992, Glutamatergic synaptic dysfunction in hyperammonemic syndromes. *Metab. Brain Dis.* 7: 1-20.

Rao, V.L.R., Giguère, J-F., Pomier Layrargues, G., and Butterworth, R.F., 1993, Increased activities of MAO_A and MAO_B in autopsied brain tissue from cirrhotic patients with hepatic encephalopathy. *Brain Res.* 621: 349-352.

Rao, V.L.R., Therrien, G., and Butterworth, R.F., 1994a, Choline acetyltransferase and acetylcholinesterase activities are unchanged in brain in human and experimental portal-systemic encephalopathy. *Metab. Brain Dis.* 9: 401-407.

Rao, V.L.R., and Butterworth, R.F., 1994b, Alterations of [^{3}H]8-OH-DPAT and [^{3}H]ketanserin binding sites in autopsied brain tissue from cirrhotic patients with hepatic encephalopathy. *Neurosci. Lett.* 182: 69-72.

Rao, V.L.R., Audet, R.M., and Butterworth, R.F., 1995, Selective alterations of extracellular brain amino acids in relation to function in experimental portal-systemic encephalopathy: results of an in vivo microdialysis study. *J. Neurochem.* 65: 1221-1228.

Reichle, R.M., and Reichle, F.A., 1975, Effect of portacaval shunt and acute hepatic ischemia on brain and liver serotonin and catecholamines. *Surg. Forum* 26: 413-414.

Reinhardt, J.F.Jr. and Wurtman, R.J., 1977, Relation between brain 5-HIAA levels and the release of serotonin into brain synapses. *Life Sci.* 21: 1741-1746.

Robinson, M.B., Heyes, M.P., Anegawa, N.J., Gorry, E., Djali, S., Mellits, E.D., and Batshaw M.L., 1992a, Quinolinate in brain and cerebrospinal fluid in rat models of congenital hyperammonemia. *Pediatr. Res.* 32: 483-488.

Robinson, M.B., Anegawa, N.J., Gorry, E., Qureshi, I.A, Coyle, J.T, Lucki, I., and Batshaw, M.L., 1992b, Brain serotonin$_2$ and serotonin$_{1A}$ receptors are altered in the congenitally hyperammonemic sparse fur mouse. *J. Neurochem.* 58: 1016-1022.

Rokicki, W, Rokicki, M., Kaminski, K., Peciak, B., and Gebska, E., 1989, Experimental investigations of the pathomechanism of portal encephalopathy. I. Activity of monoamine oxidase (MAO) in brain cortex and cerebellum of rats after portacaval shunt. *Neuropat. Pol.* 27: 199-207.

Royer, R.J., Royer-Morrot, M.J., Paille, F., Brraucand, D., Schmitt, J., Defrance, R., and Salvadori, C., 1989, Tianeptine and its main metabolite pharmacokinetics in chronic alcoholism and cirrhosis. *Clin. Pharmacokin.* 16: 186-191.

Rössle, M., Luft, M., Herz, R., Klein, B., Lehmann, M., and Gerok, W., 1984, Amino acid, ammonia and neurotransmitter concentrations in hepatic encephalopathy: serial analysis in plasma and cerebrospinal fluid during treatment with an adapted amino acid solution. *Klin. Wochenschr.* 62: 867-875.

Rössle, M., Herz, R., Klein, B., and Gerok, W., 1986, Tryptophan-Metabolismus bei Lebererkrankungen: eine pharmakokinetische und enzymatische Untersuchung. *Klin. Wochenschr.* 64: 590-594.

Sabelli, H.C., and Giardina, WJ., 1970, CNS effects of the aldehyde products of brain monoamines. *Biol. Psychiat.* 2: 119-139.

Salerno, F., Delloco, M., Incerti, P., Uggeri, F., and Beretta, E., 1984, Alterations of plasma and brain tryptophan in hepatic encephalopathy: a study in humans and in experimental animals. In (Capocaccia L, Fischer JE, and Rossi-Fanelli F, eds), *Hepatic Encephalopathy in Chronic Liver Failure.* NY, Plenum Press, pp. 95-106.

Sandyk, R., 1990, Possible role of pineal melatonin in the mechanisms of aging. *Intern. J. Neuroscience* 52: 85-92.

Sarna, G.S., Bradbury, M.W.B., and Cavanagh, J., 1977, Permeability of the blood-brain barrier after portocaval anastomosis in the rat. *Brain Res.* 138: 550-554.

Sarna, G.S., Hutson, P.H., O'Conell, M.T, and Curzon, G., 1991, Effect of tryptophan on extracellular concentrations of tryptophan and 5-hydroxyindoleacetic acid in the striatum and cerebellum. *J. Neurochem.* 56: 1564-1568.

Sawada, M., Sugimoto, T, Matsuura, S., and Nagatsu, T., 1986, (6*R*)-Tetrahydrobiopterin increases the activity of tryptophan hydroxylase in rat raphe slices. *J. Neurochem.* 47: 1544-1547.

Schaechter, J.D. and Wurtman, R.J., 1990, Serotonin release varies with brain tryptophan levels. *Brain Res.* 532: 203-210.

Schaub, R.G. and Meyers, K.M., 1975, Evidence for a small functional pool of serotonin in neurohumoral transmission. *Res. Commun. Chem. Pathol. Pharmacol.* 10: 29-36.

Schenker, S. and Mendelson, J.H., 1964, Cerebral adenosine triphosphate in rats with ammonia-induced coma. *Am. J. Physiol.* 206: 1173-1176.

Schenker, S., McCandless, D.W, Brophy, E., and Lewis, M.S., 1967, Studies on the intracerebral toxicity of ammonia. *J. Clin. Invest.* 46: 838-848.

Schenker, S., and Hoyumpa, AM.Jr., 1984, Pathophysiology of hepatic encephalopathy. *Phys. Med.* Sept: 99-121.

Schenker, S., Bergstrom, R.F., Wolen, R.L., and Lemberger, L., 1988, Fluoxetine disposition and elimination in cirrhosis. *Clin. Pharmacol. Ther.* 44: 353-359.

Schoedon, G., Troppmair, J., Fontana, A, Huber, C., Curtius, H-C., and Niederwieser, A., 1987, Biosynthesis and metabolism of pterins in peripheral blood mononuclear cells and leukemia lines of man and mouse. *Eur. J. Biochem.* 166: 303-310.

Schwartz, D.H., Hernandez, L., and Hoebel, B.G., 1990, Tryptophan increases extracellular serotonin in the lateral hypothalamus of food-deprived rats. *Brain Res. Bull.* 25: 803-807.

Sharp, T, Bramwell, S.R., Clark, D., and Grahame-Smith, D.G., 1989, In vivo measurement of extracellular 5-hydroxytryptamine in hippocampus of the anaesthetized rat using microdialysis: changes in relation to 5-hydroxytryptaminergic neuronal activity. *J. Neurochem.* 53: 234-240.

Sharp, T., and Hjorth S., 1990, Application of brain microdialysis to study the pharmacology of the 5-HT$_{1A}$ autoreceptor. *J. Neurosci. Meth.* 34: 83-90.

Sharp, T, Bramwell, S.R., and Grahame-Smith, D.G., 1992, Effect of acute administration of L-tryptophan on the release of 5-HT in rat hippocampus in relation to serotoninergic neuronal activity: an in vivo microdialysis study. *Life Sci.* 50: 1215-1223.

Shields, P.J. and Eccleston, D., 1972, Effects of electrical stimulation of rat midbrain on 5-hydroxytryptamine synthesis as determined by a sensitive radioisotope method. *J. Neurochem.* 19: 265-272.

Shields, P.J. and Eccleston, D., 1973, Evidence for the synthesis and storage of 5-hydroxytryptamine in two separate pools in the brain. *J. Neurochem.* 20: 881-888.

Shore, P.A and Giachetti, A., 1978, Reserpine: basic and clinical pharmacology. In (Iversen L.L. and Snyder SH, eds), *Handbook of Psychopharmacology*. New York, Plenum Press., pp. 197-219.

Simert, G., Nobin, A, Rosengren, E., and Vang, J., 1978, Neurotransmitter changes in the rat brain after portacaval anastomosis. *Eur. surg. Res.* 10: 73-85.

Sleight, AJ., Marsden, C.A, Martin, K.F., and Palfreyman, M.G., 1988, Relationship between extracellular 5-hydroxytryptamine and behaviour following monoamino oxidase inhibition and L-tryptophan. *Br. J. Pharmacol.* 93: 303-310.

Smith, AR., Rossi-Fanelli, F., Ziparo, V, James, J.H., Perelle, B.A, and Fischer, J.E., 1978, Alterations in plasma and CSF amino acids, amines and metabolites in hepatic coma. *Ann. Surg.* 187: 343-350.

Soeters, P.B., and de Boer, J., 1984, Why are plasma branched chain amino acid levels diminished in patients with liver cirrhosis? In (Adibi SA, Fekl W, Langenbeck U, and Schauder P, eds), *Branced Chain Amino and Keto Acids in Health and Disease*. Basel, Karger., pp. 483-496.

Sonne, J., 1996, Drug metabolism in liver disease: implications for therapeutic drug monitoring. *Ther. Drug Monit.* 18: 397-401.

Sourkes, T.L., 1977, Enzymology of aromatic amino acid decarboxylase. In (Usdin E, Weiner N, and Youdim MBH., eds), *Structure and Function of Monoamine Enzymes*. New York, Marcel Dekker Inc., pp. 477-495.

Steindl, P.E., Gottstein, J., and Blei, AT., 1995a, Disruption of circadian locomotor activity in rats after portacaval anastomosis is not gender dependent. *Hepatology* 22: 1763-1768

Steindl, P.E., Finn, B., Bendok, B., Rothke, S., Zee, P.C., and Blei, A.T., 1995b, Disruption of the diurnal rhythm of plasma melatonin in cirrhosis. *Ann. Intern. Med.* 123: 274-277.

Stoeckel, K., Pfefen, J.P., Mayersohn, M., Schoerlin, M.P., Andressen, C., Ohnhaus E.E., Frey, F., and Guentert, TW., 1990, Absorption and disposition of moclobemide in patients with advanced age or reduced liver or kidey function. *Acta Psychiatr. Scand.* Suppl 360: 94-97.

Stone, T.W., and Perkins, M.N., 1981, Quinolinic acid: a potent endogenous excitant at amino acid receptors in CNS. *Eur. J. Pharmacol.* 72: 411-412.

Stone, T.W., 1993, Neuropharmacology of quinolinic and kynurenic acids. *Pharmacol. Rev.* 45: 309-379.

Sulzer, D., and Rayport, S., 1990, Amphetamine and other psychostimulants reduce pH gradients in midbrain dopaminergic neurons and chromaffin granules: a mechanism of action. Neuron 5: 797-808.

Sulzer, D., Pothos, E., Minjung Sung, H., Maidment, N.T, Hoebel, B.G., and Rayport, S., 1992, Weak base model of amphetamine action. *Ann. N.Y. Acad. Sci.* 654: 525-528.

Sulzer, D., Maidment, N.T, and Rayport, S., 1993, Amphetamine and other weak bases act to promote reverse transport of dopamine in ventral midbrain neurons. *J. Neurochem.* 60: 527-535.

Suter, H.A and Collard, K.J., 1983, The regulation of 5-hydroxytryptamine release from superfused synaptosomes by 5-hydroxytryptamine and its immediate precursors. *Neurochem. Res.* 8: 723-730.

Swain, M.S., Blei, AT, Butterworth, R.F., and Kraig, R.P., 1991, Intracellular pH rises and astrocytes swell after portacaval anastomosis in rats. *Regulatory Intergrative Comp. Physiol.* 30: R1491-R1496.

Szerb, J.C. and Butterworth, R.F., 1992, Effect of ammonium ions on synaptic transmission in the mammalian central nervous system. *Prog. Neurol.* 39: 135-153.

Taborsky, R.G., 1971, 5-Hydroxytryptophol: evidence for its having physiological properties. *Experientia* 27: 929-930.

Takada, A, Grdisa, M., Diksic, M., Gjedde, A, and Yamamoto, YL., 1993, Rapid steady-state analysis of blood-brain transfer of L-Trp in rat, with special reference to the plasma protein binding. *Neurochem. Int.* 23: 351-359.

Tamir, H., Theoharides, TC., Gershon, M.D., and Askenase, P.W., 1982, Serotonin storage pools in basophil leukemia and mast cells: characterization of two types of serotonin binding protein and radioautographic analysis of the intracellular distribution of [^{3}H]serotonin. *J. Cell Biol.* 93: 638-647.

Tao, R. and Hjorth, S., 1992, α_2-Adrenoceptor modulation of rat ventral hippocampal 5-hydroxytryptamine release in vivo. *Naunyn-Schmiedeberg's Arch. Pharmacol.* 345: 137-143.

Tao, R., and Auerbach, S.B., 1996, Differential effect of NMDA on extracellular serotonin in rat midbrain raphe and forebrain sites. *J. Neurochem.* 66: 1067-1075.

Tappaz, M.L., and Pujol, J-F., 1980, Estimation of the rate of tryptophan hydroxylation *in vivo*: a sensitive microassay in discrete rat brain nuclei. *J. Neurochem.* 34: 933-940.

Taylor, B.K. and Basbaum, AI., 1995, Neurochemical characterization of extracellular serotonin in the rostral ventromedial medulla and its modulation by noxious stimuli. *J. Neurochem.* 65: 578-589.

Ternaux, J.P., Boireau, A, Bourgoin, S., Hamon, M., Hery, F., and Glowinski, J., 1976, *In vivo* release of 5-HT in the lateral ventricle of the rat: effects of 5-hydroxytryptophan and tryptophan. *Brain Res.* 101: 533-548.

Theander, B., Apelqvist, G., Bugge, M., Andersson, G., Hindfelt, B., and Bengtsson, F., 1996, Gender and diurnal effect on specific open-field behavioral patterns in the portacaval shunted rat. *Metab. Brain Dis. In Press.*

Thorré, K., Sarre, S., Twahirwa, E., Meeusen, R., Ebinger, G., Haemers, A, and Michotte, Y., 1996, Effect of L-tryptophan, L-5-hydroxytryptophan and L-tryptophan prodrugs on the extracellular levels of 5-HT and 5-HIAA in the hippocampus of the rat using microdialysis. *Eur. J. Pharm. Sci.* 4: 247-256.

Tracqui, P., Morot-Gaudry, Y, Staub, J.F., Brézillon, P., Perault-Staub, AM., Bourgoin, S., and Hamon, M., 1983, Model of brain serotonin metabolism. II. Physiological interpretation. *Am. J. Physiol.* 244: R206-R215.

Tricklebank, M.D., Smart, J.L., Bloxam, D.L., and Curzon, G., 1978, Effects of chronic experimental liver dysfunction and L-tryptophan on behavior in the rat. *Pharmacol. Biochem. Behav.* 9: 181-189.

Tyce, G.M., Flock, E.V, Owen, C.AJr., Stobie, G.H.C., and David, C., 1967, 5-Hydroxyindole metabolism in the brain after hepatectomy. *Biochem. Pharmacol.* 16: 979-992.

Uribe, M., Farca, A., Márquez, M.A., Garcia-Ramos, G., and Guevara, L., 1979, Treatment of chronic portal systemic encephalopathy with bromocriptine. A double-blind controlled trial. *Gastroenterology* 76: 1347-1351.

Victor, M., Adams, R.D., and Cole, M., 1965, The acquired (non-Wilsonian) type of chronic hepatocerebral degeneration. *Medicine* 44: 345-396.

Victor, M., 1974, Neurologic changes in liver disease. In (Plum F, ed), *Brain Dysfunction in Metabolic Disorders.* New York, N.Y., Raven Press, pp. 1-12.

Victor M., 1979, Neurologic disorders due to alholism and malnutrition. In (Baker A and Baker L., eds), *Clinical Neurology.* Hagerstown, Harper & Row.

Werner, E.R., Werner-Felmayer, G., Fuchs, D., Hausen, A, Reibnegger, G., and Wachter, H., 1989, Parallel induction of tetrahydrobiopterin biosynthesis and indoleamine-2,3-dioxygenase activity in human cells and cell lines by interferon-γ. *Biochem. J.* 262: 861-866.

Werner-Felmayer, G., Prast, H., Werner, E.R., Philippu, A, and Wachter, H., 1993, Induction of GTP cyclohydrolase I by bacteriel lipopolysaccharide in the rat. *FEBS Lett.* 322: 223-226.

Westerink, B.H.C., Damsma, G., Rollema, H., de Vries, J.B., and Horn, AS., 1987, Scope and limitations of in vivo brain dialysis: a comparison of its application to various neurotransmitter systems. *Life Sci.* 41: 1763-1776.

Westerink, B.H.C. and De Vries, J.B., 1991, Effect of precursor loading on the synthesis rate and release of dopamine and serotonin in the striatum: a microdialysis study in conscious rats. *J. Neurochem.* 56: 228-233.

Wetterberg, L., Arendt, J., Paunier, L., Sizonenko, P.C., van Donselaar, W, and Heyden, T., 1976, Human serum melatonin changes during the menstrual cycle. *J. Clin. Endocrinol.* Metab. 42: 185-188.

Wetterberg, L., Aperia, B., Beck-Friis, J., Kjellman, B.F., Ljunggren, J-G., Nilsonne, A, Petterson, U, Tham, A, and Undén, F., 1982, Melatonin and cortisol levels in psychiatric illness. *The Lancet* ii: 100.

Whetsell, WO.Jr., and Schwarcz, R., 1989, Prolonged exposure to submicromolar concentrations of quinolinic acid causes excitotoxic damage in organotypic cultures of rat corticostriatal system. *Neurosci. Lett.* 97: 271-275.

Whittaker, VP., and Roed, I.S., 1982, New insights into vesicle recycling in a model choliergic system. In (Bradford HF., ed), *Neurotransmitter Interaction and Compartmentation*. New York, Plenum Press., pp. 151-173.

Whitton, P.S., Biggs, C.S., Pearce, B.R., and Fowler, L.J., 1992, MK-801 increases extracellular 5-hydroxytryptamine in rat hippocampus and striatum in vivo. *J. Neurochem.* 58: 1573-1575.

Wichems, C.H., Hollingsworth, C.K., and Bennett, BA., 1995, Release of serotonin induced by 3,4-methylenedioxymethamphetamine (MDMA) and other substituted amphetamines in cultured fetal raphe neurons: further evidence for calcium-independent mechanisms of release. *Brain Res.* 695: 10-18.

Wolf, W.A., and Kuhn, D.M., 1986, Uptake and release of tryptophan and serotonin: an HPLC method to study the flux of endogenous 5-hydroxyindoles through synaptosomes. *J. Neurochem.* 46: 61-67.

Wong, D.T, Horng, J.S., Bymaster, F.P., Hauser, K.L., and Molloy, B.B., 1974, A selective inhibitor of serotonin uptake: Lilly 110140, 3-(p-trifluoromethylphenoxy)-N-methyl-3-phenylpropylamine. *Life Sci.* 15: 471-479.

Wu, P.H., and Boulton, AA., 1987, Distribution and metabolism of tryptamine in rat brain. *Can. J. Biochem.* 51: 1104-1112.

Yoshioka, M., Matsumoto, M., Togashi, H., Smith, C.B., and Saito, H., 1993, Opioid receptor regulation of 5-hydroxytryptamine release from the rat hippocampus measured by in vivo microdialysis. *Brain Res.* 613: 74-79.

Young, S.N., Lal, S., Sourkes, TL., Feldmuller, F., Aronoff, A, and Martin, J.B., 1975, Relationships between tryptophan in serum and CSF, and 5-hydroxyindoleacetic acid in CSF of man: effect of cirrhosis of liver and probenecid administration. *J. Neurol. Neurosurg. Psychiat.* 38: 322-330.

Young, S.N. and Sourkes, TL., 1977, Tryptophan in the central nervous system: regulation and significance. *Adv. Neurochem.* 2: 133-191.

Young, S.N., Anderson, G.M., and Purdy, WC., 1980, Indoleamine metabolism in rat brain studied through measurements of tryptophan, 5-hydroxyindoleacetic acid and indoleacetic acid in cerebrospinal fluid. *J. Neurochem.* 34: 309-315.

Young, S.N., and Lal, S., 1980, CNS tryptamine metabolism in hepatic coma. *J. Neural Transm.* 47: 153-161.

Young, S.N., and Anderson, G.M., 1982, Factors influencing melatonin, 5-hydroxytryptophol, 5-hydroxyindoleacetic acid, 5-hydroxytryptamine and tryptophan in rat pineal glands. *Neuroendocrinology* 35: 464-468.

Young, S.N., and Teff, K.L., 1989, Tryptophan availability, 5HT synthesis and 5HT function. *Prog. Neuro-Psychopharmacol. & Biol. Psychiat.* 13: 373-379.

Zee, P.C., Mehta, R., Turek, F.W., and Blei, AT., 1991, Portacaval anastomosis disrupts circadian locomotor activity and pineal melatonin rhythms in rats. *Brain Res.* 560: 17-22.

Zieve, L., and Olsen, R.L., 1977, Can hepatic coma be caused by a reduction of brain noradrenaline or dopamine. *Gut* 18: 688-691.

HEPATIC ENCEPHALOPATHY IN ACUTE LIVER FAILURE: ROLE OF THE GLUTAMATE SYSTEM

Adrianna Michalak, Kerstin Knecht and Roger F. Butterworth

Neuroscience Research Unit, Hôpital Saint-Luc (University of Montreal)
Montreal, Quebec, Canada H2X 3J4

INTRODUCTION

Hepatic Encephalopathy (HE) in acute liver failure is a neuropsychiatric syndrome resulting from severe inflammatory or necrotic liver disease of rapid onset. HE typically progresses through altered mental status to stupor and coma within hours or days. The most common cause of death in acute liver failure is brain herniation caused by increased intracranial pressure that results from cytotoxic brain edema. Despite intensive study in recent years, the fundamental neurobiological mechanisms responsible for HE in acute liver failure have not been fully elucidated.

AMMONIA

In experimental animal models of acute liver failure, brain ammonia concentrations are in the 1-5 mM range, concentrations that are known to result in several deleterious effects on cerebral metabolism and neurotransmission by both direct and indirect mechanisms. Such effects include the following:

(i) Millimolar concentrations of ammonia block inhibitory neurotransmission as the result of a direct effect on the inhibitory post-synaptic potential (IPSP), most likely at the level of chloride extrusion (Raabe, 1989).

(ii) Millimolar concentrations of ammonia have a direct effect on glutamate neurotransmission, an effect at the postsynaptic receptor (Fan *et al.*, 1990).

(iii) Ammonia activates the glycolytic enzyme phosphofructokinase (Lowry and Passoneau, 1966) and inhibits both pyruvate dehydrogenase (McKhann and Tower, 1961) and α-ketoglutarate dehydrogenase (Lai and Cooper, 1986).

(iv) Ammonia inhibits the uptake of glutamate into synaptic vesicles (Naito and Ueda, 1985) and into cultured astrocytes (Bender and Norenberg, 1996).

(v) Ammonia-induced alkalinization of intrasynaptic storage vesicles results in release of monoamine (but not amino acid) neurotransmitters (Erecinska *et al.*, 1987).

The extent to which any (or all) of the above mechanisms are pertinent to the CNS dysfunction characteristic of acute liver failure is unclear. For example, although ammonia in concentrations encountered in brain in experimental acute liver failure inhibits the tricarboxylic acid cycle enzyme α-ketoglutarate dehydrogenase (iii above), acute liver failure, at least at early stages, does not appear to result in impaired cerebral energy metabolism. Direct measurements of high energy phosphates in the brains of rats with acute liver failure reveal no significant alterations (Cooper and Plum, 1987) and monitoring of high energy phosphates using ^{1}H-Nuclear Magnetic Resonance also failed to reveal any changes (Bates *et al.*, 1989).

On the other hand, there is substantial evidence to suggest that ammonia-related mechanisms may result in alterations of glutamatergic neurotransmission in acute liver failure.

BRAIN AND CSF GLUTAMATE IN ACUTE LIVER FAILURE

Brain concentrations of the excitatory amino acids glutamate and aspartate are significantly reduced in acute (ischemic) liver failure in the rat (Swain *et al.*, 1992a,b) as well as in thioacetamide-induced acute liver failure in the same animal species (Figure 1). Reductions of brain glutamate parallel the deterioration of neurological status in these animals and CSF concentrations of excitatory amino acids are concomitantly increased (Swain *et al.*, 1992b). In a recent study of the correlations of altered levels of several metabolites with clinical grade of encephalopathy in acute liver failure in the rat, statistically significant positive correlations were observed between clinical grading and plasma ammonia (0.7, $p<0.01$), and brain glutamine (0.69, $p<0.01$). Negative correlations were observed between clinical grading and brain glutamate (-0.60, $p<0.01$) and aspartate (-0.66, $p<0.01$) (Mans *et al.*, 1994). A significant loss of brain glutamate was evident even at early stages of encephalopathy in acute liver failure.

Glutamate concentrations are also reduced in autopsied brain tissue from patients who died in acute liver failure (Record *et al.*, 1976).

Using the technique of *in vivo* cerebral microdialysis, several reports have consistently described increased extracellular concentrations of glutamate in experimental ischemic liver failure in the rat (Bosman *et al.*, 1992; Michalak *et al.*, 1996a; Table 1) and rabbit (de Knegt *et al.*, 1994).

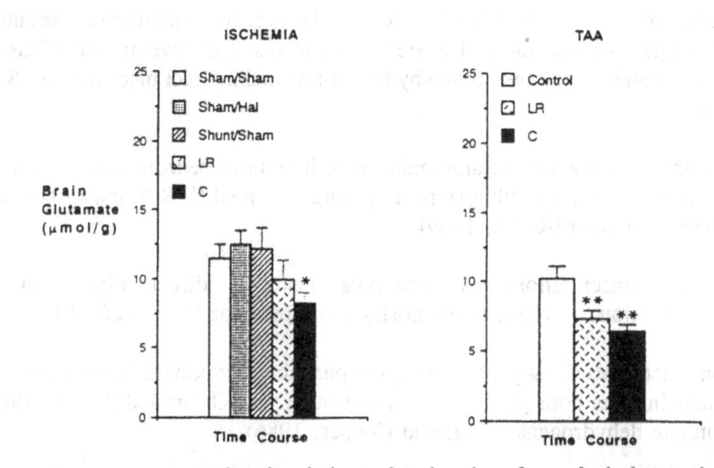

Figure 1. Brain glutamate concentrations in relation to deterioration of neurological status in rats with acute liver failure due to liver ischemia or thioacetamide (TAA) administration. C: control (vehicle injected); LR: loss of righting reflex stage of encephalopathy; C: coma. The three obligate control groups for the ischemic liver failure are indicated by sham/sham; sham/Hal (hepatic artery ligation); shunt (portacaval shunt)/sham. Values significantly different from control groups indicated by $*p<0.05$ by Analysis of Variance with post-hoc Tukey test. (Adapted from Swain *et al.*, 1992b).

Table 1. Extracellular brain concentrations of excitatory and inhibitory amino acids in acute (ischemic) liver failure

Amino acid (μM)	Sham/sham	Shunt/sham	Sham/Hal	Shunt/Hal (acute liver failure)
Glutamate	1.04±0.05	0.79±0.05	1.09±0.08	1.87±0.15*
Aspartate	0.36±0.09	0.69±0.04	1.09±0.23	0.97±0.06
GABA	0.21±0.03	0.27±0.02	0.29±0.03	0.35±0.01
Glycine	5.06±0.42	4.97±0.33	9.13±0.95	12.18±1.81*
Taurine	4.81±0.34	3.87±0.31	3.75±0.81	4.48±0.71

Sham: sham operation; Shunt: portacaval shunt; Hal: hepatic artery ligation. Values represent the mean ± S.E. of duplicate determinations from 4-6 animals per group. Values significantly different from all control groups indicated by *$p<0.05$ by ANOVA with post hoc LSD test. (Data from Michalak *et al.*, 1996a).

In contrast to these findings of altered extracellular concentrations of glutamate in experimental acute liver failure, no changes in concentrations of the inhibitory amino acids GABA, or taurine were observed. Glycine concentrations, on the other hand, were significantly increased at coma stages of encephalopathy in acute liver failure (Michalak *et al.*, 1996a, Table 1).

Brain concentrations of ammonia are increased up to 5 mM in experimental animal models of acute liver failure (Swain *et al.*, 1992a) and a positive correlation has been reported between extracellular concentrations of glutamate and arterial ammonia concentrations in acute (ischemic) liver failure in the rat (Michalak *et al.*, 1996a).

GLUTAMATE RECEPTORS IN BRAIN IN ACUTE LIVER FAILURE

Glutamate receptors in mammalian brain are either ionotropic (ligand-gated ion channels) or metabotropic (coupled to second messenger systems). Ionotropic glutamate receptors are further subdivided into N-Methyl-D-Aspartate (NMDA) and non-NMDA subtypes according to their affinity for NMDA. Non-NMDA receptors have been classified as being of the AMPA or kainate type depending upon their relative affinities for the ligands AMPA or kainate. NMDA, AMPA and kainate subclasses of glutamate receptor are distributed in a region-selective manner in mammalian brain (Monaghan *et al.*, 1989). Moreover, whereas the NMDA receptor subtype appears to be exclusively neuronal in localization, the non-NMDA (both AMPA and kainate subclasses) are localized to both neuronal and astrocytic membranes (Figure 2).

Several studies have addressed the issue of glutamate receptor changes in brain in acute liver failure. In a study published in 1984, total glutamate binding site densities, assessed using [^{3}H]-glutamate as radioligand, were unchanged in the brains of rabbits with acute liver failure caused by galactosamine (Ferenci *et al.*, 1984). Subsequent studies in the hepatectomized rat (Watanabe *et al.*, 1988) and in the rat with acute liver failure due to thioacetamide administration (Zimmerman *et al.*, 1989) likewise could find no evidence of alterations of total ^{3}H-glutamate binding. On the other hand, [^{3}H]-kainate binding sites were significantly reduced in cerebral cortical preparations from galactosamine-treated rabbits with severe encephalopathy (Ferenci *et al.*, 1984). Similar findings of a significant loss of [^{3}H]-kainate binding sites were subsequently reported in frontal cortex in ischemic liver failure in the rat (Michalak *et al.*, 1996b, Figure 3).

In contrast, densities of neuronally-localized NMDA binding sites are unchanged in ischemic liver failure in both rabbits (de Knegt *et al.*, 1993) and rats (Michalak *et al.*, 1996b).

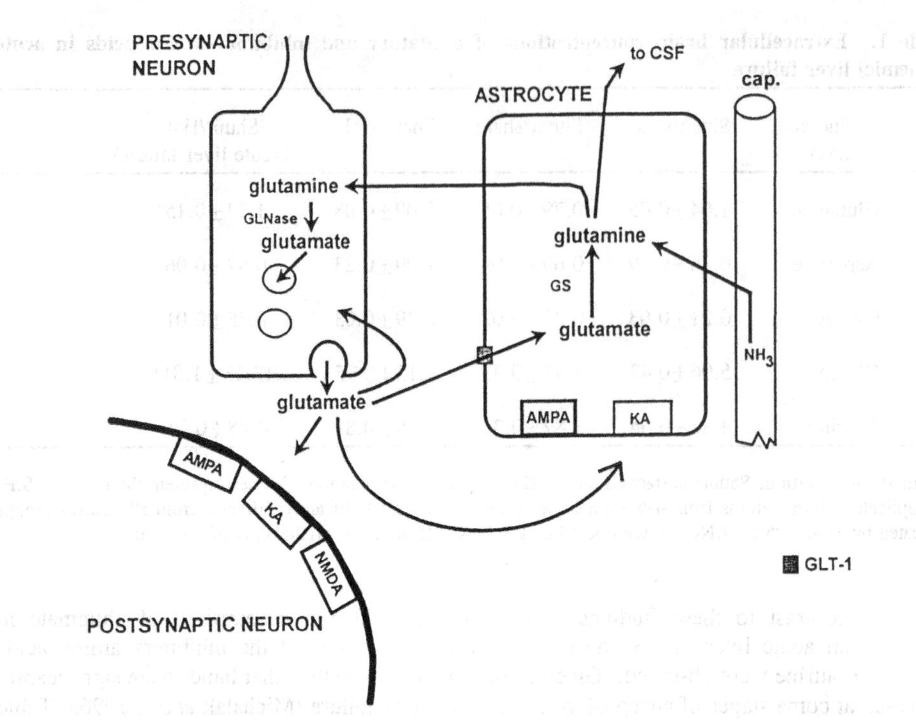

Figure 2. Key steps involved in regulation at the glutamatergic synapse. Glutamate released by the presynaptic neuron activates postsynaptic receptors of the NMDA, AMPA or KA subtypes. Glutamate may also activate AMPA or KA receptors on the perineuronal astrocyte. Removal of glutamate from the synaptic cleft is mediated by transporters into the presynaptic neuron or astrocyte. On such transporter, the astrocytic glutamate transporter GLT-1 has been cloned and sequenced. Gene expression for GLT-1 is decreased in brain in acute liver failure.

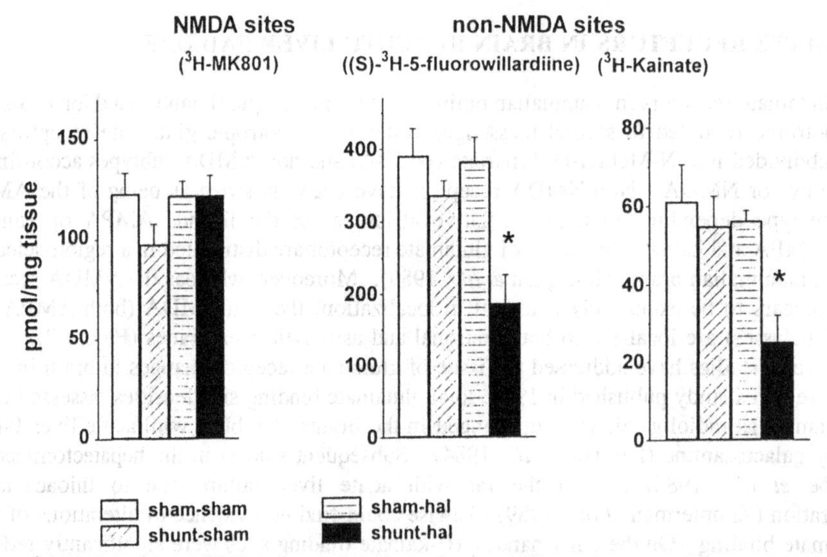

Figure 3. NMDA and non-NMDA receptors in frontal cortex: effects of acute (ischemic liver failure). Using an autoradiographic approach, binding site densities of NMDA sites (using [^{3}H-MK801), AMPA sites (using [^{3}H]-S-Fluorowillardiine) and kainate sites (using [^{3}H]-kainate) were asessed in rats at coma stages of encephalopathy following liver ischemia (portacaval anastomosis followed 24 h later by hepatic artery ligation (shunt-hal)). Data for animals in the three obligate control groups (sham-sham, shunt-sham, sham-hal). Values represent the means ± SE of dates from 4-6 animals per group. Values significantly different from control group indicated by *$p<0.02$ by Analysis of Variance with post-hoc LSD test.

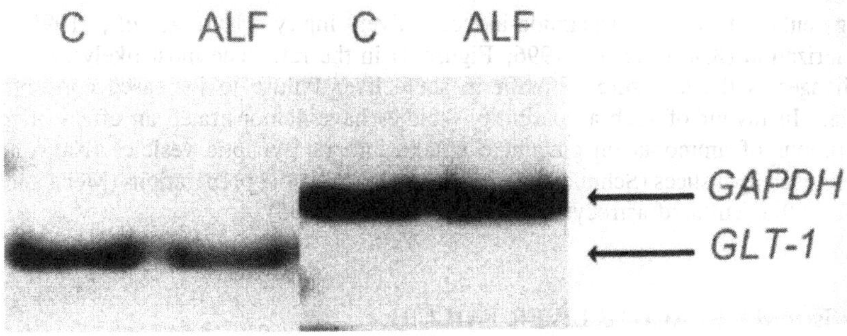

C ALF C ALF

GAPDH

GLT-1

Figure 4. GLT-1 expression (using RT-PCR) in cerebellum of rats with acute liver failure. C: Control; ALF: Acute liver failure; GAPDH: glyceraldehyde phosphate dehydrogenase (housekeeping gene). From Knecht *et al.* 1996.

On the other hand, results of a recent study reveal a selective loss of the AMPA subclass of non-NMDA binding sites in the brains of rats with ischemic liver failure (Michalak *et al.*, 1996b; Figure 3). This selective loss of AMPA sites could be the consequence of exposure of the brains of these animals to increased ammonia concentrations generated in acute liver failure. In favour of such a possibility, previous studies had demonstrated a selective depression of AMPA currents by exposure of hippocampal pyramidal neurons to 3 mM ammonia (Fan and Szerb, 1993). In a separate series of electrophysiological studies, millimolar concentrations of ammonia led to a reduction in the degree of depolarization of cerebral cortical wedges induced by AMPA (Moroni *et al.*, 1995) suggesting that ammonia had the capacity to modify the structural or functional characteristics of the neuronal AMPA receptor. Ammonia-related changes of AMPA receptors provides one possible explanation for the decreased binding of AMPA ligands in brain in acute liver failure (Michalak *et al.*, 1996b).

Glutamate's excitatory actions are not confined to neurons. Rather it interacts with both neurons and astrocytes which share similar types of ionotropic and metabotropic receptors with the exception of the N-Methyl-D-Aspartate (NMDA) receptor which is localized primarily on neuronal membranes. When applied on cultured astrocytes, glutamate regulates the opening of receptor channels, activates second messenger systems and causes the release of neuroactive compounds (Teichberg, 1991). A growing body of experimental evidence suggests that astrocytes perform several functions related to the regulation of the neuronal environment. Astrocytes respond to neuronally released neurotransmitters with increases in intracellular Ca^{2+} (Porter and McCarthy, 1995) which, in turn, may affect many different astrocytic functions secondary to the activation of Ca^{2+}-sensitive enzymes and other proteins. For example, AMPA receptor agonists cause transient increases in intracellular Ca^{2+} which, via the Na^+/Ca^{2+} exchanger and the Na^+/K^+ pump, sustains K^+ uptake by astrocytes (Muller *et al.*, 1992). A significant loss of AMPA sites therefore could result in impaired astrocytic processes such as the regulation of K^+ conductances (Jabs *et al.*, 1994) or neuron-astrocytic signalling.

BRAIN GLUTAMATE TRANSPORT IN ACUTE LIVER FAILURE

Removal of glutamate released into the synaptic cleft by the presynaptic neuron relies on high affinity uptake systems located both on neuronal and astrocytic membranes (Figure 1). The increased concentrations of glutamate in extracellular fluid of brain in acute liver failure, therefore, could be the consequence of a failure in capacity of one or other of these transporters. A recent study using synaptosomal (nerve ending) preparations from rats with acute liver failure due to thioacetamide administration revealed a significant reduction in high affinity glutamate uptake (Oppong *et al.*, 1995). More recently, two groups have independently reported a reduction in gene expression for the astrocytic glutamate transporter GLT-1 in acute liver failure resulting either from thioacetamide-induced liver injury (Huo *et al.*, 1995) or liver devascularization (Knecht *et al.*, 1996; Figure 4) in the rat. The most likely explanation for these changes is the exposure of brain in acute liver failure to increased concentrations of ammonia. In favour of such a possibility, studies have demonstrated an effect of millimolar concentrations of ammonia on glutamate uptake into rat synaptic vesicles (Naito and Ueda, 1985), hippocampal slices (Schmidt *et al.*, 1990), synaptosomal preparations (Mena and Cotman, 1985) as well as cultured astrocytes (Norenberg *et al.*, 1985).

BRAIN EDEMA IN ACUTE LIVER FAILURE

The results of several recent studies suggest that ammonia may play an important role in the pathogenesis of brain edema in acute liver failure. Increased brain water content has been described in dogs with urease-induced hyperammonemia (Levin *et al.*, 1989) as well as in rats with ammonia infusions (Takahashi *et al.*, 1991). Furthermore, treatment of cerebral cortical slices with ammonia in pathophysiological (millimolar) concentrations results in significant cell swelling (Ganz *et al.*, 1989). Similar results have been described following the exposure of cultured astrocytes to ammonia (Norenberg *et al.*, 1991).

There is recent evidence to suggest that ammonia-induced brain swelling may be mediated, at least in part, by accumulation of glutamine in the astrocyte. Since brain is devoid of all effective urea cycle, it relies on glutamine formation for effective removal of excess ammonia and the enzyme responsible, glutamine synthetase, is highly enriched in astrocytes. A significant correlation exists between the rise in brain glutamine and brain water content in rats following ammonia infusions (Takahashi *et al.*, 1991) and it was suggested that the increased brain water content in these animals was the consequence of the osmotic effects of increased cellular glutamine. In favour of such a possibility, subsequent studies whereby hyperammonemic animals were treated with methionine sulfoximine, an inhibitor of glutamine synthesis, showed a prevention of the increases of brain glutamine and of brain water in these animals. Studies in postmortem brain tissue from patients who died in acute liver failure reveal significantly increased glutamine concentrations (Record *et al.*, 1976) and brain glutamine concentrations are increased several-fold in experimental acute liver failure in the rat (Swain *et al.*, 1992a,b).

Brain edema in acute liver failure could also result from exposure of the astrocyte to increased concentrations of glutamate. As previously mentioned, deterioration of cerebral function parallels increased extracellular glutamate concentrations in several animal models of acute liver failure. Furthermore, the time course of this increase reflects the time course of the establishment of brain edema in these animals (Swain *et al.*, 1992a). Glutamate, when injected directly into brain in submillimolar quantities, causes marked astrocytic swelling (Van Harreveld and Fifkova, 1971). Moreover, a novel anion exchange inhibitor was shown to inhibit astrocytic swelling in traumatic-hypoxic brain injury caused by glutamate and it was suggested that the mechanism responsible for astroglial swelling involved the exchange transport inhibitor-sensitive glutamate uptake system (Kimmelberg *et al.*, 1989). Moreover, administration of the AMPA receptor antagonist NBQX significantly reduces glutamate-induced brain edema (Westergren and Johansson, 1992). These findings suggest that modifications of the astrocytic glutamate system, therefore, could be implicated in the pathogenesis of brain edema in acute liver failure. Further studies are required in order to assess this possibility.

ACUTE AMMONIA NEUROTOXICITY AND NMDA RECEPTORS

It has been suggested that acute ammonia neurotoxicity is mediated by activation of NMDA receptors. In favour of such a mechanism, MK-801, an NMDA receptor antagonist has been shown to prevent the death of mice and rats administered lethal doses of ammonia (Marcaida *et al.*, 1992; Seiler *et al.*, 1992). MK-801 prevents the deleterious effects of acute ammonia toxicity including ATP depletion, activation of Na^+/K^+-ATPase (Kosenko *et al.*, 1994) as well as proteolysis of the microtube-associated protein MAP-2 (Felipo *et al.*, 1993), all of which are NMDA-receptor mediated. Ammonia has also been shown to prevent activation of NMDA receptors by glutamate in rat cerebellar neurons in culture (Marcaida *et al.*, 1995).

Furthermore, it is well known that chronically hyperammonemic animals manifest a reduced sensitivity to acute ammonia loading and it has been suggested that it may result from down-regulation of NMDA receptors in brain in chronic hyperammonemia. In favour of this possibility, it has been consistently demonstrated that the brains of hyperammonemic rats (Peterson *et al.*, 1990; Rao *et al.*, 1991) and mice (Ratnakumari *et al.*, 1993) contain reduced densities of NMDA binding sites.

CONCLUSIONS

There is a growing body of evidence to suggest that modifications of glutamatergic function and of neuron-astrocytic trafficking of glutamate are implicated in the pathogenesis of the CNS consequences (encephalopathy, edema) of acute liver failure. Whole brain glutamate concentrations are reduced in both human and experimental acute liver failure and concentrations of glutamate in the extracellular fluid of brain (a reflection of synaptic availability of the neurotransmitter) are increased in several animal models of acute liver failure. This increased extracellular glutamate appears to result from failure of the astrocytic and neuronal glutamate transporters to reuptake neuronally-released glutamate from the synaptic cleft, a mechanism which may result from a neurotoxic effect of ammonia. Acute liver failure in the rat results in a selective loss of the AMPA/kainate subclass of glutamate receptors from cortical and hippocampal structures, a finding which may reflect alterations of the neuronal and/or astrocytic glutamate systems. Since both are involved in the maintenance of neuronal hyperexcitability, modifications of AMPA/kainate-mediated events could be involved in the pathogenesis of hepatic encephalopathy in acute liver failure. The selective loss of neuronal AMPA/kainate sites in acute liver failure together with unchanged NMDA sites and increased extracellular glutamate could result in relative increases of NMDA-receptor mediated events in acute liver failure.

The time course of establishment of significant brain edema in acute liver failure in the rat parallels the increase in extracellular glutamate and glutamate infusions are known to cause edema possibly by activation of AMPA receptors on astrocytes. Further studies are required in order to more fully elucidate the role of the glutamate system in the pathogenesis of hepatic encephalopathy and (possibly also) brain edema in acute liver failure. Subsequent pharmacological manipulation of the glutamate system could then result in new therapeutic approaches to these serious neurological complications of acute liver failure.

ACKNOWLEDGMENTS

Studies from the authors research unit were funded by grants from The Medical Research Council of Canada (PG 11118). AM is recipient of a research fellowship from The Canadian Liver Foundation. The authors thank Dominique D. Roy and Jean-Pascal de Waele for their assistance with the preparation of this manuscript.

REFERENCES

Bates, T.E., Williams, S.R., Kauppinen, R.A., and Godian, D.G., 1989, Observation of cerebral metabolites in an animal model of acute liver failure *in vivo*: ^{1}H and ^{31}P nuclear magnetic resonance study. *J. Neurochem.* 53:102-110.

Bender, A.S. and Norenberg, M.D., 1996, Effects of ammonia on L-glutamate uptake in cultured astrocytes. *Neurochem. Res.* 21:567-573.

Bosman, D.K., Deutz, N.E.P., Maas, M.A.W., van Eijk, H.M.H., Smit, J.J.H., de Haan, J.G., and Chamuleau, R.A.F.M., 1992, Amino acid release from cerebral cortex in experimental acute liver failure, studied by *in vivo* microdialysis. *J. Neurochem.* 59:591-599.

Cooper, A.J.L. and Plum, F., 1987, Biochemistry and physiology of brain ammonia. *Physiol. Rev.* 67:440-519.
de Knegt, R.J., Kornhuber, J., Schalm, S.W., Rusche, K., Riederer, P., and Tan, J., 1993, Binding of the ligand [^{3}H]MK-801 to the MK-801 binding site of the N-methyl-D-aspartate receptor during experimental encephalopathy from acute liver failure and from acute hyperammonemia in the rabbit. *Metab. Brain Dis.* 8:81-94.
de Knegt, R.J., Schalm, S.W., van der Rijt, C.C.D., Fekkes, D., Dalm, E. and Hekking-Weyma, I., 1994, Extracellular brain glutamate during acute liver failure and during acute hyperammonemia simulating acute liver failure: an experimental study based on *in vivo* brain dialysis. *J. Hepatol.* 20:19-26.
Erecinska, M, Pastuszko, A., Wilson, D.F., and Nelson, D., 1987, Ammonia-induced release of neurotransmitters from rat brain synaptosomes: differences between the effects on amines and amino acids. J. Neurochem. 49:1258-1265.
Fan, P., and Szerb, J.C., 1993, Effects of ammonium ions on synaptic transmission and on responses to quisqualate and N-methyl-D-aspartate in hippocampal CA1 pyramidal neurons *in vitro*. *Brain Res.* 632:225-231.
Fan, P., Lavoie, J., Le, N.L.O., Szerb, J.C., Butterworth, R.F., 1990, Neurochemical and electrophysiological studies on the inhibitory effect of ammonium ions on synaptic transmission in slices of rat hippocampus: evidence for a postsynaptic action. *Neuroscience* 39:327-334.
Felipo, V., Grau, E., Miñana, M.D. and Grisolía, S., 1993, Ammonium injection induces an N-methyl-D-aspartate receptor-mediated proteolysis of the microtubule-associated protein MAP-2. *J. Neurochem.* 60:1626-1630.
Ferenci, P., Pappas, S.C., Munson, P.J., Henson, K. and Jones, E.A., 1984, Changes in the status of neurotransmitter receptors in a rabbit model of hepatic encephalopathy. *Hepatology* 4:186-191.
Ganz, R., Swain, M., Traber, P., CalCanto, M., Butterworth, R.F., and Blei, A.T., 1989, Ammonia-induced swelling of rat cerebral cortical slices: implications for the pathogenesis of brain edema in acute hepatic failure. *Metab. Brain Dis.* 4:213-244.
Huo, Z., Neary, J.T., Petito, C.K. and Norenberg, M.D., 1995, The glutamate transporter GLT-1 is down regulated in hyperammonemic and acute liver failure. *Soc. Neurosci. Abs.* 21:108.
Jabs, R., Kirchhoff, F., Kettenmann, H. and Steinhauser, C., 1994, Kainate activates Ca^{2+}-permeable glutamate receptors and blocks voltage-gated K^+ currents in glial cells of mouse hippocampal slices. *Pfugers Arch.* 426:310-319.
Kimelberg, H.K., Pang, S. and Treble, D.H., 1989, Excitatory amino-acid stimulated uptake of Na in primary astrocyte cultures. *J. Neurosci.* 9:1141-1149.
Kosenko, E., Kaminsky, Y., Miñana, M.D., Grisolía, S. and Felipo, V., 1994, Brain ATP depletion induced by acute ammonia intoxication in rats is mediated by activation of the NMDA receptor and of Na^+/K^+-ATPase. *J. Neurochem.* 63:2172-2178.
Knecht, K., Michalak, A., Rose, C., and Butterworth, R.F., 1996, Decreased glutamate transporter [GLT-1] gene expression in brain in acute liver failure. *Hepatology* 24:248A
Lai, J.C.K. and Cooper, A.J.L., 1986, Brain α-ketoglutarate dehydrogenase: kinetic properties, regional distribution and effects of inhibitors. *J. Neurochem.* 47:1376-1386.
Levin, L.H., Koehler, R.C., Brusilow, S.W., Jones, J., Traystman, R.J., 1989, Elevated brain water during urease-induced hyperammonemia in dogs. In: *Intracranial Pressure*, J.T. Hoff, A.L. Betz, eds, Springer-Verlag, Berlin, pp. 1032-1034.
Lowry, O.H. and Passonneau, J.V., 1966, Kinetic evidence for multiple binding sites on phosphofructokinase. *J. Biol. Chem.* 241:2268-2279.
Mans, A.M., DeJoseph, M.R., and Hawkins, R.A., 1994, Metabolic abnormalities and grade of encephalopathy in acute hepatic failure. *J. Neurochem.* 63:1829-1838.
Marcaida, G., Miñana, M.D., Burgal, M., Grisolía, S. and Felipo, V., 1995, Ammonia prevents activation of NMDA receptors by glutamate in rat cerebellar neuronal cultures. *Eur. J. Neurosci.* 7:2389-2396.
Marcaida, G., Felipo, V., Hermenegildo, C., Miñana, M.D. and Grisolía, S., 1992, Acute ammonia toxicity is mediated by the NMDA type of lgutamate rceptors. FEBS Lett. 296:67-68.
McKhann, G.M. and Tower, D.B., 1961, Ammonia toxicity and cerebral oxidative metabolism. *Am. J. Physiol.* 200:420-424.
Mena, E.E., and Cotman, C.W., 1985, Pathologic concentraitons of ammonium ions block L-glutamate upake. *Exp. Neurol.* 59:259-263.
Michalak, A., Rose, C., Butterworth, J. and Butterworth R.F., 1996, Neuroactive amino acids and glutamate (NMDA) receptors in frontal cortex of rats with experimental acute liver failure. *Hepatology* 24:908-913.
Michalak, A. and Butterworth, R.F., 1996, Selective loss of binding sites for the non-NMDA (glutamate) receptor ligands [^{3}H]-kainate and (S)-[^{3}H]-5-fluorowillardiine in the brains of rats with acute liver failure. *Hepatology* (in press)
Monaghan, D.T., Bridges, R.J. and Cotman, C.W., 1989, The excitatory amino acid receptors: their classes, pharmacology, and distinct properties in the function of the central nervous system. *Ann. Rev. Pharmacol. Toxicol.* 29:365-402.
Moroni, F., Mannaioni, G., Cherici, G., Leonardi, P., Carlà, V. and Lombardi. G., 1995, Excitatory amino acid neurotransmission and ammonia toxicity. In: *Advances in Hepatic Encephalopathy and Metabolic Nitrogen*

Exchange, L. Capocaccia, M. Merli, O. Riggio, eds., Boca Raton, Florida: CRC Press, Chap. 22, 130-139.

Muller, T., Moller, T., Berger, T., Schnitzer, J. and Kettenmann, H., 1992, Calcium entry through kainate receptors and resulting potassium-channel blockade in Bergmann glial cells. *Science* 256:1563-1566.

Naito, S. and Ueda, T., 1985, Characterization of glutamate uptake into synaptic vesicles. *J. Neurochem.* 44:99 109.

Norenberg, M.D., Baker, L., Norenberg, L.O.B., Blicharska, J., Bruce-Gregario, H.H., Neary, J.T., 1991, Ammonia-induced astrocyte swelling in primary culture. *Neurochem. Res.* 16:833-836.

Norenberg, M.D., Mozes, L.W., Papendick, R.E. and Norenberg, L.O.B., 1985, Effect of ammonia on glutamate,GABA and rubidium uptake by astrocytes. *Ann. Neurol.* 18:149.

Oppong, K.N.W., Bartlett, K., Record, C.O. and Al Mardini, H., 1995, Synaptosomal glutamate transport in thioacetamide-induced hepatic encephalopathy in the rat. *Hepatology* 22:553-558.

Peterson, C., Giguère, J.F., Cotman, C.W. and Butterworth, R.F., 1990, Selective loss of N-methyl-D-aspartate-sensitive [^{3}H]-glutamate binding sites in rat brain following portacaval anastomosis. *J. Neurochem.* 55:386-390.

Porter, J.T. and McCarthy, K.D., 1995, GFAP-positive hippocampal astrocytes *in situ* respond to glutamatergic neuroligands with increases in $[Ca^{2+}]_i$. *Glia* 13:101-112.

Raabe, W., 1989, Ammonium decreases excitatory synaptic transmission in cat spinal cord *in vivo*. *J. Neurophysiol.* 62:1461-1473.

Rao, V.L.R., Agrawal, A.K. and Murthy, C.R.K., 1991, Ammonia-induced alterations in glutamate and muscimol binding to cerebellar synaptic membranes. *Neurosci. Lett.* 130:251-254.

Ratnakumari, L., Qureshi, I.A. and Butterworth, R.F., 1993, Loss of [^{3}H]MK-801 binding sites in brain in congenital ornithine transcarbamylase deficiency. *Metab. Brain Dis.* 10:249-255.

Record, C.O., Buxton, B., Chase, R., Curzon, G., Murray-Lyon, I.M. and Williams, R., 1976, Plasma and brain amino acids in fulminant hepatic failure and their relationship to hepatic encephalopathy. *Eur. J. Clin. Invest.* 6:387-394.

Schmidt, W., Wolf, G., Grungreiff, K., Meier, M. and Reum, T., 1990, Hepatic encephalopathy influences high affinity uptake of transmitter glutamate and aspartate into the hippocampal formation. *Metab. Brain. Dis.* 5:19-32.

Seiler, N., Sarhan, S., Knoedgen, B., Hornsperger, J.M. and Sablone, M., 1993, Enhanced endogenous ornithine concentrations protein against tonic seizures and coma in acute ammonia intoxication. *Pharmacol. Toxicol.* 72:116-123.

Swain, M., Butterworth, R.F. and Blei, A.T., 1992, Ammonia and related amino acids in the pathogenesis of brain edema in acute ischemic liver failure in rats. *Hepatology* 15:449-453.

Swain, M.S., Bergeron, M., Audet, R., Blei, A.T. and Butterworth, R.F., 1992, Monitoring of neurotransmitter amino acids by means of an indwelling cisterna magna catheter. A comparison of two rodent models of fulminant hepatic failure. *Hepatology* 16:1028-1035.

Takahashi, H., Koehler, R.C., Brusilow, S.W., Jones, J., Traystman, R.J., 1991, Inhibition of brain glutamine accumulation prevents cerebral edema in hyperammonemic rats. *Am. J. Physiol.* 281:H826-H829.

Teichberg, V.I., 1991, Glial glutamate receptors: likely actors in brain signaling. *FASEB J.* 5:3086-3091.

Van Harreveld, A. and Fifkova, E., 1971, Light- and electro-microscopic changes in central nervous tissue after electrophoretic injection of glutamate. *Exp. Mol. Pathol.* 15:61-81.

Watanabe, A., Fujiwara, M., Shiota, T. and Tsuji, T., 1988, Amino acid neurotransmitters and their receptors in the brain synaptosomes of acute hepatic failure rats. *Biochem. Med. Metab. Biol.* 40:247-252.

Westergren, I and Johansson, B.B., 1992, Blockade of AMPA receptors reduces brain edema following opening of the blood-brain barrier. *J. Cerebr. Blood Flow and Metab.* 13:693-608.

Zimmerman, C., Ferenci, P., Pifl, C., Yurdaydin, C., Ebner, J., Lassmann, H., Roth, E. and Hortnagle, H., 1989, Hepatic encephalopathy in thioacetamide-induced acute liver failure in rats: characterization of an improved model and study of amino-acidergic neurotransmission. *Hepatology* 9:594-601.

GLUTAMATE AND MUSCARINIC RECEPTORS IN THE MOLECULAR MECHANISMS OF ACUTE AMMONIA TOXICITY AND OF ITS PREVENTION

María-Dolores Miñana, Marta Llansola, Carlos Hermenegildo, Carmen Cucarella, Carmina Montoliu, Elena Kosenko, Santiago Grisolía and Vicente Felipo

Instituto de Invetigaciones Citológicas
Fundación Valenciana de Investigaciones Biomédicas
Amadeo de Saboya, 4
46010 Valencia, Spain

1. Introduction

Hyperammonemia increases ammonia levels in the brain, and induces functional disturbances in the central nervous system. Increases of ammonia in the brain affect the function of neurons and disturb neuronal interactions (1). Injection of normal animals with large doses of ammonium salts leads to the rapid death of animals. However, the mechanism by which ammonia causes these deletereous effects has not been clarified.

Glutamate is the main excitatory neurotransmitter in mammals. However, when it is in excess, glutamate is neurotoxic, leading to neuronal degeneration and death. Excitatory amino acid neurotoxicity has been shown to contribute to the pathogenesis of different neurodegenerative situations, including brain ischemia, amyotrophic lateral esclerosis, and Huntington's disease. Altered glutamatergic neurotransmission has been also involved in the pathogenesis of Alzheimer's and Parkinson's disease.

There are several types of glutamate receptors. Some of them (ionotropic) are associated to the opening of ion channels; the ionotropic glutamate receptors include NMDA and kainate/AMPA receptors. Other glutamate receptors (metabotropic) are coupled to G-proteins and modulate the activity of certain enzymes (e.g. phospholipase C or adenylate cyclase).

In many systems, glutamate neurotoxicity is mediated by excessive activation of the NMDA type of glutamate receptors (2,3) and concomitant increase in free intracellular Ca^{2+} concentration.

Hyperammonemia and hepatic encephalopathy result in altered glutamatergic neurotransmission. Neurotransmission can be altered at different steps, including the synthesis or release of the neurotransmitter, its uptake from the synaptic cleft, or the amount (synthesis, turnover) or function of the receptors. There is also an interplay between different neurotransmitter systems, so that glutamatergic neurotransmission can be also altered as a consequence of previous alterations in other neurotransmitter systems. Hyperammonemia affects glutamatergic neurotransmission at different steps.

Alterations in the extracellular concentration of glutamate in brain, of other excitatory amino acids and in glutamate receptors have been reported.

2. Effects of hyperammonemia and of hepatic encephalopathy on extracellular glutamate in brain in vivo

Studies in vitro have shown that high ammonia levels affect the release and the uptake of glutamate in different systems (4-10). These ammonia-induced alterations could lead to changes in the concentration of glutamate in the extracellular space in the brain, leading to altered activation of glutamate receptors.

The effects of hyperammonemia and of hepatic encephalopathy on the extracellular concentration of glutamate in different areas of the brain or in cerebrospinal fluid have been studied in vivo using different animal models. Most of the studies have been carried out using in vivo brain microdialysis. A summary of these studies is shown in Table 1.

Moroni et al. (11) showed that acute ammonia intoxication (i.p. injection of 8 mmol/kg of ammonium acetate) leads to increased release of glutamate from the brain surface of the rat (cerebral cortex).

Table 1. Effects of hyperammonemia and of hepatic encephalopathy on extracellular glutamate in brain in vivo

ANIMAL	MODEL	REGION	EFFECT	Ref / year
Rat	Inyection (i.p.) ammonium acetate	Cerebral cortex	Increased	11 / 1983
Rat	Portacaval shunt	Striatum	No effect	12 / 1983
Rabbit	Galactosamine	Hippocampus	Increased	13 / 1984
Human	Liver cirrhosis with hepatic encephalop.	Cerebrospinal fluid (CSF)	Increased	14 / 1984
Rat	Portacaval shunt	Cortex Striatum	Slight Increase No effect	15 / 1987
Rat	Portacaval shunt	CSF	Increased	16 / 1991
Rat	Acute liver ischemia	Cerebral cortex	Increased	17 / 1992
Rat	Continuous ammonia infusion	Striatum Brain cortex	Increased No effect	18 / 1992
Rat	Liver ischemia	CSF	Increased	19 / 1992
	Thioacetamide		Slight increase	
Rabbit	Acute liver failure	Cerebral cortex	Increased	20 / 1994
	Continuous ammonia infusion		Increased	
Rat	Portacaval shunt + ammonium acetate	Frontal cortex	No effect	21 / 1995

A summary of reports studying the effects of different models of hyperammonemia and hepatic encephalopathy on the extracellular content of glutamate in brain in vivo.

Rao et al.(21) showed that i.p. administration of 3.85 mmol/kg of ammonium acetate to portacaval shunted rats did not affect extracellular glutamate in frontal cortex.

Continuous ammonia infusion (0.75 mmol/hour) increases extracellular glutamate in striatum but not in cortex (18) of rats. In rabbits, continuous infusion of ammonia (20) increases extracellular glutamate in cerebral cortex.

The effect of portacaval shunt on glutamate has been also studied. Tossman et al. did not found any alteration of extracellular glutamate in striatum of portacaval shunted rat while it was a slight increase in cortex (12,15). A lack of effect of portacaval shunt on extracellular glutamate in frontal cortex was reported by Rao et al.(21).

The effects of two hepatotoxins have been also studied. Thioacetamide induces a slight, non siginificant, increase in glutamate in rat cerebrospinal fluid (19). Galactosamine increases extracellular glutamate in hippocampus in rabbit (13).

More severe treatments such as acute liver ischemia in rat increase extracellular glutamate in cerebral cortex (17) and in cerebrospinal fluid (19). Induction of acute liver failure in rabbits also increase extracellular glutamate in cerebral cortex (20).

In human patients with liver cirrhosis, it has been reported that glutamate is increased in cerebrospinal fluid of patients with hepatic encephalopathy but not in those without hepatic encephalopathy (14).

It seems therefore that mild hyperammonemia or liver failure without hepatic encephaloapthy (e.g. portacaval shunt alone) did not affect, or affect only slightly, the extracellular concentration of glutamate in brain. However, situations of more severe hyperammonemia or liver failure showing hepatic encephalopathy seem to be associated with increased extracellular glutamate in brain.

3. Effects of hyperammonemia on NMDA receptors

Glutamate neurotoxicity is usually mediated by activation of NMDA receptors (2,3). A selective loss of brain NMDA binding sites has been reported in different models of hyperammonemia.

Peterson et al.(22) showed that portacaval anastomosis in the rat, resulting in sustained hyperammonemia, leads to selective loss of NMDA-sensitive glutamate binding sites in several regions of cerebral cortex, hippocampus, striatum and thalamus.

Rao et al (23) induced hyperammonemia in rats by intraperitoneal injection of ammonium acetate and found a selective decrease in NMDA binding sites in cerebellum.

A loss of [^{3}H]MK-801 binding sites has been reported (24) to occur in most areas of the brain of chronically hyperammonemic sparse-fur mice (spf), mutant mice with a congenital defect of ornithine transcarbamylase (see chapter from Qureshi in this book).

Marcaida et al. (25) induced chronic moderate hyperammonemia in rats by feeding an ammonium-containing diet. This treatment resulted in decreased binding of [^{3}H]-MK-801 to NMDA receptors. However the reduced binding was not due to reduced content of NMDA receptor protein but to altered function of the receptor. The decrease in MK-801 binding sites was also produced in cultured neurons by long-term treatment with ammonia. It was shown that ammonia impairs NMDA receptor function, hindering the opening of the ion channel and the entry of Ca^{2+} into the neuron. The function of the NMDA receptor (the opening of the ion channel) was restored by activating protein kinase C (25), suggesting that high ammonia levels impair NMDA receptor function by altering protein kinase C-mediated phosphorylation.

Prenatal exposure of rats to high ammonia levels induces long-lasting impairment of NMDA receptor function in the pups. Normal function is not recovered until several weeks after normalizing ammonia levels (26). NMDA receptor plays an important role in brain plasticity and in learning and memory. The long-lasting ammonia-induced impairment of NMDA receptor function can be involved therefore in the origen of mental retardation found in neonatal hyperammonemia due to congenital deficiencies of urea cycle enzymes, to asphixia or to other causes leading to neonatal transient hyperammonemia (27-29).

4. Acute ammonia toxicity is mediated by activation of NMDA receptors

We supposed that the selective loss of NMDA receptor binding sites in chronic hyperammonemia would be an adaptative response to prevent the deletereous effects of excessive activation of NMDA receptors induced by high ammonia levels.

This would be in agreement with the following facts:

a) Glutamate-induced neurodegeneration is usually mediated by activation of NMDA receptors.

b) Extracellular glutamate in brain is increased in severe hyperammonemia (Table 1).

c) Moderate hyperammonemia results in selective loss of NMDA sensitive binding sites.

On these basis, we supposed that acute toxicity induced by large doses of ammonium salts could be mediated by excessive activation of NMDA receptors. To test this hypothesis we tested whether antagonists of NMDA receptors, acting on different sites of the receptor, are able to prevent ammonia-induced death of animals. Some of the results obtained are summarized in Table 2.

We found that MK-801, a selective NMDA receptor antagonist that blocks the associated ion channel, prevent acute ammonia toxicity (ammonia-induced death) in mice and rats (30). The protective effect of MK-801 has been later confirmed by Seiler et al (32) but not by Itzhak and Norenberg (33). The lack of effect found by Itzhak and Norenberg should be due to the fact that they inject MK-801 30 min before ammonia, while in the reports of Marcaida et al (30) or Seiler et al (32), it was injected 10 or 15

Table 2. Effect of different NMDA receptor antagonists on ammonia-induced death of mice. Groups of mice were injected i.p. with the indicated doses and compounds. Fifteen min later, mice were injected i.p. with 14 mmol/kg of ammonium acetate. The number of animals injected and those surviving after 24 hours are indicated. Data have been taken from references 30 and 31. Some additional data are included.

COMPOUND	Dose (mg/kg)	Survivors/injected	Survival (%)
NONE	----	10 / 218	5
MK-801	2	38 / 50	76
Ketamine	20	9 / 20	45
Ketamine	50	32 / 43	75
PCP	25	25 / 32	78
Memantine	30	11 / 32	34
CGP 40116	50	6 / 10	40
CGP 40116	100	15 / 20	75
CGS 19755	20	20 / 24	83
AP-5	150	6 / 10	40
AP-5	500	4 / 5	80
CPP	20	23 / 30	77

min before ammonia. In our hands, MK-801 prevents ammonia-induced death of mice when injected 15 min before ammonia but not when injected 30 min before ammonia.

To confirm that acute ammonia toxicity is mediated by activation of NMDA receptors, we tested whether other antagonists, acting on different sites of the receptor, are able to prevent ammonia-induced death of mice (31). As shown in Table 2, MK-801, phencyclidine and ketamine, which block the ion channel of NMDA receptors, prevent death of 75-78% of mice. CPP, AP-5, CGS 19755 and CGP 40116, competitive antagonists acting on the glutamate (and NMDA) binding site, also prevent death of at least 75% of mice.

It has been reported that alcohols prevent ammonia toxicity in animals (34) and also that they act as antagonists of NMDA receptors (35). It seems that alcohols act on the glycine binding site of the NMDA receptor (35). There is an excellent correlation between the ability of different alcohols to prevent ammonia toxicity in animals and their capacity to block NMDA receptors (31). All these results support the idea that acute ammonia toxicity is mediated by activation of NMDA receptors.

This idea is also supported by the excitotoxic damage found in sparse-fur mice, an animal model of congenital hyperammonemia. Robinson et al (36) found a significant loss of medium spiny neurons and increased numbers of reactive oligodendroglia and microglia in the striatum of sparse fur mice. These neuropathological observations are consistent with an excitotoxic influence on brain injury in these mice.

5. The protective effect of carnitine against acute ammonia toxicity and glutamate neurotoxicity is mediated by activation of metabotropic glutamate receptors

Carnitine protects animals against acute ammonia toxicity (37). It was tested, by using primary cultures of cerebellar neurons, the possibility that carnitine prevents ammonia toxicity by preventing glutamate neurotoxicity. Addition of 1 mM glutamate to the medium leads to the death of most (ca. 80%) cultured neurons. However, when the neurons were previously incubated with carnitine, the neurotoxicity of glutamate was prevented (38). Addition of 0.5 mM carnitine prevented death of 50% of the neurons and all cells were protected when 3 mM carnitine was added. The large concentrations of carnitine required are in agreement with the large doses required to completely prevent ammonia toxicity in animals. These results are consistent with the idea that carnitine could prevent ammonia toxicity by preventing glutamate neurotoxicity.

To assess whether the protective effect of carnitine against glutamate neurotoxicity is due to altered binding of glutamate to its receptors, the effect of carnitine on [^{3}H]glutamate binding to synaptic membranes was determined. It was found that carnitine increases the affinity of glutamate for quisqualate (including metabotropic) receptors while does not affect or reduces slightly the binding to NMDA or kainate receptors (38).

This suggested that the protective effect of carnitine could be mediated by increased activation of metabotropic glutamate receptors. It was found that, in fact, preincubation with AP-3, an antagonist of metabotropic receptors, abolished the protective effect of carnitine (38). Moreover, tACPD, an agonist of metabotropic receptors, also prevent glutamate or NMDA neurotoxicity in cultured cerebellar neurons (38), cortical neurons (39) and in rat retina in vivo (40).

These results indicate that the protective effect of carnitine against glutamate neurotoxicty is mediated by activation of metabotropic glutamate receptors.

6. Carnitine and choline derivatives prevent ammonia toxicity in mice and glutamate neurotoxicity in primary cultures of neurons

It has been shown that betaine and TMAO, two compounds that share with carnitine, a trimethylamine group, also prevent acute ammonia toxicity in mice. This protective effect was attributed to an osmotic effect (41).

Table 3. **Protective effect of different compounds against acute ammonia toxicity.** Groups of mice were injected intraperitoneally with the indicated doses of each compound. Fifteen min later mice were injected i.p. with 14 mmol/kg of ammonium acetate. The number of animals injected and surviving are given. Data from reference 42.

COMPOUND	DOSE	SURVIVAL	
	mmol/kg	Survivors/injected	%
NONE	---	17/142	12
L-carnitine	16	24/ 28	86
D-carnitine	16	21/ 31	68
Betaine	16	12/ 20	60
TMAO	8	32/ 50	64
Choline	1.6	43/ 65	66
Acetylcholine	0.28	17/ 30	57
Acetylcholine	0.55	63/ 88	71
Carbachol	0.0028	14/ 30	46
Carbachol	0.0055	23/ 49	51
Acetylcarnitine	6	41/ 54	76
Isovalerylcarnitine	4	17/ 21	80

However, we considered of interest to test whether the protective effect of betaine and TMAO against ammonia toxicity in animals could also be due to prevention of glutamate neurotoxicity.

We also tested whether other compounds containing a trimethylamine group are able to prevent acute ammonia toxicity in mice and/or glutamate neurotoxicity in cultured neurons.

The protective effect of different compounds containing a trimethylamine group against acute ammonia toxicity is shown in Table 3. Acetylcholine and carbachol prevented ammonia-induced death of mice at very low doses, e.g. injection of 0.55 mmol/kg of acetylcholine prevented death of 71% of mice. For carnitine, betaine, TMAO, choline, acetylcarnitine and isovalerylcarnitine, the doses required were larger, but all of them prevented death of 60-86% of mice. Acetylcarnitine affords significant protection when injected at 4-8 mmol/kg, but not at lower or higher doses. A similar effect was found for isovalerylcarnitine, which only prevents ammonia-induced death of mice when injected at 4-6 mmol/kg (42).

These results indicate that compounds sharing the trimethylamine group also share the capacity to prevent acute ammonia toxicity in mice, although the doses required to afford protection varied widely for the different compounds.

It was then tested whether these compounds prevent glutamate toxicity in primary cultures of cerebellar neurons. The protective effect of different concentrations of carbachol, choline, acetylcarnitine, TMAO, acetylcholine and betaine against glutamate neurotoxicity is shown in Fig. 1. All these compounds prevent glutamate toxicity nearly completely when used at suitable concentrations. The results shown in Fig. 1 reveal two kinds of responses. Acetylcholine, choline and acetylcarnitine afford partial protection at very low concentrations; 0.2 nM acetylcholine, choline or acetylcarnitine prevent death of 45-50% of neurons. There is a plateau in the protection afforded by these compounds up to 0.1 to 1 μM and then the protective effect increases again. Carbachol, TMAO and betaine did not afford protection at concentrations lower than 1 μM and prevent completely glutamate toxicity at 0.1 to 1 mM concentrations.

These results suggest that at least two different mechanisms would be involved in the protective effect of trimethylamine-containing compounds against glutamate neurotoxicity. One mechanism would be activated by very low (less than 1 nM) concentrations of acetylcholine, choline or acetylcarnitine, and would be active only in abouth one half of the neurons. The second mechanism would be activated in all neurons by carbachol, TMAO, betaine, acetylcholine, choline and acetylcarnitine. The underlying signal transduction pathways involved in each molecular mechanism remain to be clarified.

7. Carnitine and trimethylamine-containign compounds prevent glutamate but not NMDA toxicity in primary cultures of neurons

Glutamate toxicity in cerebellar neurons in culture is mediated by activation of NMDA receptors and is completely prevented by preincubation with MK-801, an antagonist of NMDA receptors.

As mentioned above, the protective effect of carnitine against glutamate neurotoxicity seems to be mediated by increased activation of metabotropic receptors. Glutamate can bind to both NMDA and metabotropic glutamate receptors; however, NMDA can not bind to metabotropic receptors. It is then likely that carnitine could prevent glutamate but not NMDA-induced neurotoxicity.

The protective effects of carnitine and of other trimethylamine-containing compounds against glutamate and NMDA neurotoxicity is shown in Table 4. NMDA toxicity was completely prevented by MK-801, an antagonist of the receptor. Trans-ACPD, an agonist of metabotropic glutamate receptors also prevent NMDA toxicity, confirming that activation of metabotropic receptors prevent NMDA-induced neuronal death. Acetylcholine did not afford any protection against NMDA neurotoxicity. Carnitine, choline, acetylcarnitine, betaine and carbachol afford only a very slight protection. Only TMAO affords a significant protection against NMDA toxicity (Table 4). These results indicate that trimethylamine-containing compounds are very efficient in preventing glutamate-induced but not NMDA-induced neuronal death, supporting the idea that their protective effects could be mediated by increased activation of metabotropic glutamate receptors by glutamate.

Table 4. **Effects of trimethylamine-containing compounds on neuronal death induced by glutamate or NMDA**

Primary cultures of cerebellar neurons were used for assays of glutamate toxicity 9-12 days after seeding. Monolayers were washed three times with Locke's solution without magnesium. The compounds to be tested were then added. The concentrations used were the following: carnitine 5 mM; betaine 1 mM; TMAO 1 mM; choline 1 mM; acetylcholine 1 mM; carbachol 1 mM; acetylcarnitine 1 μM ; trans-ACPD 0.1 mM and MK-801 20 nM. Neurons were incubated with these compounds for 15 min and then 1 mM glutamate or 0.5 mM NMDA was added to all plates. Neuronal survival was determined four hours later. Survival in control neurons not exposed to glutamate was 84 ± 4%. Data from reference 42.

COMPOUND	Glutamate	NMDA
	Surviving neurons (% of total)	
None	20 ± 8	28 ± 7
Carnitine	70 ± 8	47 ± 8
Betaine	69 ± 7	46 ± 5
TMAO	75 ± 4	64 ± 12
Choline	65 ± 5	41 ± 5
Acetylcholine	68 ± 4	23 ± 11
Carbachol	73 ± 3	40 ± 6
Acetylcarnitine	69 ± 3	48 ± 8
Trans-ACPD	84 ± 6	65 ± 5
MK-801	80 ± 5	83 ± 6

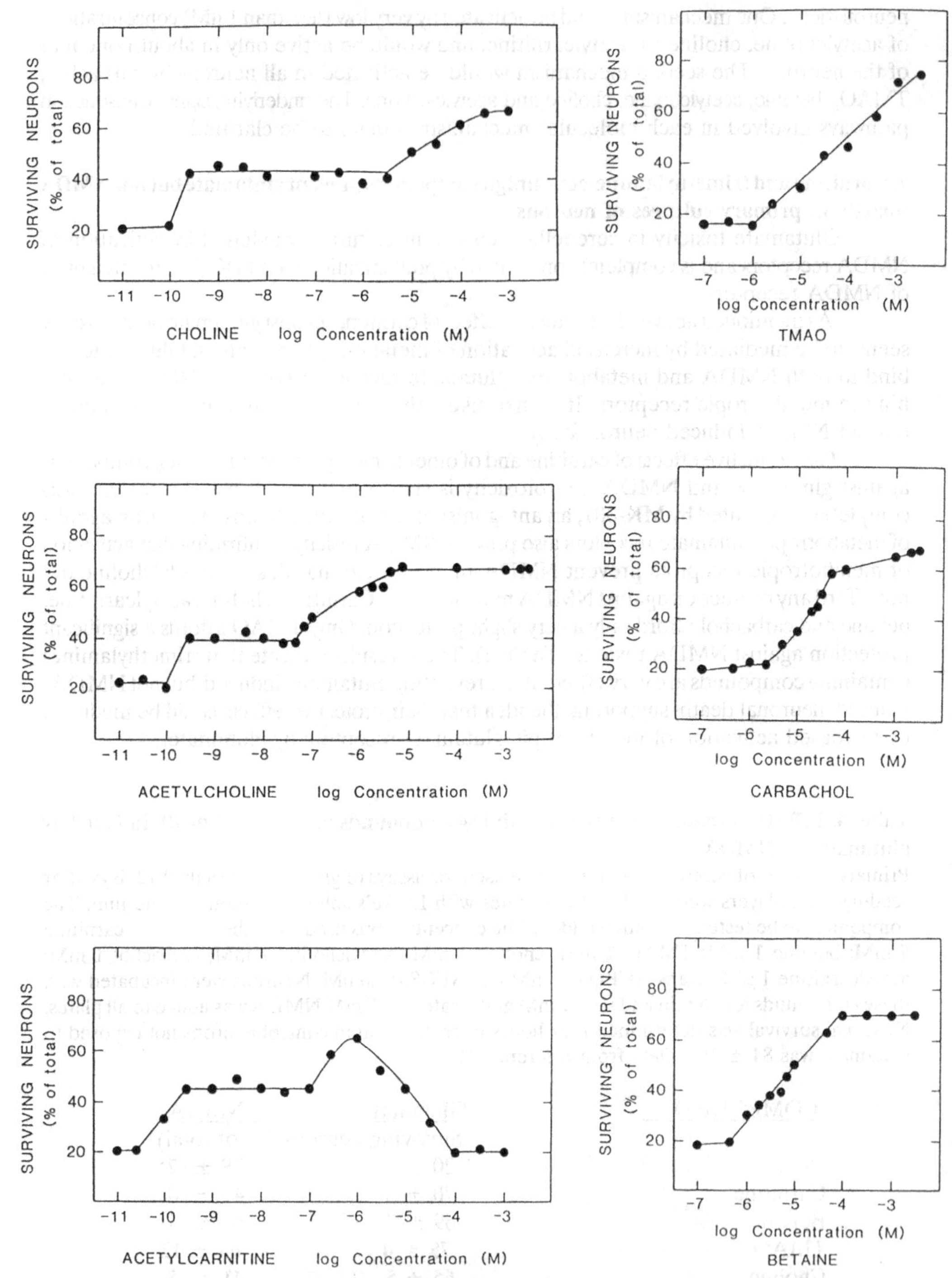

Figure 1. **Protective effects of different concentrations of acetylcarnitine, acetylcholine, choline, carbachol, betaine and TMAO against glutamate toxicity in primary cultures of neurons.** Primary cultures of cerebellar neurons were used 9-12 days after seeding to assess the protective effect of acetylcarnitine, acetylcholine, choline, carbachol, betaine and TMAO, against glutamate neurotoxicity. Monolayers were incubated with the indicated concentrations of the above compounds for 15 min. Then, 1 mM glutamate was added to all samples and incubation was continued for 4 hours. Cell viability was then assayed. From (42).

8. The protective effect of trimethylamine-containing compounds is prevented by antagonists of metabotropic glutamate receptors or of muscarinic cholinergic receptors

It was tested whether, as is the case for carnitine, the protective effect of the above trimethylamine-containing compounds is prevented by the antagonist of metabotropic glutamate receptors AP-3. As shown in Table 5, none of the compounds tested prevent glutamate neurotoxicity after preincubation with AP-3, which also prevents the protective effect of tACPD, an agonist of metabotropic glutamate receptors.

Some of the compounds tested (e.g. acetylcholine, carbachol) act as agonists of cholinergic receptors. To assess whether the protective effect of these compounds is mediated by activation of cholinergic receptors, we tested if atropine, an antagonist of muscarinic cholinergic receptors, prevents the protective effect against glutamate toxicity. As shown in Table 5, the protective effects of acetylcholine, carbachol, choline, betaine and carnitine are abolished by pretreatment with atropine. The protective effects of acetylcarnitine and TMAO are reduced in the presence of atropine.

These results indicate that both antagonists of metabotropic glutamate receptors or antagonists of muscarinic receptors prevent the protective effect of trimethylamine-containing compounds against glutamate neurotoxicity. It is not clear, at this moment, how antagonists for both type of receptors can prevent the protective effect. In control experiments we found that atropine does not interfere with the activation of metabotropic glutamate receptors; also, AP-3 does not interfere with muscarinic receptors. It seems that it could be an interplay between the signal transduction pathways stimulated by both type of receptors.

Table 5. **Prevention by AP-3 and atropine of the protective effect of trimethylamine-containing compounds against glutamate neurotoxicity**

Primary cultures of cerebellar neurons were used for assays of glutamate toxicity 9-12 days after seeding. Some plates were preincubated with AP-3 (0.2 mM) for 30 min or with atropine (20 nM) for 10 min. The compounds to be tested were then added. The concentrations used were the following: carnitine 5 mM; betaine 1 mM; TMAO 1 mM; choline 1 mM; acetylcholine 1 mM; carbachol 1 mM; acetylcarnitine 1 μM and trans-ACPD 0.1 mM. Neurons were incubated with these compounds for 15 min and then 1 mM glutamate was added to all plates. Survival in control neurons not exposed to glutamate was 84 ± 4%. Data from reference 42.

COMPOUND	PREINCUBATION WITH		
	Nothing	AP-3	Atropine
	Surviving neurons (% of total)		
None	20 ± 8	40 ± 9	26 ± 7
Carnitine	70 ± 8	41 ± 7	43 ± 3
Betaine	69 ± 7	48 ± 7	38 ± 6
TMAO	75 ± 4	35 ± 14	64 ± 6
Choline	65 ± 5	33 ± 3	38 ± 6
Acetylcholine	68 ± 4	44 ± 7	36 ± 7
Carbachol	73 ± 3	52 ± 3	43 ± 6
Acetylcarnitine	69 ± 3	45 ± 6	50 ± 7
Trans-ACPD	84 ± 6	28 ± 5	26 ± 4

9. Atropine prevents the protective effect of some trimethylamine-containing compounds against acute ammonia toxicity in mice

As atropine prevents the protective effect against glutamate neurotoxicity of most of the trimethylamine-containing compounds tested, and we believe that the protective effect of these compounds against acute ammonia toxicity in mice is due to prevention of glutamate neurotoxicity, we tested whether injection of atropine into mice prevents the protective effect of trimethylamine-containing compounds against ammonia-induced death of mice.

As shown in Table 6, atropine did not prevent the protective effects of betaine or carnitine, but reduced significantly the protective effect of acetylcholine and abolished the protection afforded by carbachol, choline and acetylcarnitine against ammonia toxicity in animals. These results indicate that primary cultures of cerebellar neurons can be a useful model to study the molecular mechanism of ammonia toxicity and of its prevention. These studies could allow to propose possible protective agents against ammonia toxicity in animals.

Table 6. **Effect of previous injection of atropine on the protective effect of different compounds against acute ammonia toxicity**

Groups of mice were injected with the indicated compounds with or without previous injection of atropine (100 μg/kg of body weight, i.p., 10 min before the compound tested). The indicated compounds were injected intraperitoneally. The doses injected were, in mmol/kg of body weight: 0.55 for acetylcholine; 1.6 for choline; 16 for carnitine; 0,0028 for carbachol; 8 for betaine and 6 for acetylcarnitine. 14 mmol/kg of ammonium acetate were injected i.p. fifteen min later. The number of animals surviving and injected are given. Asterisks indicate the compounds for which the protective effect is significantly reduced by previous injection of atropine. Data from reference 42.

COMPOUND	ATROPINE	SURVIVAL	
		Survivors/injected	%
NONE	NO	12/ 78	15
	YES	11/ 40	27
ACETYLCHOLINE	NO	16/ 23	69
	YES	8/ 26	30*
CHOLINE	NO	23/ 37	62
	YES	5/ 30	16*
CARNITINE	NO	17/ 20	85
	YES	18/ 19	94
CARBACHOL	NO	13/ 28	46
	YES	4/ 28	14*
BETAINE	NO	14 / 20	70
	YES	18/ 22	82
ACETYLCARNITINE	NO	8/ 12	67
	YES	1/ 12	8*

ACKNOWLEDGMENTS. Supported in part by a grant (PM95-0174) from the Ministerio de Educación y Ciencia, Programa de Promoción General del Conocimiento, of Spain. C. Hermenegildo is a Severo Ochoa fellow from the Ayuntamiento de Valencia. C. Cucarella received a fellowship from the Consellería de Educación y Ciencia of Generalitat Valenciana.

REFERENCES

1. Raabe, W. Effects of NH_4^+ on the function of the CNS. Adv. Exp. Med. Biol. 272 (1990) 99-120
2. Choi, D. W. Ionic dependence of glutamate neurotoxicity. J. Neurosci. 7 (1987) 369-379
3. Novelli, A., Reilly, J. A., Lysko, P. and Henneberry, R. C. Glutamate becomes neurotoxic via the N-methyl-D-aspartate receptor when intracellular energy levels are reduced. Brain Res. 451 (1988) 205-212
4. Mena, E.E. and Cotman, C. W. Pathologic concentrations of ammonium ions block l-glutamate uptake. Exp. Neurol. 89 (1985) 259-263
5. Erecinska, M., Pastuszko, A., Wilson, D.F. and Nelson, D. Ammonia-induced release of neurotransmitters from rat brain synaptosomes: differences between the effects of amines and amino acids. J. Neurochem. 49 (1987) 1258-1265
6. Schmidt, W., Wolf, G., Grüngreiff, K., Meier, M. and Reum, T. Hepatic encephalopathy influences high-affinity uptake of transmitter glutamate and aspartate into the hippocampal formation. Metab. Brain Dis. 5 (1990) 19-31
7. Hilgier, W., Haugvicova, R. and Albrecht, J. Decreased potassium-stimulated release of[^{3}H]D-aspartate from hippocampal slice distinguishes encephalopathy related to acute liver failure from that induced by simple hyperammonemia. Brain Res. 567 (1991) 165-168
8. Rao, V.L.R. and Murthy, C.R.K. Hyperammonemic alterations in the uptake and release of glutamate and aspartate by rat cerebellar preparations. Neurosci. lett. 130 81991) 49-52
9. Butterworth, R.F., Le, O., Lavoie, J. and Szerb, J.C. Effect of portacaval anastomosis on electrically stimulated release of glutamate from hippocampal slices. J. Neurochem. 56 (1991) 1481-1484
10. Albrecht, J., Hilgier, W. and Walski, M. Ammonia added in vitro, but not moderate hyperammonemia in vivo, stimulates glutamate uptake and H^+-ATPase activity in synaptic vesicles of rat brain. Metab. Brain Dis. 9 (1994) 257-266
11. Moroni, F., Lombardi, G., Moneti, G. and Cortesini, C. The release and neosynthesis of glutamic acid are increased in experimental models of hepatic encephalopathy. J. Neurochem. 40 81983) 850-854
12. Tossman, U., Eriksson, S., Delin, A., Hagenfeldt, L., Law, D. and Ungerstedt, U. Brain amino acids measured by intracerebral dialysis in portacaval shunted rats. J. Neurochem. 41 (1983) 1046-1051
13. Hamberger, A. and Nyström, B. Extra- and intracellular amino acids in the hippocampus during development of hepatic encephalopathy. Neurochem. Res. 9 (1984) 1181-1192
14. Watanabe, A., Takei, N., Shiota, T., Nakatsukasa, H., Fujiwara, M., Sakata, T. and Nagashima, H. Glutamic acid and glutamine levels in serum and cerebrospinal fluid in hepatic encephalopathy. Biochem. Med. 32 (1984) 225-231
15. Tossman, U., Delin, A., Eriksson, S. and Ungerstedt, U. Brain cortical amino acids measured by intracerebral dialysis in portacaval shunted rats. Neurochem. Res. 3 (1987) 265-269
16. Therrien, G. and Butterworth, R.F. Cerebrospinal fluid amino acids in relation to neurological status in experimental portal-systemic encephalopathy. Metab. Brain Dis. 6 (1991) 65-74
17. Bosman, D. K., Deutz, N.E.P., Maas, M.A.W., van Eijk, H.M.H., Smit, J.J.H., de Haan, J.G. and Chamuleau, A.F.M. Amino acid release from cerebral cortex in experimental acute liver failure, studied by in vivo cerebral corrtex microdialysis. J. Neurochem. 59 (1992) 591-599
18. Suzuki, K., Matsuo, N., Moriguchi, T., Takeyama, N., Kitazawa, Y. and Tanaka, T. Changes in brain ECF amino acids in rats with experimentally induced hyperammonemia. Metab. Brain. Dis. 7 (1992) 63-75
19. Swain, M. S., Bergeron, M., Audet, R., Blei, A. T. and Butterworth, R. F. Monitoring of neurotransmitter amino acids by mean of an indwelling cisterna magna catheter: a comparison of two rodent models of fulminant liver failure. Hepatology 16 (1992) 1028-1035

20. De Knegt, R.J., Schalm, S. W., van der Rijt, C.C.D., Fekkes, D., Dalm, E. and Hekking-Weyma, I. Extracellular brain glutamate during acute liver failure and during acute hyperammonemia simulating acute liver failure. J. Hepatol. 20 (1994) 19-26
21. Rao, V.L.R., Audet, R.M. and Butterworth, R.F. Selective alterations of extracellular brain amino acids in relation to function in experimental portal-systemic encephalopathy: results of an in vivo microdialysis study. J. Neurochem. 65 (1995) 1221-1228
22. Peterson, C., Giguere, J.F., Cotman, C.W. and Butterworth, R.F. Selective loss of N-methyl-D-aspartate-sensitive L-[^{3}H]glutamate binding sites in rat brain following portacaval anastomosis. J. Neurochem. 55 (1990) 386-390
23. Rao, V.L.R., Agrawal, A.K. and Murthy, C.R.K Ammonia-induced alterations in glutamate and muscimol binding to cerebellar synaptic membranes. Neurosci. Lett. 130 (1991), 251-254
24. Ratnakumari, L., Qureshi, I.A. and Butterworth, R.F. Loss of [^{3}H]MK-801 binding sites in brain in congenital ornithine transcarbamylase deficiency. Metab. Brain Dis. 10 (1995) 249-255
25. Marcaida, G., Miñana, M.D., Burgal, M., Grisolía, S. and Felipo, V. Ammonia prevents activation of NMDA receptors by glutamate in rat cerebellar neuronal cultures. Eur. J. Neurosci. 7 (1995) 2389-2396
26. Miñana, M.D., Marcaida, G., Grisolía, S. and Felipo, V. Prenatal exposure of rats to ammonia impairs NMDA receptor function and affords delayed protection against ammonia toxicity and glutamate neurotoxicity. J. Neuropathol. Exp. Neurol. 54 (1995) 644-650
27. Yoshino, M., Sakaguchi, Y., Kuriya, N. et al A nationwide survey on transient hyperammonemia in newborn infants in Japan: prognosis of life and neurological outcome. Neuropediatrics 22 (1991) 198-202
28. Msall, M., Batshaw, M.L., Suss, R., Brusilow, S.W. and Mellits, E.D. Neurological outcome in children with inborn errors of urea synthesis. Outcome of urea cycle enzymopathies. N. Engl. J. Med. 310 (1984) 1500-1505
29. Colombo, J.P. N-Acetylglutamate synthetase (NAGS) deficiency. Adv. Exp. Med. Biol. 364 (1994) 135-143
30. Marcaida, G., Felipo, V., Hermenegildo, C., Miñana, M.D. and Grisolía, S. Acute ammonia toxicity is mediated by the NMDA type of glutamate receptors. FEBS Lett. 296 (1992) 67-68
31. Hermenegildo, C., Marcaida, G., Montoliu, C., Grisolía, S., Miñana, M. D. and Felipo, V. NMDA receptor antagonists prevent acute ammonia toxicity in mice. Neurochem. Res. 21 (1996) 1237-1244
32. Seiler, N., Sarthan, S., Knoedgen, B., Hornsperger, J.M. and Sablone, M. Enhanced endogenous ornithine concentrations protect against tonic seizures and coma in acute ammonia intoxication. Pharmacol. Toxicol. 72 (1993) 116-123
33. Itzhak, Y. and Norenberg, M.D. Attenuation of ammonia toxicity in mice by PK 11195 and pregnenolone sulfate. Neurosci. Lett. 182 (1994) 251-254
34. O'Connor, J.E., Guerri, C. and Grisolía, S. Protective effect of ethanol on acute ammonia intoxication in mice. Biochem. Biophys. Res. Commun. 104 (1982) 410-415
35. Weight, F.E., Lovinger, D.M., White, G. and Peoples, R.W. Alcohol and anesthetic actions on excitatory amino acid-activated ion channels. in Rubin, E., Miller, K.W. and Roth, S, eds. Molecular and Cellular Mechanisms of Alcohols and Anesthetics. Ann. N. Y. Acad. Sci. 625 (1991) 97-107
36. Robinson, M.B., Hopkins, K., Batshaw, M.L., McLaughlin, B.A., Heyes, M.P. and Oster-Granite, M.L. Evidence of excitotoxicity in the brain of the ornithine carbamoyltransferase deficient sparse fur mouse. Dev. Brain Res. 90 (1995) 35-44
37. O'Connor, J.E., Costell, M. and Grisolía, S. Protective effect of L-carnitine on hyperammonemia. FEBS Lett. 166 (1984) 331-334
38. Felipo, V., Miñana, M.D., Cabedo, H. and Grisolía, S. L-carnitine increases the affinity of glutamate for quisqualate receptors and prevents glutamate neurotoxicity. Neurochem. Res. 19 (1994) 373-377
39. Kho, J.Y., Palmer, E. and Cotman, C.W. Activation of the metabotropic glutamate receptor attenuates N-methyl-D-aspartate neurotoxicity in cortical cultures. Proc. Natl. Acad. Sci. USA 88 (1991) 9431-9435
40. Siliprandi, R., Lipartiti, M., Fadda, E., Sautter J. and Manev, H. Activation of metabotropic receptor protects retina against N-methyl-D-aspartate toxicity. Eur. J. Pharmacol. 219 (1992) 173-174
41. Kloiber, O., Banjac, B. and Drewes, L.R. Protection against acute hyperammonemia: the role of quaternay amines. Toxicology 49, (1988) 83-90
42. Miñana, M.D., Hermenegildo, C., Llansola, M., Montoliu, C., Grisolía, S. and Felipo, V. Carnitine and choline dervatives containing a trimethylamine group prevent ammonia toxicity in mice and glutamate toxicity in primary cultures of neurons. J. Pharmacol. Exp. Ther. 279 (1996) 194-199

STUDIES ON THE PHARMACOLOGICAL PROPERTIES OF OXINDOLE (2-HYDROXYINDOLE) AND 5-HYDROXYINDOLE: ARE THEY INVOLVED IN HEPATIC ENCEPHALOPATHY?

Flavio Moroni, Raffaella Carpenedo, Guido Mannaioni, Alessandro Galli, Alberto Chiarugi, Vincenzo Carlà and Gloriano Moneti

Department of Pharmacology, University of Florence, Viale Morgagni 65, 50134 Firenze, Italy

INTRODUCTION

It has been repeatedly described that plasma or CSF tryptophan concentrations increase in experimental animal models of liver impairment and in patients suffering from hepatic encephalopathy or hepatic coma (Hirayama, 1971; Curzon et al. 1973; Sourkes, 1978; ONO et al. 1996). It has also been demonstrated that the administration of large doses of tryptophan to patients affected by hepatic disorders or to dogs with a portocaval shunt may lead to coma (Sherlock, 1975; Rossi-Fanelli et al. 1982). On the basis of the widely agreed assumption that increased brain tryptophan concentrations signify increased 5OH-tryptamine turnover, several years ago, a number of investigators proposed that an increased stimulation of 5OH-tryptamine receptors plays a key role in the neurological and psychiatric symptoms associated with liver diseases (Cummings et al. 1976). Tryptophan may be metabolized not only into 5OH-tryptamine, but also into quinolinic or kynurenic acids, neuroactive compounds which are able to interact with glutamate receptors of the NMDA type (see: Stone, 1993 for a review). Approximately ten years ago, we observed that quinolinic acid was indeed increased in the rat brain with portocaval anastomosis or in patients who had died in hepatic coma (Moroni et al. 1986; Moroni et al. 1986a). We therefore proposed that "..quinolinic acid should be added to the list of compounds possibly involved in the pathogenesis and symptomatology of brain disorders associated to liver failure." Other groups have recently confirmed that quinolinic acid is indeed increased in the blood and brain of rat models suffering from either acute or chronic liver failure. The concentration of quinolinic acid in the brain, however, does not seem to correlate with the neurological symptoms observed in these liver disorders. Furthermore, it is possible that quinolinic acid synthesis occurs mostly in macrophages or other peripheral tissues, suggesting that its importance in the pathogenesis of hepatic encephalopathy may be "minor" (Bergquist et al. 1995; Basile et al. 1995).

In the last several years, our group has been particularly interested in understanding the role that the above-mentioned tryptophan metabolites may have in physiology or pathology, and we have been investigating the regulation of the activities of a number of enzymes responsible for quinolinate or kynurenate formation in the mammalian brain (Moroni et al. 1984; Moroni et al. 1986; Moroni et al. 1988; Moroni et al. 1991). We characterized several selective inhibitors of most of the enzymes involved in the kynurenine pathway which are responsible for the biosynthesis of quinolinic acid and then of NAD. These inhibitors were quite potent *in vitro*, but we noticed that they were not able to significantly decrease quinolinic acid formation when administered to rats or mice *in vivo*. Such results could be explained by assuming the existence of unknown metabolic pathways which lead to the synthesis of 3-OH anthranilic acid, the direct precursors of quinolinic acid through kynurenine independent pathways (Carpenedo et al. 1994; Chiarugi et al. 1995: Chiarugi, et al. 1996). In order to uncover such metabolic pathways, we administered indole derivatives to rats and mice and we then evaluated the formation of anthranilic and 3-OH anthranilic acid. In the course of these studies, we noticed that the administration of oxindole (2-indolinone) (20-200 mg/kg i.p.) had profound neurodepressant effects, while similar doses of the isomer 5-hydroxyindole caused convulsions and death.

Research in old literature and discussion with a chemist who was involved in studies on tryptophan metabolism for several decades (Dr. Allegri, Padua, Italy) informed us that oxindole was being administered to mice, rats, hamster, rabbits, cats, dogs and humans in the early sixties and that its potent neurodepressant action was observed and described (Orcutt et al. 1964). The convulsant actions of 5-hydroxyindole have not been previously reported. It has, however, been recently demonstrated that this compound may modulate the function of $5HT_3$-receptors (Kooyman et al. 1993; Kooyman et al. 1994). The possibility that oxindole or 5-hydroxyindole could be present in mammalian tissues in physiology or

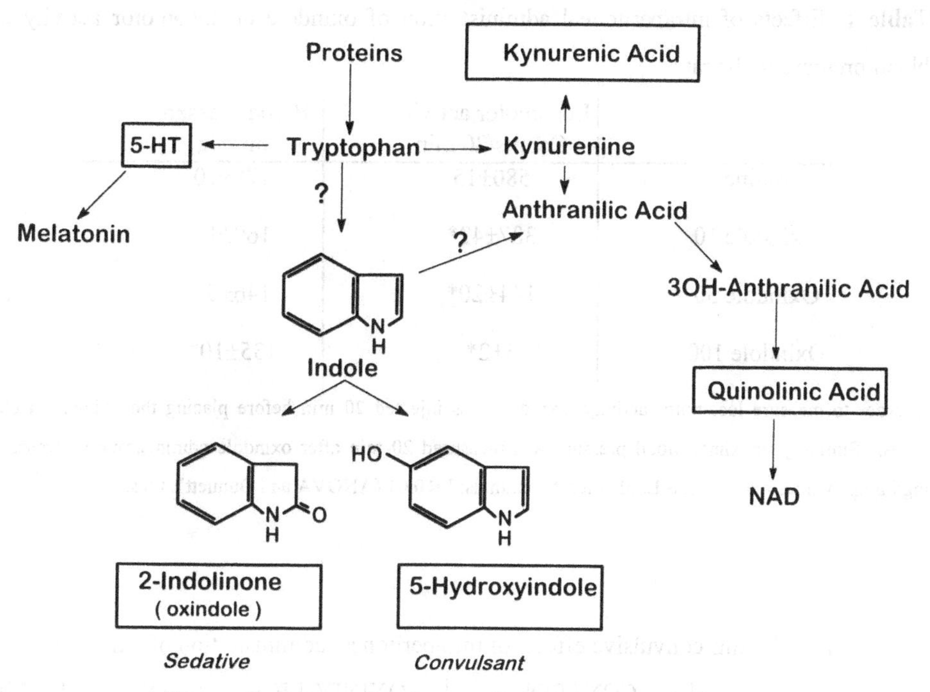

Figure 1. Proposed pathway of tryptophan metabolism.

pathology was never mentioned in any of these previous studies since both compounds were considered by products of tryptophanase activity, a bacterial enzyme not found in mammalian tissues ((King, et al. 1966; van Pée and Lingens, 1984). In view of the potent pharmacological effects observed after oxindole or 5-hydroxyindole administration, we thought it important to clarify: 1) the behavioral effects and the pharmacological properties of these indole derivatives; 2) whether or not such neuro-active molecules are present in mammalian tissues; 3) whether or not they accumulate in the course of hepatic encephalopathy; 4) what the mechanism is of their pharmacological actions.

We report here a series of preliminary results on these issues. Unfortunately, the basic mechanism of the pharmacological action of oxindole and of 5-OH-indole remains to be clarified.

STUDIES ON THE BEHAVIORAL EFFECTS OF OXINDOLE AND 5-HYDROXYINDOLE

Spontaneous locomotor activity of mice or rats was evaluated using an Animex activity meter apparatus (model LKB FARAD). The number of interruptions of photocells was then monitored for 20 min after placing each animal in a clean cage. Blood pressure was

Table 1. Effects of intraperitoneal administration of oxindole on locomotor activity and blood pressure in the rat

	Locomotor activity Counts/20 min	Blood pressure mmHg
Saline	580±15	178±10
Oxindole 10	387±42*	160±13
Oxindole 30	144±20*	146±5*
Oxindole 100	5±2*	135±10*

In order to measure locomotor activity, oxindole was injected 20 min before placing the animals in clean cages. Similarly, maximal blood pressure was measured 20 min after oxindole administration. Doses are mg/kg i.p. Values are mean± S.E. of at least 6 animals; P< 0.01 (ANOVA and Dunnett's t test).

Table 2. Anti-convulsive effects of intraperitoneal administration of oxindole

	CONTROLS	OXINDOLE 30	OXINDOLE 100
PTZ	5/5	2/5	0/5*
STRYCHNINE	5/5	--	3/4
PICROTOXINE	5/5	0/5	--
ß-MERCAPTO PROPIONATE	21/25	5/15*	0/5

Data represent the number of animals showing seizures (clonic or tonic) relative to the total number of animals. Doses are mg/kg i.p. Doses of the convulsants were: pentametilentetrazole 100 mg/kg; β-mercaptopropioniate 30 mg/kg; strychnine 1.6 mg/kg.

Table 3. Convulsive effects of intraperitoneal administration of 5-hydroxyindole

	CLONIC	TONIC	DEATH
5-OH indole 50	0/6	0/6	0/6
5-OH indole 80	3/5*	0/5	0/5
5-OH indole 100	4/5*	4/5*	4/5*

Data represent the number of animals showing seizures (clonic or tonic) or death relative to the total number of animals. Doses are mg/kg i.p. $^2\chi$ test, P<0.01.

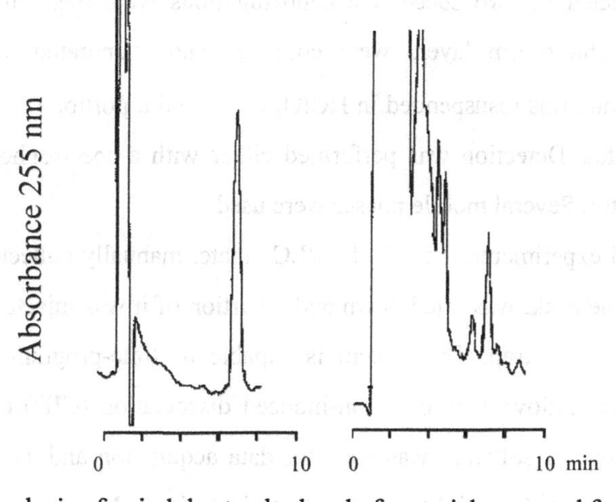

Figure 2. HPLC analysis of oxindole standard and of material extracted from the brain.
A is an HPLC tracing of the standard (50 picomol/100 μl) and B of the brain extract. Mobile phase was a 0.05 M acetate buffer plus 15 % acetonitrile. The column was a 25 cm long, C_{18} reverse phase.

evaluated in the rat tail with a blood pressure recorder (Basile, Varese, model 8006). As reported in table 1, animals treated with oxindole (10-100 mg/kg i.p.) had significantly reduced locomotor activity; they were calm and easy to manage and at 100 mg/kg their righting reflex was completely abolished for approximately two hrs. Blood pressure was also significantly decreased.

Besides reducing blood pressure and causing sedation and coma, oxindole (30-100 mg/kg i.p.) prevented chemically-induced tonic convulsions. As reported in table 2, the convulsions induced by chemicals affecting the GABA system were antagonized by doses of oxindole (30 and 100 mg/kg) which were inactive against convulsant agents acting on the glycine system. A significant protection from convulsant-induced death was also observed.

When 5-hydroxyindole (30-100 mg/kg) was administered i.p. to rats or mice, the animals had tonic-clonic convulsions which started between 5 and 10 min after its administration and at the larger dose lasted until the animal death (Table 3).

IDENTIFICATION AND MEASUREMENT OF OXINDOLE IN MAMMALIAN TISSUES

Experiments were performed in male Wistar rats, male white Swiss mice and male guinea pigs. The animals were decapitated and the blood or other organs (brain, liver, kidney) were rapidly removed, weighed and frozen. Approximately 1 g of each tissue was then homogenized in 2 volumes of 0.4 N $HClO_4$ (or $HClO_4$ 1 N for the blood). The supernatants collected by two successive centrifugations were then mixed with 8 ml of chloroform. The chloroform layers were collected and evaporated under a stream of nitrogen. The residue was resuspended in $HClO_4$ 0.4 N and a portion of it was injected into the HPLC apparatus. Detection was performed either with a spectrophotometer or with a coulometric detector. Several mobile phases were used.

In selected experiments, 1.5 ml of HPLC eluate, manually collected at the retention time of the oxindole peak, was dried down and a portion of it was injected into a Saturn 4D GC/MS quadrupole ion trap. The system is capable of time-programmable isolation of selected parent ions followed by collision-induced dissociation (CID) of specific product ions. Saturn version 5.2 software was used for data acquisition and Toolkit software was used for the application of multiple scan functions in a given chromatographic run (MS/MS and MS/MS/MS experiments). The gas chromatograph was a Varian Star 3400 CX equipped with a temperature programmable injector which permits large volume injection.

The first identification of oxindole was performed by comparing the retention times of the standard with those of one of the peaks present when purified homogenates of mammalian organs were injected into the HPLC. The U.V. absorbance at 255 nm was recorded. As shown in the figure, such retention times were identical and this occurred no matter of the mobile phase used. Spiking experiments were performed using different mobile phases and confirmed that the peak present in the homogenates and that of the standard had identical retention times. In most of our determinations, we used U.V. detection since the method is simpler yet has sufficient sensitivity for determining oxindole content in a single rat brain. Figure 2 shows the HPLC chromatographic pattern obtained when standards or brain samples were injected. When the collected HPLC eluate fractions from rat brain homogenates were dried, resuspended in acetonitrile and injected into the GC/MS, presence of the oxindole peak was definitively confirmed. Figure 3 (top) reports the proposed fragmentation pattern of authentic oxindole and Figure 3A shows the total ion chromatogram (TIC) and the extracted ion chromatogram of m/z 133 obtained from rat brain homogenates: a peak at the same gas-chromatographic retention time of authentic oxindole was recorded on m/z 133 trace. The corresponding EI mass spectrum (Figure 3B) was identical to that of oxindole. It is interesting to note the reduction in chemical noise due to the matrix used under different analytical conditions. While a peak at the retention time of oxindole is not clearly evident, in the TIC trace of the full scan MS acquisition, in MS/MS acquisition mode (figure 3C) and in the MS/MS/MS acquisition mode (Figure 3E), a distinct

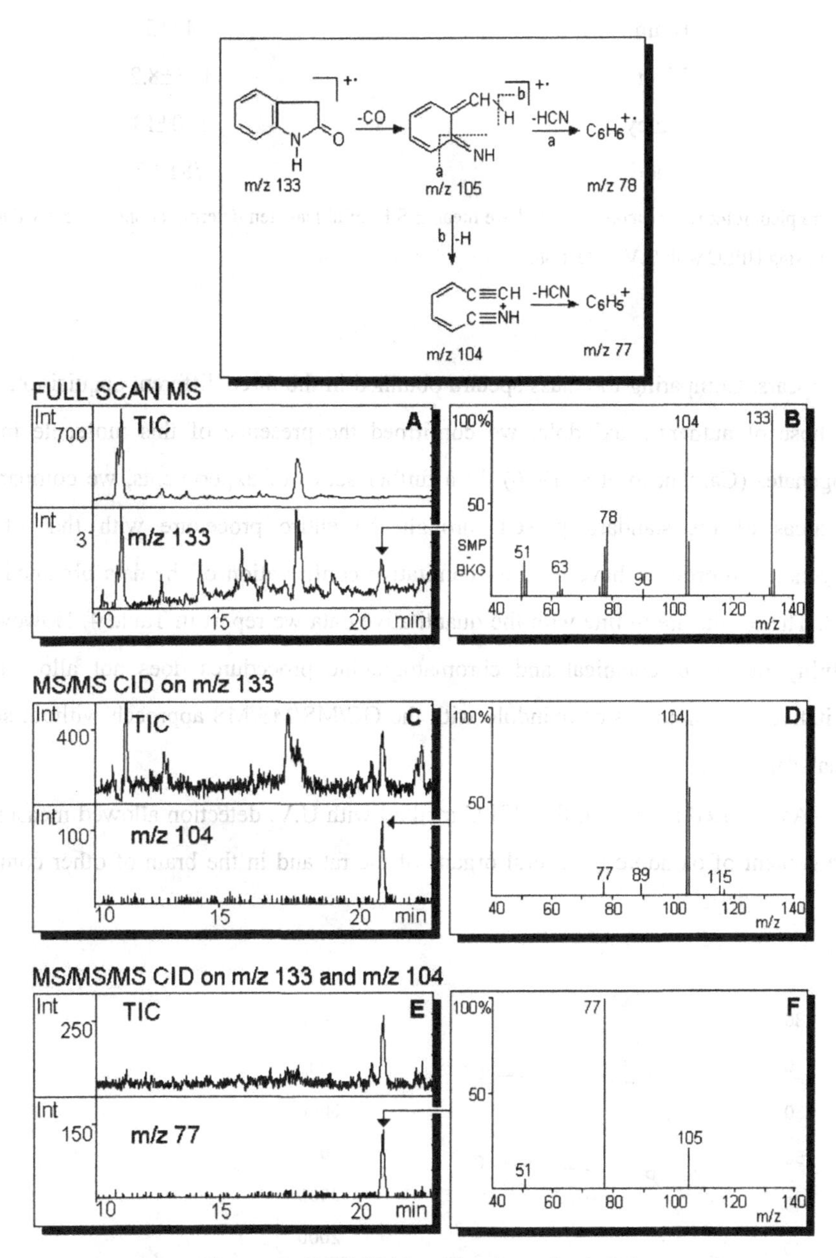

Figure 3. GC/MS identification of oxindole

The proposed fragmentation pattern of authentic oxindole (top). Figure 3A, 3C and 3E report the total ion chromatograms (above tracing) and the extracted ion chromatograms (bottom tracing) obtained by injecting the biological sample (extracted and purified as described in the text) into a Saturn 4D quadrupole ion trap and recording the results obtained using GC/MS, GC/MS/MS and GC/MS/MS/MS modes respectively. B, D and F are the mass spectra corresponding to the peaks indicated by the arrows and are identical to the peaks obtained by injecting authentic oxindole.

Table 4. Oxindole content in rat tissues

Brain	42±5
Liver	113±8.2
Kidney	110±13
Blood	78±8.7

Values are picomol/g wt or picomol/ml and are mean ± S.E. of at least ten determinations. These values were obtained using HPLC with U.V. detection.

peak appears. Comparing the mass spectra obtained in the three different acquisition modes with those of authentic oxindole, we confirmed the presence of this molecule in brain homogenates (Carpenedo et al 1996). In a further series of experiments, we compared the peak areas of the standard passed through the entire procedure with that of brain homogenates in order to have a semi-quantitative confirmation of the data obtained in the HPLC. The results are in line with the quantitative data we report in Table 4. However, the variability of the biochemical and chromatographic procedures does not allow precise quantitative measurements of oxindole with the GC/MS/MS/MS approach without suitable internal standards.

As reported in table 4, the HPLC method with U.V. detection allowed measurement of the content of oxindole in several organs of the rat and in the brain of other commonly

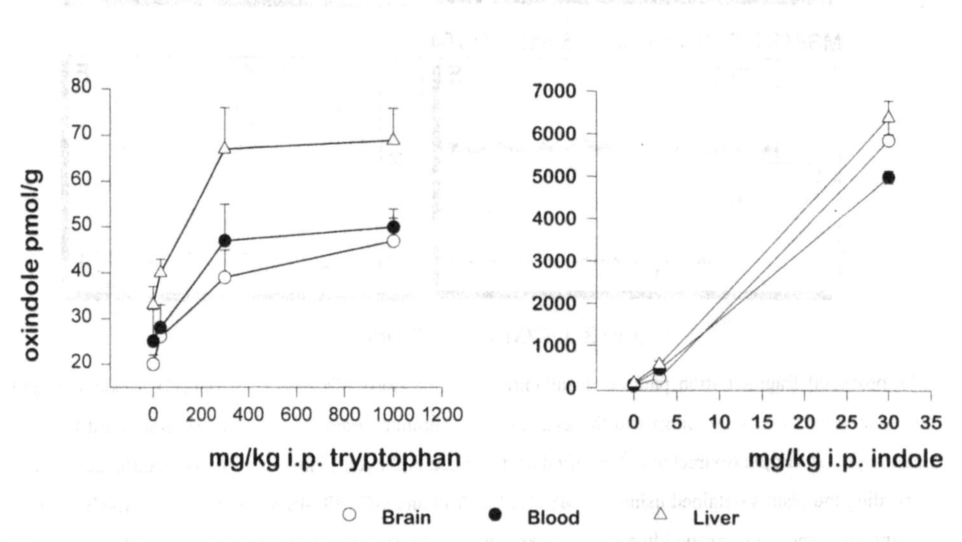

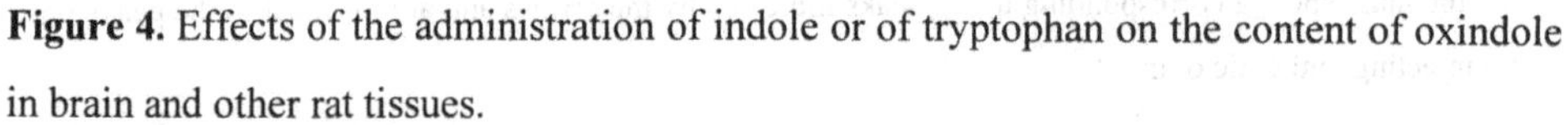

Figure 4. Effects of the administration of indole or of tryptophan on the content of oxindole in brain and other rat tissues.

Each point is the mean ± S.E. of at least 6 animals per group.

used laboratory animals. In the rat brain the concentration of oxindole was similar to that in blood, while larger concentrations were found in the liver and kidney. The brain of mice contained relatively elevated concentrations of oxindole (90±8 picomol/g), while guinea pigs had brain oxindole concentrations (4.4±1.1) one order of magnitude lower than those of the rats. When tryptophan was administered to rats, a dose dependent increase of oxindole was found in the liver, blood or brain, thus confirming that the amino acid may be the precursor of oxindole (see figure 4). Figure 4 also reports that systemic administration of indole causes a much larger increase of oxindole in various organs, supporting the possibility that most of oxindole formation occurs through indole oxidation.

MECHANISMS OF THE PHARMACOLOGICAL ACTIONS OF OXINDOLE AND OF 5-HYDROXYINDOLE

As previously mentioned, the administration of oxindole (20-200 mg/kg) to rats or mice caused a profound reversible coma, while similar doses of 5-hydroxyindole caused convulsions and death. In order to clarify the mechanism of action of these indoles, we tested them in binding studies and in simple electrophysiological paradigms. Binding experiments were performed in order to evaluate possible interactions of oxindole with GABAa, GABAb, BDZ, or strychnine binding sites. Unfortunately, as reported in table 5 the results were negative.

Table 5. Lack of effects of oxindole on the binding of different ligands

	$[^3H]$ GABA		$[^3H]$ Strychnine	$[^3H]$ Flunitrazepam
	GABAa	GABAb		
Oxindole (100 μM)	100±2	97±5	87±4	98±4
Diazepam (10 μM)	110±7	---	75±6	0
GABA (100 μM)	0	0	91±5	145±12

Values are mean percentage ± S.E.. Binding conditions: 1) GABAa binding was performed by utilizing whole brain membranes, 3nM of the ligand and 100 μM of GABA in order to evaluate the non-specific binding; GABAb binding: whole brain membranes, 5 nM of the ligand, 40μM of isoguvacine and 100 μM baclofen for non-specific binding; 2) $[^3H]$Strychnine (2nM), spinal cord membranes and 1 mM of glycine; 3) $[^3H]$flunitrazepam 1nM, cortical membranes and diazepam (10μM).

Other experiments were performed in order to study oxindole action on glutamate receptors of AMPA and NMDA types. Cortical wedges were prepared as previously described (Mannaioni et al. 1994; Lombardi et al. 1994) and superfused with oxindole concentrations of up to 300 μM. Oxindole did not change depolarization caused by AMPA or NMDA, suggesting that ionotropic glutamate receptors are not involved in the oxindole neurodepressant action. Similar results were also obtained in a different electrophysiological set-up: in *in vitro* hippocampal slices. In this model, test pulses (80-110 μs duration; 0.017-0.05 Hz) were delivered through bipolar nichrome electrodes positioned in the CA1 stratum radiatum. Evoked extracellular potentials were recorded with glass microelectrodes (2-10 M Ω) filled with 3 M NaCl and placed in the pyramidal cell layer of the CA1 area. Stimulus/response curves were constructed at the beginning of each experiment by gradually increasing the stimulus strength. The test stimulus pulse was then adjusted to produce a population spike at an amplitude of 50 % of the maximum and, unless otherwise stated, was kept constant throughout the experiment. Population spikes and excitatory post-synaptic potentials were then measured as the peak-to-peak amplitude of the first negative phase of the response. No changes in the population spikes or excitatory post synaptic potentials were found in this preparation during the application of oxindole (30-300 μM). On the contrary, as reported in Figure 5, 5-OH-indole significantly increased the population spike amplitude. The dentritic potentials were also increased and this effect was easily reversible upon washing the preparations.

These experiments suggest that 5-hydroxyindole improves synaptic transmission in the CA1 area, possibly explaining the convulsant action of the molecule. The superfusion of the preparation with $5HT_3$ antagonists did not change the potentiation of the synaptic responses described above, thus ruling out the involvement of $5HT_3$ receptors in the electrophysiological effects of 5OH indole in the CA1 area. Experiments are currently in progress in order to better understand the basic mechanism of this interesting modulation of synaptic activity.

CHANGES OF BRAIN OXINDOLE CONTENT IN FULMINANT HEPATIC FAILURE

It is widely accepted that gut derived compounds are largely responsible for the neurological symptoms present in the course of liver diseases (Jones et al. 1984; Fraser and Arieff, 1985; Jones et al. 1993). Among gut originated, neurologically active compounds, particular attention has been devoted to ammonia, mercaptans, GABA, octopamine or other

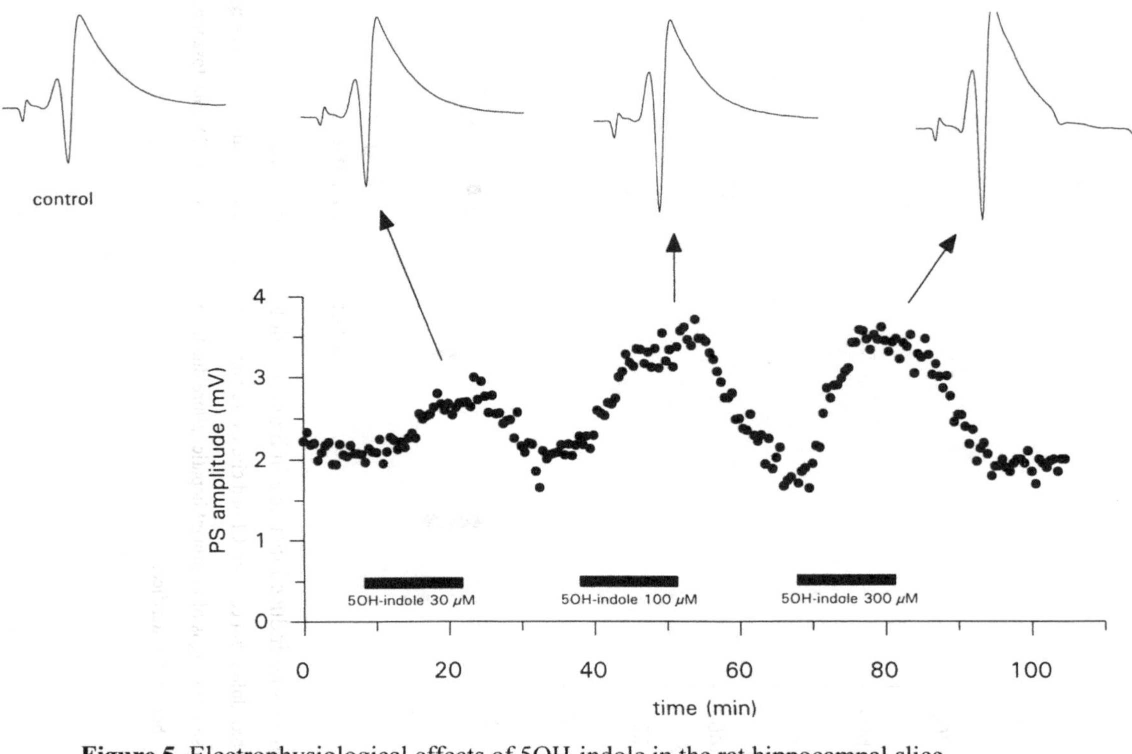

Figure 5. Electrophysiological effects of 5OH-indole in the rat hippocampal slice.

Dose dependent effects of 5-OH indole (5 OH) in the rat CA1 region. The upper portion of the figure reports examples of population spikes under control conditions, and after perfusion with 5-OH indole at the reported micromolar concentrations (bottom). PS is population spike.

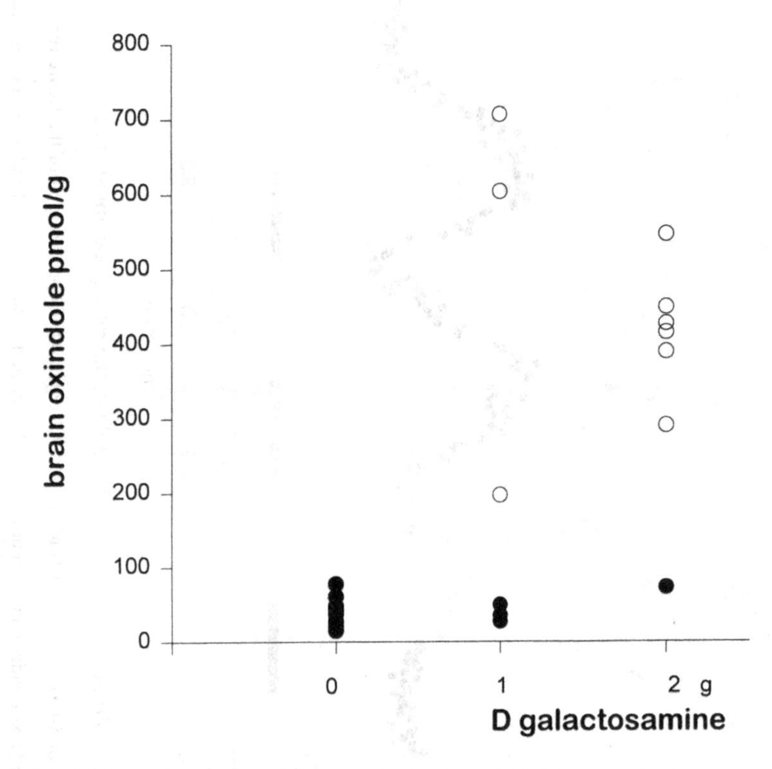

Figure 6. D-galactosamine-induced increase in brain oxindole concentrations

Each point represents oxindole brain content. Closed circles are animals without signs of neurological damage. Empty circles are rats showing signs of fulminant hepatic failure due to the reported dose of D-galactosamine administered 48-60 hrs before the sacrifice.

amines. Blood accumulation of such molecules may affect central nervous system function. However, GABA does not increase in plasma or CSF of hepatic coma patients (Moroni et al. 1987), amines do not easily cross the blood brain barriers, mercaptans do not lead to coma and ammonia administration causes convulsions and death, but not a reversible coma. In the last few years, other substances have been added to the list of compounds possibly responsible for the neurological symptoms of hepatic encephalopathy. Several laboratories focused their attention on endogenous benzodiazepine receptor ligands (endozapines) (Olasmaa et al. 1989; Basile et al. 1990). It is now accepted that the concentrations of compounds able to displace [^{3}H]diazepam binding from the benzodiazepine receptors increase in the blood or brain of experimental models of hepatic encephalopathy, and administration of benzodiazepine receptor antagonists reduces the neurological symptoms in selected patients in hepatic coma (Basile et al. 1991).

We now report that the administration of low doses of oxindole to rats causes loss of the righting reflex, hypotension, reflex modifications and a reversible coma with features commonly observed in patients affected by hepatic encephalopathy. We therefore measured oxindole content in the blood and brain of galactosamine treated rats, one of the available models of FHF (Zeneroli et al. 1982). Figure 6 reports that the brain concentrations of oxindole increased by 10-20 fold in animals having neurological symptoms of hepatic encephalopathy.

It is reasonable to assume that at least one step of oxindole synthesis requires the function of an enzymatic activity (tryptophanase) which is particularly abundant in bacteria; therefore, gut flora may be important in the accumulation of blood and brain oxindole. Tryptophan could be metabolized into indole by bacterial enzymes. It is then absorbed and metabolized into oxindole in the brain or in other peripheral tissues. Under basal conditions, oxindole may be further metabolized (into 5 OH oxindole which may be then conjugated with glucuronic acid or with sulphate) and excreted, but when liver function is impaired, its accumulation in blood and brain may be partially responsible for CNS depression.

CONCLUSIONS

Hepatic encephalopathy is associated with a 10-20 fold increase in the brain concentration of oxindole (see figure 5), a neurodepressant agent. It is reasonable to propose that this compound originates from tryptophan metabolism and that one of the enzymes leading to its formation is tryptophanase, which is particularly abundant in bacteria. This enzyme leads to the production of indole which is then absorbed from the gut and probably metabolized in the liver. Under physiological conditions, the amount of oxindole or of 5-hydroxyindole present in the blood or brain is quite low (10^{-7} M). When liver function is impaired, sufficient concentration of indole may reach systemic circulation and may be oxidized into both oxindole or 5-hydroxyindole in several tissues. An elevated concentration of oxindole in CNS causes a profound neurodepressant syndrome or coma. Elevated concentrations of the convulsant agent 5-hydroxyindole may also participate in altered CNS function of patients affected by FHF. The basic mechanism of the sedative oxindole action is still unknown. Similarly, the convulsant action of 5-hydroxyindole has not yet been described and is due to a still unknown interaction with brain functions. We ruled out effects of these molecules on ionotropic glutamate receptors of AMPA and NMDA types, and we are currently evaluating oxindole and 5-hydroxyindole interaction with other receptor types or ion channels. Oxindole does not displace labeled GABA from its GABAa or GABAb receptors or labeled flunitrazepam from the BDZ binding sites; therefore, we assume that these sites are not involved in its mechanism of action. However, the GABA receptor complex may certainly have other recognition sites that could be affected by the two indole metabolites we have identified in mammalian tissues. The experiments on the anticonvulsant actions of oxindole seems to point to the GABA receptors as the site of its pharmacological effects.

In conclusion, oxindole should be considered one of the main components of the already long list of molecules whose accumulation is responsible for the neurological symptoms observed when the liver function is impaired.

REFERENCES

Basile, A.S., L. Panell, T. Jaouni, S.H. Gammal, H. Fales, E.A. Jones and P. Skolnick, 1990, Brain concentration of benzodiazepines are elevated in an animal model of hepatic encephalopathy, *Proc. Natl. Acad. Sci. USA* 97, 5263.

Basile, A.S., K. Saito, H. Li and M.P. Heyes, 1995, The relationship between plasma and brain quinolinic acid levels and the severity of hepatic encephalopathy in animal models of fulminant hepatic failure, *J. Neurochem.* 64, 2607.

Basile, A.S., E.A. Jones and P. Skolnick, 1991, The pathogenesis and treatment of hepatic encephalopathy: evidence for the involvement of benzodiazepine receptor ligands, *Pharmacol. Rev.* 42, 27.

Bergquist, P.B.F., M.P. Heyes, M. Bugge and F. Bengtsson, 1995, Brain quinolinic acid in chronic hepatic encephalopathy, *J. Neurochem.* 65, 2235.

Carpenedo, R., A. Chiarugi, P. Russi, G. Lombardi, V. Carlà, R. Pellicciari, L. Mattoli and F. Moroni, 1994, Inhibitors of kynurenine hydroxylase and kynureninase increase cerebral formation of kynurenic acid and have sedative and anticonvulsant activities, *Neuroscience* 61, 237.

Chiarugi, A., R. Carpenedo, M.T. Molina, L. Mattoli, R. Pellicciari and F. Moroni, 1995, Comparison of the neurochemical and behavioral effects resulting from the inhibition of kynurenine hydroxylase and/or kynureninase. *J. Neurochem.* 65, 1176-1183.

Chiarugi, A., R. Carpenedo and F. Moroni, 1996, Kynurenine disposition in blood and brain of mice: effects of selective inhibitors of kynurenine hydroxylase and of kynureninase, *J. Neurochem.* 67, 692.

Cummings, M.G., H.J. James and P.B. Soeters, 1976, Regional brain studies of indoleamine metabolism in the rat in acute hepatic failure, *J. Neurochem.* 27, 741.

Curzon, G., B.D. Kantamaneni, J. Winch, A. Rojas-Bueno, I.M. Murray-Lyon and R. Williams, 1973, Plasma and brain tryptophan changes in experimental acute hepatic failure, *J. Neurochem.* 21, 137.

Fraser, C.L. and A.I. Arieff, 1985, Hepatic encephalopathy, *N. Engl. J. Med.* 313, 865.

Hirayama, C. 1971, Tryptophan metabolism in liver disease, *Clin. Chim. Acta* 32, 191.

Jones, E.A., D.E. Shafer, P. Ferenci and S.C. Pappas, 1984, The neurobiology of hepatic encephalopathy, *Hepatology* 4, 1235.

Jones, E.A., C. Yurdaydin, A.S. Basile, J.E. Maddison, W.E. Watson, G.A. Johnston, C.H. Dejong, N.E. Deutz, P.B. Soeters, V. Felipo, E. Grau, M.D. Minana, S. Grisolia, K.D. Mullen, Z.Q. Gu, G. Nowak, C. Fromm, A.G. Holt, D.B. Jones, A. Puspok, A. Herneth, P. Steindl, P. Ferenci, S. Sarhan, B. Knodgen, C. Grauffel, N. Seiler and S. Sherlock, 1993, The GABA hypothesis--state of the art Glutamatergic neurotransmission in hepatic encephalopathy, *Adv. Intern. Med.* 38, 245.

King, L.J., D.V. Parke and R.T. Williams, 1966, The metabolism of [2-^{14}C]indole in the rat, *Biochem. J.* 98, 266.

Kooyman, R.A., J.A. van Hooft, P.M.L. Vanderheijden and H.P.M. Vijverberg, 1994, Competitive and non-competitive effects of 5-hydroxyndole on $5HT_3$ receptors in N1E-115 neurpblastoma cells, *Br. J. Pharmacol.* 112, 541.

Kooyman, R.A., J.A. van Hooft and H.P.M. Vijverberg, 1993, 5-Hydroxyindole slows desensitization of the 5HT3 receptor-mediated ion current in N1E-115 neuroblastoma cells, *Br. J. Pharmacol.* 108, 287.

Lombardi, G., G. Mannaioni, P. Leonardi, G. Cherici, V. Carlà and F. Moroni, 1994, Ammonium acetate inhibits ionotropic receptors and differentially affects metabotropic receptors for glutamate, *J. Neural Transm.* 97, 187.

Mannaioni, G., M. Alesiani, V. Carlà, B. Natalini, M. Marinozzi, R. Pellicciari and F. Moroni, 1994, Sulfate esters of hydroxy amino acids as stereospecific glutamate receptor agonists, *Eur. J. Pharmacol.* 251, 201.

Moroni, F., G. Lombardi, V. Carlà and G. Moneti, 1984, The excitotoxin quinolinic acid is present and unevenly distributed in the rat brain, *Brain Res.* 295, 352.

Moroni, F., G. Lombardi, V. Carlà, S. Lal, P.E. Etienne and N.P.V. Nair, 1986a, Increase in the content of quinolinic acid in cerebrospinal fluid and frontal cortex of patients with hepatic failure, *J. Neurochem.* 47, 1667.

Moroni, F., G. Lombardi, V. Carlà, D. Pellegrini, G.L. Carassale and C. Cortesini, 1986b, Content of quinolinic acid and of other tryptophan metabolites increases in brain regions of rats used as experimental models of hepatic encephalopathy, *J. Neurochem.* 46, 869.

Moroni, F., O. Riggio, V. Carlà, V. Festuccia, F. Ghinelli, I.R. Marino, M. Merli, L. Natali, G. Pedretti, F. Fiaccadori and L. Capocaccia, 1987, Hepatic Encephalopathy:lack of changes of GABA content in plasma and cerebrospinal fluid, *Hepatology* 7, 816.

Moroni, F., P. Russi, G. Lombardi, M. Beni and V. Carlà, 1988, Presence of kynurenic acid in the mammalian brain, *J. Neurochem.* 51, 177.

Moroni, F., P. Russi, M.A. Gallo-Mezo, G. Moneti and R. Pellicciari, 1991, Modulation of quinolinic and kynurenic acid content in the rat brain: effects of endotoxins and nicotinylalanine, *J. Neurochem.* 57, 1630.

Olasmaa, M., A. Guidotti, E. Costa, J.D. Rothstein, M.E.. Goldman, R.J. Weber and S.M. Paul, 1989, Endogenous benzodiazepines in hepatic encephalopathy, *Lancet* 1, 491.

Ono, J., D.G. Huston, R.S. Dombro, U.E. Levi, A. Livingstone and R. Zeppa, 1996, Tryptophan and hepatic coma, *Gastroenterology* 74, 196.

Orcutt, J.A., J.P. Prytherch, M. Konicov and S.M. Michaelson, 1964, Some new compounds exhibiting selective CNS-depressant activities. Part1, Preliminary observations, *Arch. Int. Pharmacodyn. 152*, 121.

Rossi-Fanelli, F., H. Freund, R. Krause, A.R. Smith, H. James, S. Castorina-Ziparo and J.E. Fischer, 1982, Induction of coma in normal dogs by infusion of aromatic amino acids and its prevention by the addition of branched chain amino acids, *Gastroenterology* 83, 664.

Sherlock, S. 1975, *Diseases of the liver and biliary system* (Blackwell, Oxford)
Sourkes, T.L. 1978, Tryptophan in hepatic coma, *J. Neural Transm.* S14, 79.
Stone, T.W. 1993, Neuropharmacology of quinolinic and kynurenic acids. *Pharmacol. Rev.* 45, 309.
Van Pée, K.H. and F. Lingens, 1984, Metabolism of tryptophan in pseudomonas aureofaciens, in: *Progress in tryptophan and serotonin research*, eds. H.G. Schlossberger, W. Kochen, B. Linzen and H. Steinhart (de Gruyter,W. Berlin) p. 753.
Zeneroli, M.D., E. Iuliano, G. Racagni and M. Baraldi, 1982, Metabolism and brain uptake of GABA in galactosamine induced hepatic encephalopathy in rats, *J. Neurochem.* 38, 1219.

THE INVOLVEMENT OF AMMONIA WITH THE MECHANISMS THAT ENHANCE GABA-ERGIC NEUROTRANSMISSION IN HEPATIC FAILURE

E. Anthony Jones[1] and Anthony S. Basile[2]

[1]Department of Gastrointestinal and Liver Diseases, Academic Medical Center, Amsterdam, The Netherlands
[2]Laboratory of Neuroscience, NIDDK, National Institutes of Health Bethesda, MD 20892

INTRODUCTION

There are currently two primary hypotheses regarding the pathogenic mechanisms contributing to the development of hepatic encephalopathy (HE). Ammonia has been implicated in the pathogenesis of the encephalopathies associated with hepatic failure since the 1950's[1]. While challenged by other hypotheses over time, the ammonia hypothesis of the pathogenesis of HE has remained dominant. The other main hypothesis postulates a role for increased GABAergic neurotransmission in the development of HE, a concept supported by a large body of evidence that has been accumulating since 1980[2]. Over the years, these hypotheses have had a uneasy, and apparently mutually exclusive relationship. However, recently reported information now makes it appear possible that both elevated levels of ammonia and increased GABAergic neurotransmission are involved in the pathogenesis of HE[3,4]. Thus, it now appears that these two hypotheses are not mutually incompatible, but essential for the development of the encephalopathy. Furthermore, the new findings suggest a concept that unifies both hypotheses.

THE AMMONIA HYPOTHESIS

Originally, there were three components to the ammonia hypothesis. First, elevated plasma levels of ammonia occur in liver failure. Studies of cirrhotics ingesting ammoniagenic compounds, such as amino acids, urea, and ammonia releasing resins[1], suggested that ammonia accumulation and HE are associated. Encephalopathies develop in parallel with hyperammonemia in congenital defects of urea cycle enzymes and valproate hepatotoxicity[5,6]. However, the plasma ammonia concentrations that occur in these syndromes are higher than those usually associated with acute or chronic liver failure. In addition, CSF levels of the ammonia metabolites glutamine and α-ketoglutaramate correlate well with the clinical severity of HE[7,8]. Moreover, therapies which decrease intestinal ammonia absorption are often followed (after several hours) by an amelioration of HE in patients with cirrhosis[9].

Nonetheless, plasma ammonia levels do not correlate well with the occurrence or severity of HE[10]. A variety of factors may contribute to this variability, including ammonia production by contracting muscle, differential ammonia tolerance, altered ammonia compartmentation resulting from pH and electrolyte imbalances, and technical problems associated with taking proper blood samples[11]. Indeed, plasma ammonia levels may be normal in liver failure in the presence of elevated CNS levels of ammonia[12]. Finally, hemodialysis of patients in hepatic coma due to acute or chronic liver failure improves neurological function in less than 50% of the patients[13].

Secondly, ammonia can readily enter the brain. Early studies of the difference in arterio-venous concentrations of ammonia across the brain suggested that there was no ammonia uptake, possibly due to the inability of the ammonium ion to cross the blood-brain barrier[14]. Subsequent investigations where the pH of the ammonia probe was carefully maintained[15] indicated that ammonia entered the CNS primarily in its gaseous (non-ionized) form[16,17]. In the CNS, ammonia is fixed by conversion to glutamine by astrocytic glutamine synthetase, with a concomitant reduction in brain levels of the primary substrate of glutamine synthetase, glutamate[18]. This may result in altered glutamatergic neurotransmission, which is presently a field of intense study[19].

Finally, a major component of the ammonia hypothesis is based on unequivocal evidence that ammonia is neurotoxic[20]. A well known manifestation of this toxicity is the ability of ammonia to induce seizures. In congenital hyperammonemias, plasma ammonia concentrations are typically in the range of 0.5-2 mM, and the associated behavioral changes can be classified as a preconvulsive state, or seizures. In contrast, plasma ammonia concentrations are usually in the range of 0.1-0.4 mM in HE, and the associated behavioral changes are consistent with a global increase in neuronal inhibition. Insights into the role that ammonia plays in these two behavioral syndromes may be gained by considering the electrophysiological effects induced by different concentrations of ammonia. At concentrations of 4-8 mM, ammonia inhibits EPSP formation and axonal conductance through a depolarization block[21]. However, these concentrations of ammonia are so high that they are pathophysiologically irrelevant. At the sort of concentrations (0.5-3 mM) that occur in congenital hyperammonemias, ammonia inactivates Cl^- extrusion pumps[22]. The resulting elevation of intracellular Cl^- concentration blocks the formation of the hyperpolarizing inhibitory post-synaptic potential (IPSP), impairing postsynaptic inhibitory processes throughout the brain[21,23]. Ultimately, the resting membrane potential increases, depolarizing neurons, and transiently inducing excitatory phenomena such as seizures. This behavioral effect not only contrasts with the manifestations of HE, but with the lethargy and EEG slowing induced by the acute administration of ammonia, which, if the infusion is continued, is followed by seizures and post-ictal coma[24]. Furthermore, cats with portacaval shunts appear to have normal IPSPs, despite chronically elevated plasma ammonia concentrations[21]. This observation has been attributed to the development of Cl^- pump tolerance to the persistently increased levels of ammonia[21]. However, a change in Cl^- pump activity has never been confirmed by direct measurement, and the CNS becomes more sensitive to when exposed to acute ammonia rechallenges[21]. These observations argue against the development of neuronal Cl^- pumps tolerance under conditions of chronic ammonia excess. While seizures are common in congenital hyperammonemia syndromes[25], they are unusual in HE associated with chronic liver failure. Thus, currently available data do not adequately explain why the initial failure of IPSP formation following ammonia administration causes lethargy, rather than seizures. Furthermore, there is a paucity of information on the neuroelectrophysiological effects of ammonia at the concentrations commonly observed in HE (0.1-0.4 mM), and whether they can <u>enhance</u> inhibitory neurotransmission

In summary, the above evidence indicates that ammonia is a key factor in the pathogenesis of HE. A significant body of information indicates that brain and plasma

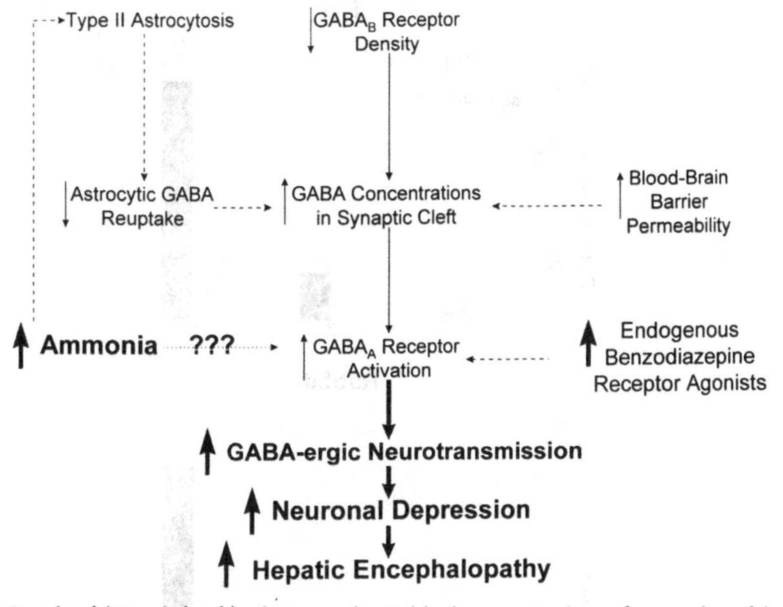

Figure 1. Postulated interrelationships between elevated brain concentrations of ammonia and increased GABAergic neurotransmission in the pathogenesis of HE. GABAergic neurotransmission may be enhanced by the presence of endogenous BZ receptor agonists, the increased availability of GABA in synaptic clefts due to ammonia-induced abnormalities in glial function, leading to decreased glial GABA reuptake, loss of presynaptic feedback inhibition of GABA release due to a decrease in $GABA_B$ receptors, and/or increased blood-to-brain transfer of GABA. Recent investigations also suggest that ammonia directly enhances GABAergic neurotransmission.

ammonia levels are elevated in liver failure, and that ammonia can modulate neuronal function. However, evidence that hyperammonemia is solely responsible for the development of HE is lacking. Moreover, the precise nature of the relationship between elevated brain levels of ammonia and HE remains unclear, as are the mechanisms by which ammonia can contribute to HE. The primary discrepancy is that the clinical features of HE (impaired motor function and decreased consciousness) appear to be most consistent with a global increase in inhibitory neurotransmission rather than a net increase in excitatory neurotransmission.

THE GABAERGIC NEUROTRANSMISSION HYPOTHESIS

In order to address whether ammonia can alter inhibitory neurotransmission, thereby contributing to the manifestations of HE, it is necessary to consider the GABAergic neurotransmission hypothesis. This is necessary because GABA is the principal inhibitory neurotransmitter of the mammalian brain and increased GABA-mediated neurotransmission impairs motor function and decreases consciousness, two of the cardinal clinical features of HE. That an increase in GABAergic tone associated with hepatic failure contributes to HE is supported by at least four lines of evidence (Figure 1), most of which occur independent of the presence of ammonia .

Elevated levels of benzodiazepine (BZ) receptor agonists are one mechanism by which GABAergic neurotransmission is increased in hepatic failure. The concentrations of BZ receptor ligands with agonist properties are elevated in the brain, plasma and cerebrospinal fluid of several animal models of HE due to fulminant hepatic failure (the thioacetamide-

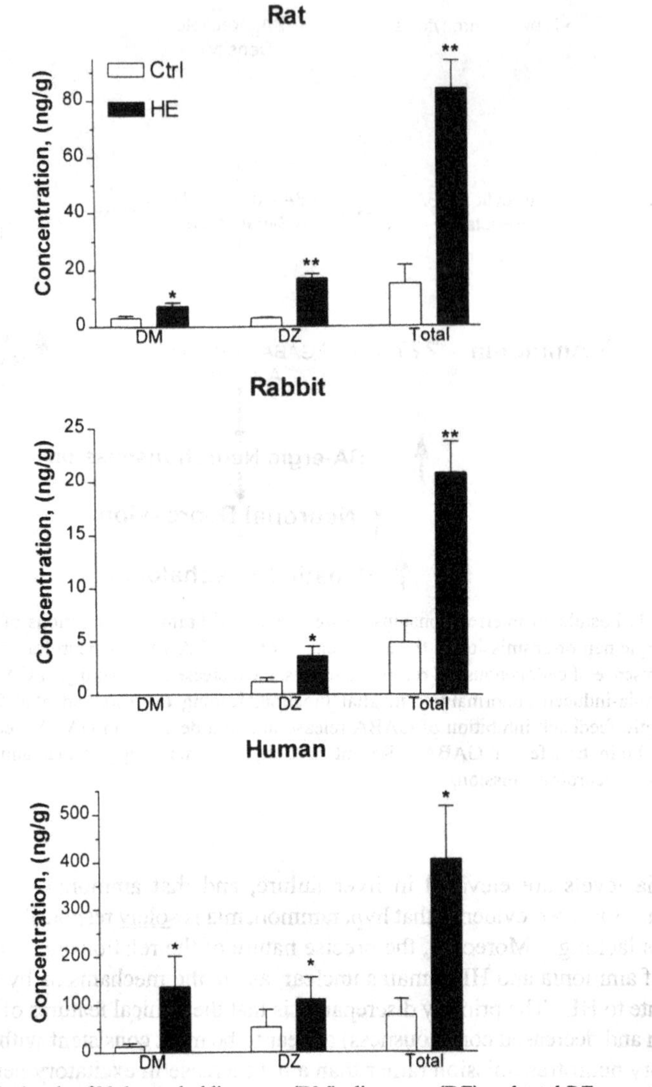

Figure 2. Summary of the levels of N-desmethyldiazepam (DM), diazepam (DZ) and total BZ receptor ligand activity in the brains of rats, rabbits, and humans with fulminant hepatic failure. Concentrations are in absolute ng/g tissue wet weight for DM and DZ (determined by mass spectroscopy), and in ng/g of DZ equivalents for total BZ receptor ligand activity (determined radiometrically). BZ levels in HE were significantly greater than control values (animal models: * = $p<0.05$; ** = $p<0.01$ Students t-test; humans * = $p<0.05$, Mann-Whitney U test).

treated rat, and galactosamine-treated rat and rabbit)[26] (Figure 2). Similarly, elevated levels of BZ receptor ligands have been found in human plasma and brain[26,27]. These ligands have the pharmacological properties of agonists at the BZ receptor, and some have been identified as the 1,4 substituted benzodiazepines N-desmethyldiazepam and diazepam, although the identity of the bulk of these agents remains unknown[26,27]. Moreover, there is some evidence that these ligands arise from gut flora[28]. The concentrations of the BZ receptor agonists are such that approximately 20% of the BZ receptors are occupied in the rabbit with galactosamine-induced fulminant hepatic failure. That degree of receptor occupancy is sufficient to protect against grand-mal seizures[26]. Indeed, in rats with thioacetamide-induced

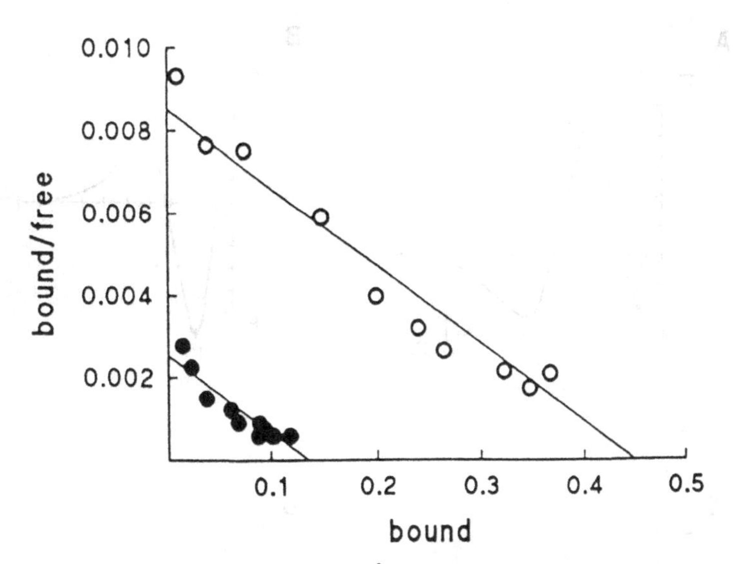

Figure 3. Scatchard plots illustrating the binding of [^{3}H]GABA to $GABA_B$ receptors in cerebral cortical membranes from control rats (○) and rats with acute HE due to thioacetamide-induced fulminant hepatic failure (●). From reference 32, by permission.

fulminant hepatic failure, there is a substantial decrease in the seizure threshold to convulsants such as 3-mercaptoproprionic acid[29]. Moreover, the motor deficits associated with hepatic failure in thioacetamide-treated rats are ameliorated by the administration of BZ antagonists at doses that have no effect on the motor activity of normal rats[26]. Additional evidence that BZ receptor agonists contribute to the pathogenesis of HE by increasing GABAergic neurotransmission is provided by the ability of BZ receptor antagonists to rapidly (<15 min) improve HE in 40-60% of the humans with this syndrome[26,30,31].

Another mechanism by which GABAergic neurotransmission can be increased in hepatic failure would be an increase in the amount of GABA in the synaptic cleft. This may occur due to increased neuronal GABA release. Many GABAergic synapses regulate neurotransmitter release by negative feedback involving presynaptic "autoreceptors". Neurotransmitter (GABA) is released from the presynaptic bouton to the extent that it may flow out of the immediate environs of the synaptic cleft. At this time, the neurotransmitter will encounter GABA receptors on the outer sides of the presynaptic terminal and bind to them. Activation of these receptors results in the suppression of further neurotransmitter release. A recent study of radioligand binding to the $GABA_B$ receptors in the cerebral cortex of rats with TAA-induced fulminant hepatic failure indicates that the density of $GABA_B$ receptors was decreased to 30% of normal in the model (Figure 3) by unknown mechanisms[32]. These receptors are known to presynaptically modulate the release of a number of neurotransmitters, including glutamate and GABA. Thus, the levels of GABA in the synaptic environment may be increased as a result of increased synaptic release.

Free GABA levels in the extracellular fluid of the CNS can also be increased by transfer across a leaky blood-brain barrier[33]. There is evidence for increased GABA concentrations of gut origin in the plasma of some patients with hepatic failure[34]. In order to determine if this material could enter the CNS in hepatic failure, the brain uptake index of GABA in a rabbit model of fulminant hepatic failure was measured . The data were corrected for the rapid metabolism of the tracer and slow brain washout and recirculation . The brain uptake index for GABA was higher in animals with stage II or III HE than in controls, and was significantly higher in stage III than stage II HE. Thus, with the progression of <u>acute</u> liver

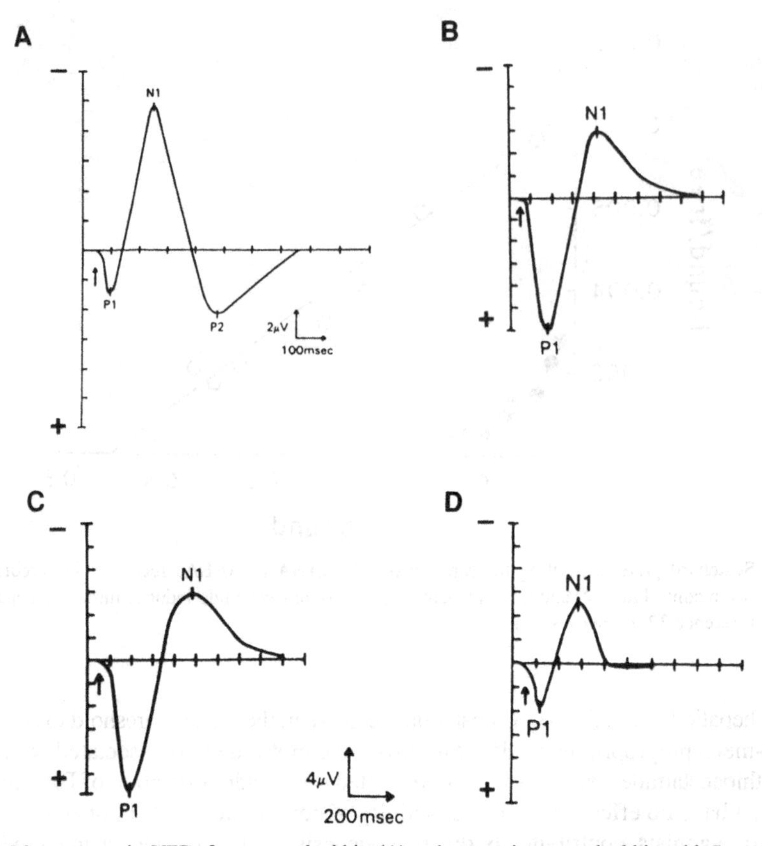

Figure 4. Mean composite VERs from normal rabbits (A), galactosamine-treated rabbits with Stage IV HE (B), normal rabbits administered pentobarbital © or ammonium chloride (D). Note the similarity in VER patterns of the rabbit with HE and the pentobarbital treated rabbit, with a significant increase in P_1 amplitude and loss of the P_2 component. Ammonia had no effect on P_1 amplitude. 4 μV voltage calibration applies to panels B-C., 2 μV calibration to panel A only. From references 28,39, by permission.

failure in the model studied, there was an increased transfer of GABA from plasma to brain extracellular fluid.

In contrast to the above mechanisms for increasing the levels of GABA, there is some evidence that ammonia may be involved in a fourth mechanism for enhancing GABAergic neurotransmission. Ammonia is known to impair astrocytic function, leading to the development of type II astrocytes[35]. There is evidence that GABA uptake by cultured astrocytes decreased 26% following exposure to 2 or 10 mM ammonia concentrations for 4 days[36]. Furthermore, a microdialysis study indicates that GABA release is either increased, or its reuptake is decreased in portacaval shunted rats[37]. Following neuronal activation by the infusion of KCl through the microdialysis probe, GABA levels increased in the shunted animals to 2 fold above control levels. This phenomenon may be attributable to the higher concentrations of ammonia observed in the portacaval-shunted animals. While this mechanism provides an indirect way by which ammonia can increase GABAergic neurotransmission, the question arises whether ammonia, at pathophysiologically relevant concentrations, can be implicated in mechanisms responsible for directly increasing GABAergic neurotransmission?

During the 1980's, attempts were made to determine whether the altered neuroelectrophysiology associated with HE was similar to that induced by ammonia. This was done by comparing the patterns of visual evoked responses (VER) recorded from either rats or rabbits with HE due to hepatotoxin-induced fulminant hepatic failure with corresponding patterns in control animals with normal livers that had been rendered hyperammonemic or had been treated with GABAergic agents[24,38,39]. These studies indicated that the abnormal VER patterns recorded from animals in stage IV HE (coma) bore a very close resemblance to those of animals treated with comagenic doses of pentobarbital or diazepam (Figure 4). However, hyperammonemia in animals with normal livers resulted in an altered VER pattern that did not closely resemble that observed in HE.

There seem to be several potential reasons why a possible enhancement of ammonia on GABAergic neurotransmission may have been missed in these studies. First, there was no attempt to reproduce ammonia levels in animals with normal livers that closely corresponded to those that occur in liver failure. The reason for this was the failure to see any significant changes in either overt behavior or the EEG at ammonia concentrations less than ≈ 1.5 mM[24,39]. Thus, the VER may not be a sufficiently sensitive tool to detect an ammonia-induced enhancement of GABAergic neurotransmission. Moreover, the ammonia levels achieved in these studies were in the range observed in congenital hyperammonemias[25] and employed in the electrophysiological studies that defined the excitatory properties of ammonia[21]. Indeed, slight additional increases in the dose of ammonium chloride resulted in the development of seizures in a majority of the animals tested. Thus, the VER changes recorded in association with hyperammonemia in these studies may reflect the development of the excitatory component of hyperammonemias. Second, VERs, like other evoked potentials, are a summation of the inhibitory and excitatory potentials of large populations of neurons in response to a given (photic) stimulus. It is not possible to infer from the VER the degree of excitation or inhibition of specific neurons. Consequently, the VER may not accurately reflect the neuroelectrophysiological events at the level of individual neurons. It has been subsequently found that in order to observe the direct effects of ammonia on GABAergic neurotransmission it is necessary to record the currents in single, isolated neurons under conditions where the ammonia concentrations are closely controlled. Electrophysiological measures of the effects of pathophysiologically relevant concentrations of ammonia on the activity of individual neurons *in situ* in neural tissue or of large neuronal populations in the intact animal are subject to interference by anesthetics and other neurotransmitter systems. Moreover, the techniques used (such as EEG) may not be sufficiently sensitive to detect relatively small, but pathophysiologically important enhancements in GABAergic neurotransmission that may be caused by ammonia that may contribute to the manifestations of HE, particularly in its pre-comatose stages.

CONCLUSIONS

The cumulative weight of evidence acquired through basic scientific studies and clinical observation indicate that elevated levels of ammonia and increased GABAergic neurotransmission play important roles in the pathogenesis of HE. There are many pathways by which both ammonia and GABAergic neurons can act independently to contribute to the manifestations of HE and other hyperammonemic syndromes. However, there is now accumulating evidence to show that ammonia can act to enhance GABAergic neurotransmission by both indirect and direct means. Examples of the former include decreased astrocytic reuptake of GABA, and the latter the direct interaction of ammonia with the $GABA_A$ receptor. The employment of sensitive electrophysiological and biochemical (e.g., positron emission tomography) techniques in well planned studies of neuronal function in the intact CNS should yield additional information regarding the extent of ammonia-GABA interaction during the early phases of encephalopathy. Not only may such studies provide better procedures for the diagnosis of HE, but also insights into its pathogenesis which may lead to the development of new therapeutic modalities for treating this syndrome.

REFERENCES

1. G. Gabuzda, G.B Phillips, and C.S. Davidson, Reversible toxic manifestations in patients with cirrhosis of the liver given cation-exchange resins, *New Engl. J. Med.* 246:124 (1952).
2. D.F. Schafer and E.A. Jones, Hepatic encephalopathy and the γ-aminobutyric-acid neurotransmitter system. *Lancet* i:18 (1982).
3. K. Takahashi, H. Kameda, M. Kataoka, K. Sanjou, N. Harata, and N. Akaike, Ammonia potentiates $GABA_A$ response in dissociated rat cortical neurons, *Neurosci. Lett.* 151:51 (1993).
4. J-H. Ha and A.S. Basile, Modulation of ligand binding to components of the $GABA_A$ receptor complex by ammonia: implications for the pathogenesis of hyperammonemic syndromes, *Brain Res.* 720:35 (1996).
5. D.L. Coulter and R.J. Allen, Secondary hyperammonemia: A possible mechanism of valproate encephalopathy. *Lancet* i:1310 (1980).
6. D.B. Flannery, Y.E. Hsia, and B. Wolf, Current status of hyperammonemia syndromes, *Hepatol.* 2: 495 (1982).
7. F. Vergara, F. Plum, and T.E. Duffy, α-Ketoglutaramate: increased concentrations in the cerebrospinal fluid of patients in hepatic coma, *Science* 183:81 (1974).
8. L.T. Oei, J. Kuys, A.J.P. Lombarts, C. Goor, L.J. Endtz, Cerebrospinal fluid glutamine levels and EEG findings in patients with hepatic encephalopathy, *Clin. Neurol. Neurosurg.* 81: 59 (1979).
9. H.O. Conn, and M.M. Lieberthal, *The Hepatic Coma Syndromes and Lactulose.* Williams & Wilkins, Baltimore, (1978).
10. J. Stahl, Studies of the blood ammonia in liver disease: Its diagnostic, prognostic and therapeutic significance. *Ann. Int. Med.* 58: 1 (1963).
11. H.O. Conn, Cirrhosis, in: *Diseases of the Liver*, L. Schiff and E.R. Schiff, eds., Lippincott, Philadelphia, (1987).
12. M. Ehrlich, F. Plum, and T.E. Duffy, Blood and brain ammonia concentrations after portacaval anastomosis: effects of acute ammonia loading, *J. Neurochem.* 34: 1538 (1980).
13. P. Opolon, Large-pore hemodialysis in fulminant hepatic failure, in: *Artificial Liver Support*, G. Brunner and F.W. Schmidt, eds., Springer Verlag, Berlin, (1980).
14. L. T. Webster and G.J. Gabuzda, Ammonium uptake by the extremities and brain in hepatic coma, *J. Clin. Invest.* 39:414 (1958).
15. A.H. Lockwood, R.D. Finn, J.A. Campbell, and T.B. Richman, Factors that affect the uptake of ammonia by the brain: the blood-brain pH gradient, *Brain Res.* 181:259 (1980)
16. M.E. Raichle, and K.B. Larson, The significance of the NH_3-NH_4^+ equilibrium on the passage of ^{13}N ammonia from blood to brain, *Circ. Res.* 48:913 (1981).
17. A.H. Lockwood, J.M. MacDonald, R.E. Reiman, A.S. Gelbard, J.S. Laughlin, T.E. Duffy, and F. Plum, The dynamics of ammonia metabolism in man: effects of liver disease and hyperammonemia, *J. Clin. Invest.* 63: 449 (1979).
18. B. Hindfelt, F. Plum and T.E. Duffy, Effect of acute ammonia intoxication on cerebral metabolism in rats with portacaval shunts, *J. Clin. Invest.* 59:386 (1977).
19. R.F. Butterworth, Neurobiology of hepatic encephalopathy, *Sem. Liver Dis.* In press, (1996).
20. C. Torda, Ammonium ion content and electrical activity of the brain during the preconvulsive and convulsive phases induced by various convulsants. J. *Pharm. Exp. Ther.* 107: 197 (1953).
21. W. Raabe, Neurophysiology of ammonia intoxication, in: *Hepatic Encephalopathy. Pathophysiology and Treatment*, R.Butterworth and G. Pomier Layrargues, eds., Humana Press, Clifton, NJ, (1989).

22. H.D. Lux, Ammonium and chloride extrusion: Hyperpolarizing synaptic inhibition in spinal motoneurons, *Science* 173:555 (1971).
23. H.D. Lux, E. Loracher, and E. Neher, The action of ammonium on postsynaptic inhibition of cat spinal motoneurons, Exp. Brain Res., 11:431 (1970).
24. S.C. Pappas, P. Ferenci, D.F. Schafer, and E.A. Jones, Visual evoked potentials in a rabbit model of hepatic encephalopathy. II Comparison of hyperammonemic encephalopathy, postictal coma, and coma induced by synergistic neurotoxins, *Gastroenterol.* 86:546 (1984).
25. J.F. Iles and J.J.B. Jack, Ammonia: assessment of its action on postsynaptic inhibition as a cause of convulsions, *Brain* 103:555 (1983).
26. A.S. Basile, E.A. Jones, and P. Skolnick, The pathogenesis of hepatic encephalopathy: evidence for the involvement of benzodiazepine receptor ligands, *Pharmacol. Rev.* 43:27 (1991).
27. A.S. Basile, R. Hughes, P. Harrison, R. Murata, L. Pannel, E.A. Jones, R. Williams, and P. Skolnick, Brain concentrations of 1,4 benzodiazepines are elevated in patients with fulminant hepatic failure, *New Engl. J. Med.* 325: 473 (1991).
28. C. Yurdaydin, T.J. Walsh, H. Engler, J-H. Ha, Y. Li, E.A. Jones, and A.S. Basile, The role of gut bacteria in the accumulation of benzodiazepine receptor ligands in a rat model of hepatic encephalopathy, Brain Res. 679:42 (1995).
29. M.R. Ferreira, S.H. Gammal, and E.A. Jones, Hepatic encephalopathy: evidence of increased GABA-mediated neurotransmission in a rat model of fulminant hepatic failure, *Hepato-Gastroenterol.* In press (1996).
30. G. Masterton and R.E. O'Carroll, Psychological assessment in liver disease, *Bailliere's Clin. Gastroenterol.* 9:791 (1995).
31. J.F. Cadranel, M. El Younsi, B. Pidoux, P. Zylberberg, Y. Benhamou, D. Valla, and P. Opolon. Flumazenil therapy for hepatic encephalopathy in cirrhotic patients: a double-blind pragmatic randomized, placebo study, *Eur. J. Gastro. Hep.* 7:325 (1995).
32. S.S. Oja, P. Saransaari, U. Wysmyk, J. Albrecht, Loss of $GABA_B$ binding sites in the cerebral cortex of rats with acute hepatic encephalopathy. *Brain Res.* 629:355 (1993).
33. M.L. Bassett, K.D. Mullen, B. Scholz, J.D. Fenstermacher, and E.A. Jones, Increased brain uptake of γ-aminobutyric acid in a rabbit model of hepatic encephalopathy. Gastroenterol. 98:747 (1990).
34. G.Y. Minuk, A. Winder, E.D. Burgess, and E.J. Sargeant, Serum γ-aminobutyric acid levels in patients with hepatic encephalopathy, *Hepatogastroent.* 32:171 (1985).
35. M.D. Norenberg, The astrocyte in liver disease, in: *Advances in Cellular Neurobiology*, S. Fedoroff and L. Hertz, eds., Academic Press, NY, (1981).
36. M.D. Norenberg, L.W. Mozes, R.E. Papendick, L.O.B. Norenberg, Effect of ammonia on glutamate, GABA and rubidium uptake by astrocytes. [abstract] *Ann. Neurol.* 18:149 (1985).
37. U. Tossman, A. Delin, S. Eriksson, and U. Ungerstedt, Brain cortical amino acids measured by intracerebral dialysis in portacaval shunted rats, Neurochem. Res. 12:265 (1987).
38. D.F. Schafer, S.C. Pappas, L.E. Brody, R.Jacobs, and E.A. Jones, Visual evoked potentials in a rabbit model of hepatic encephalopathy, I. Sequential changes and comparisons with drug-induced comas, *Gastroenterol.* 86:540 (1984).
39. D.B. Jones, K.D. Mullen, M. Roessle, T. Maynard, and E.A. Jones, Hepatic encephalopathy: application of visual evoked responses to test hypotheses of its pathogenesis in rats, *J. Hepatol.* 4:118 (1987).

DIRECT ENHANCEMENT OF GABA-ERGIC NEUROTRANSMISSION BY AMMONIA

Jeoung-Hee Ha[1,2], Scott Knauer[1,3], Eric Moody[1,3], E. Anthony Jones[4] and Anthony S. Basile[1]

[1]Laboratory of Neuroscience, NIDDK, National Institutes of Health Bethesda, MD 20892
[2]Department of Pharmacology, Yeungnam Univ. School of Medicine Taegu, Korea
[3]Department of Anesthesiology, Johns Hopkins Univ. School of Medicine Baltimore, MD
[4]Department of Gastrointestinal and Liver Diseases, Academic Medical Center, Amsterdam, The Netherlands

INTRODUCTION

Ammonia (NH_4^+) has been implicated since the 1950's as the primary pathogenic agent contributing to the encephalopathies associated with hepatic failure[1]. NH_4^+ is clearly neurotoxic, but the molecular mechanisms by which ammonia exerts its toxic actions remain the subject of active investigation. Because the primary neurologic manifestations of these encephalopathies are consistent with central nervous system depression, increased activity of neuronal pathways using the principle inhibitory neurotransmitter, γ-aminobutyric acid (GABA) appeared likely to contribute to the pathogenesis of these syndromes. Despite ample evidence for the presence of both increased GABAergic neurotransmission and elevated NH_4^+ concentrations in the brain during hepatic failure, these two pathogenic mechanisms appear to be mutually exclusive. However, recent investigations suggest that these two pathogenic mechanisms are linked, in that NH_4^+ may enhance GABAergic neurotransmission by directly interacting with the $GABA_A$ receptor at pathophysiologically relevant concentrations. These new findings not only have important implications for the mechanisms contributing to the encephalopathies associated with hepatic failure and congenital hyperammonemia syndromes, but may provide a locus for the development of new treatment modalities.

ACTIONS OF NH_4^+ ON NEURONAL ELECTROPHYSIOLOGY

Early studies of the effects of NH_4^+ on neuronal electrophysiology were performed on neurons in relatively intact preparations[2,3]. The first study of the effects of NH_4^+ on the function of single neurons reported a reduction in the amplitude of inhibitory post-synaptic

Advances in Cirrhosis, Hyperammonemia, and Hepatic Encephalopathy
Edited by Felipo and Grisolía, Plenum Press, New York, 1997

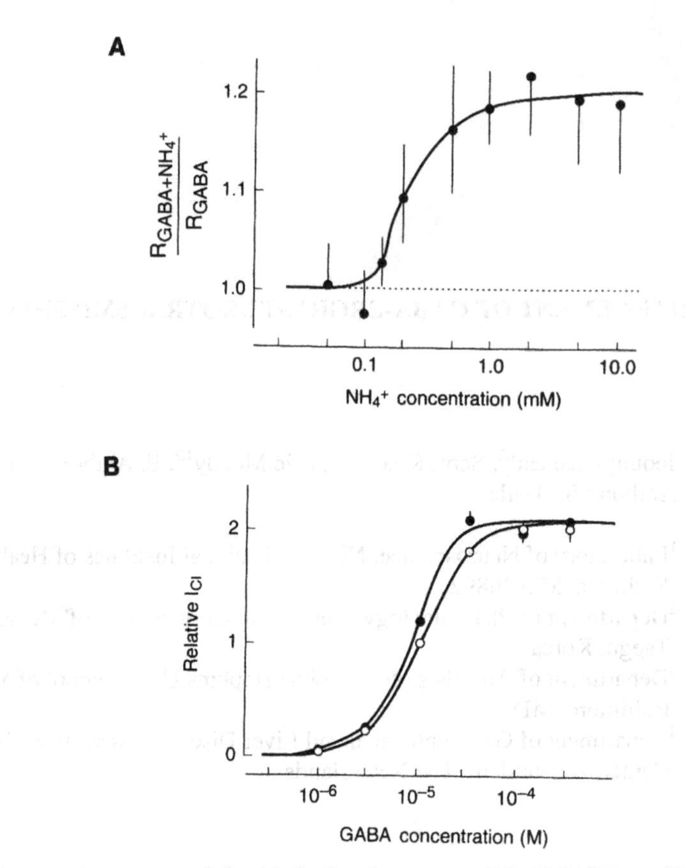

Figure 1. Concentration-response relationship for the enhancement of 10 μM GABA-gated I_{Cl} by NH_4^+ (Panel A). Dissociated cortical neurons were maintained at a holding potential of -50 mV, and were pretreated for 60 sec with increasing concentrations of NH_4^+. The concentration-response relationships for the amplitude of the GABA-gated I_{Cl} of dissociated cortical neurons in the presence or absence of 1 mM NH_4^+ are shown in panel B. All currents were normalized to the peak current amplitude induced by 10 μM GABA. Panels A and B from reference 9, by permission.

potentials (IPSP) at normal resting membrane potentials in cat spinal motoneurons[2]. Because Cl^- is the principle ion carrying the IPSP current in mammalian neurons, these results suggested that the intracellular Cl^- concentration increased in the presence of NH_4^+. Subsequent investigations[4] indicated that NH_4^+ (1mM) blocked the active extrusion of Cl^-. Blocking this pump increases intracellular Cl^- concentrations, reducing the concentration gradient for Cl^- entry into the neuron, and thereby suppressing the IPSP amplitude. As a result, the neuron is not hyperpolarized (or depressed) by a typical inhibitory stimulus. However, it should be noted that the ability of NH_4^+ to block neuronal IPSPs shows considerable regional variability[5]. The second effect of NH_4^+ is to depolarize neurons at concentrations greater than 2 mM[3]. This effect results from the potassium-like actions of NH_4^+, such that increased extracellular NH_4^+ levels are the electrophysiological equivalent of an elevation in extracellular potassium, which subsequently depolarizes neurons. These NH_4^+ -induced depolarizations are further enhanced by the ability of NH_4^+ to inhibit potassium uptake by astrocytes, thereby directly increasing extracellular potassium concentrations.

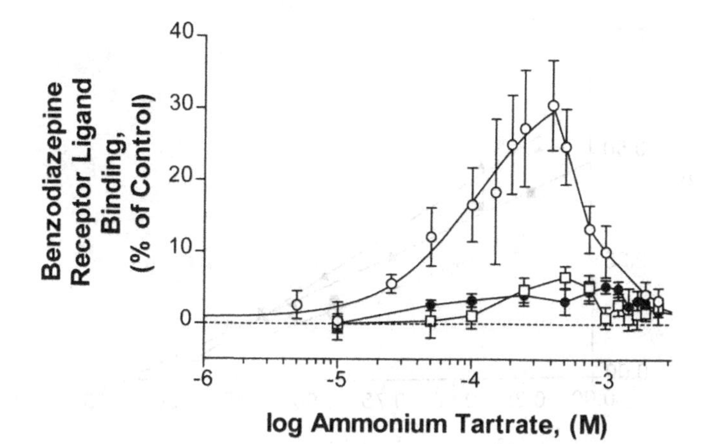

Figure 2. Modulation of radioligand binding to benzodiazepine receptors in cerebral cortex by ammonium tartrate. Ammonium tartrate (5-500 μM) increased [^{3}H]flunitrazepam (○) binding by 32%, with an EC_{50} value of 98 μM. Further increasing the ammonium tartrate concentration from 500 μM to 2.5 mM reduced [^{3}H]flunitrazepam binding to baseline levels, with an IC_{50} of 733 μM. In contrast, ammonium tartrate did not significantly alter the binding of [^{3}H]flumazenil (□) or [^{3}H]Ro 15-4513 (●, E_{max}: 6 and 5%, respectively). From reference 10, with permission.

Although it is clear that NH_4^+ has the ability to suppress IPSP formation and depolarize neurons, the question remains if and when these events occur during the evolution of hepatic and hyperammonemic encephalopathies. The changes in neuronal electrophysiology reported above were observed following the application of 1-5 mM concentrations of NH_4^+. In contrast, plasma and CSF NH_4^+ levels in patients with clinically significant and animals with behaviorally relevant manifestations of encephalopathy secondary to liver failure or congenital hyperammonemia syndromes range from 70-850 μM, and only occasionally exceed 1 mM[6-8]. In addition to the relatively high concentrations of NH_4^+ used in these preparations, little effort was taken to determine whether NH_4^+ had any direct effect on the function of neurotransmitter receptors. This issue becomes increasingly important given that the manifestations of hepatic encephalopathy at NH_4^+ concentrations below 1 mM (e.g., lethargy) are inconsistent with neuroexcitatory actions of NH_4^+ reported above.

An insight into the depressant actions of NH_4^+ at pathophysiologically relevant concentrations was provided by a study of isolated cortical neurons maintained in culture[9]. The use of isolated neurons in this investigation is particularly important, since the concentrations of NH_4^+ can be precisely determined in this preparation, and the potentially conflicting influences of multisynaptic excitatory and inhibitory circuits on the neurons under study can be eliminated. GABA- gated Cl^- currents were recorded from these neurons in the presence of 0.75-10 mM concentrations of NH_4^+ using whole cell clamp techniques. NH_4^+ (in the form of ammonium acetate) alone had little effect on membrane currents. However, the Cl^- current induced by 10 μM GABA was enhanced to a maximum of approximately 120% by 1 mM NH_4^+, with an EC_{50} of 200 μM (Figure 1A). The potency of GABA in gating the Cl^- currents in these neurons was increased 15% by 1 mM NH_4^+ (EC_{50}: 8.5 vs 10 μM) without altering the maximum current (Figure 1B). This effect of NH_4^+ was selective for GABA, as NH_4^+ had no effect on currents induced by glycine or glutamate. Moreover, in these experiments, NH_4^+ had no effect on the reversal potential of the GABA-gated Cl^- current. This indicates that NH_4^+ had no effect on the intracellular Cl^- concentration, and thus,

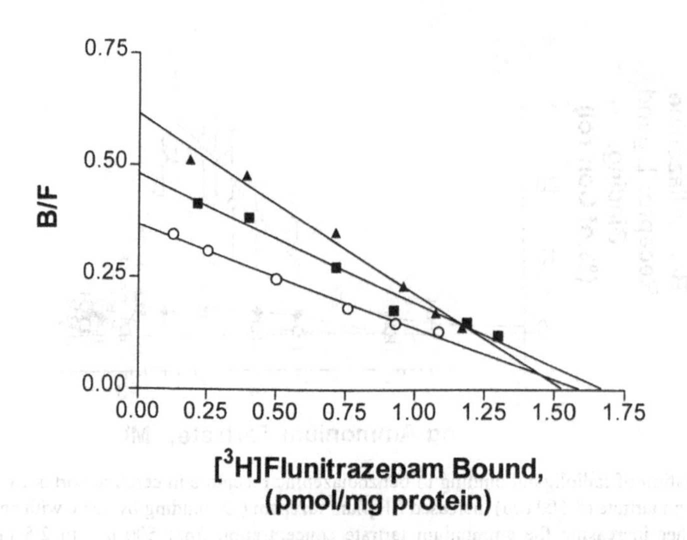

Figure 3. Ammonium tartrate increases [^{3}H]flunitrazepam binding by decreasing the K_d, as illustrated in these Scatchard-Rosenthal plots. The K_d and B_{max} for [^{3}H]flunitrazepam binding under basal conditions (O) were 2.4 nM and 1.7 pmol/mg protein, respectively. In the presence of 500 µM ammonium tartrate (▲), the K_d was significantly reduced to 1.1 nM, without altering the B_{max} (1.5 pmol/mg protein). Raising the ammonium tartrate concentration to 2.5 mM (■) caused the K_d to increase to 1.9 nM, while the B_{max} was not significantly altered (1.7 pmol/mg protein). All K_d and B_{max} values were determined using non-linear regression analysis. From reference 10, with permission.

the activity of the Cl^- extrusion pumps. In conclusion, these results suggest that pathophysiologically relevant concentrations of NH_4^+ can selectively enhance GABA-gated Cl^- currents in individual neurons by increasing the affinity of GABA for the $GABA_A$ receptor.

DIRECT ACTIONS OF NH_4^+ ON THE $GABA_A$ RECEPTOR

The ability of NH_4^+ to significantly enhance GABA-gated Cl^- currents led to an investigation of the direct actions of NH_4^+ on radioligand binding to components of the $GABA_A$ receptor[10]. These studies were performed using standard radioligand binding techniques for the $GABA_A$ and benzodiazepine receptors derived from the cerebral cortex and cerebellum of normal Sprague-Dawley rats. [^{3}H]Muscimol and [^{3}H]flunitrazepam were used as the principle radioligands for the $GABA_A$ and benzodiazepine receptors, respectively. Neutral ammonium salts (ammonium tartrate and acetate) were used as NH_4^+ sources.

Ammonium salts caused a biphasic increase followed by a decrease in the binding of the agonist [^{3}H]flunitrazepam to the benzodiazepine receptor in the cerebral cortex (Figure 2). NH_4^+ increased the maximal binding of [^{3}H]flunitrazepam by 31%. In contrast, NH_4^+ had no significant effect on the binding of the benzodiazepine receptor antagonist [^{3}H]flumazenil or the partial inverse agonist [^{3}H]Ro 15-4513 (Figure 2). As the concentration of NH_4^+ salts was increased above 500-750 µM, the precentage enhancement of agonist ligand binding to the benzodiazepine receptor in the cerebral cortex declined until no significant increase in ligand binding was observed at an NH_4^+ concentration of 2.5 mM (Figure 2). Saturation analysis indicated that the enhancement of [^{3}H]flunitrazepam binding induced by ammonium

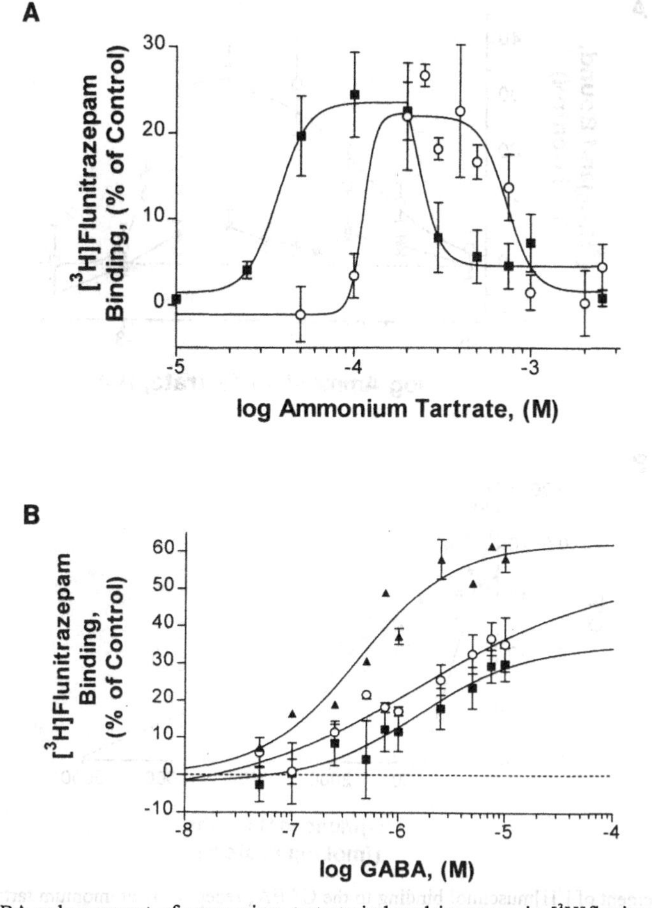

Figure 4. GABA enhancement of ammonium tartrate-induced increases in $[^3H]$flunitrazepam binding to benzodiazepine receptors in the cerebral cortex (Panel A). The potency of ammonium tartrate (O, EC_{50} = 113 µM) in increasing $[^3H]$flunitrazepam binding was significantly increased in the presence of 20 µM GABA (■, EC_{50} = 37 µM). Similarly, GABA shifted the IC_{50} for ammonium tartrate to the left (228 vs 725 µM, +/- 20 µM GABA, respectively). The E_{max} was not altered (24 vs 22%, +/- 20 µM GABA, respectively). Reciprocally, ammonium tartrate enhances the potency of GABA in increasing $[^3H]$flunitrazepam binding (Panel B). Ammonium tartrate (500 µM, ▲, EC_{50} = 420 nM) increased the potency of GABA-enhanced $[^3H]$flunitrazepam binding (O, EC_{50} = 1.6 µM), without altering the E_{max}, (60% and 62%, control vs. ammonium tartrate, respectively). Raising the ammonium tartrate concentration to 2.5 mM (■), returned the EC_{50} for GABA-enhanced $[^3H]$flunitrazepam binding to control levels (1.6 µM), and significantly decreased the E_{max} (37%). From reference 10, with permission.

tartrate was manifested as an increase in the affinity of $[^3H]$flunitrazepam for the benzodiazepine receptor (Figure 3). The K_d of $[^3H]$flunitrazepam for the benzodiazepine receptor was reduced by approximately 60% in the presence of 500 µM ammonium tartrate, without any significant change in the density (B_{max}) of $[^3H]$flunitrazepam binding sites. Both NH_4^+ and GABA interacted with the benzodiazepine receptor to increase $[^3H]$flunitrazepam binding. The potency of ammonium salts in enhancing $[^3H]$flunitrazepam binding to the cortex could be further increased 2.5-3.5 fold in the presence of 20 µM GABA (Figure 4A), without altering the E_{max}. Conversely, discrete concentrations of NH_4^+ increased the potency

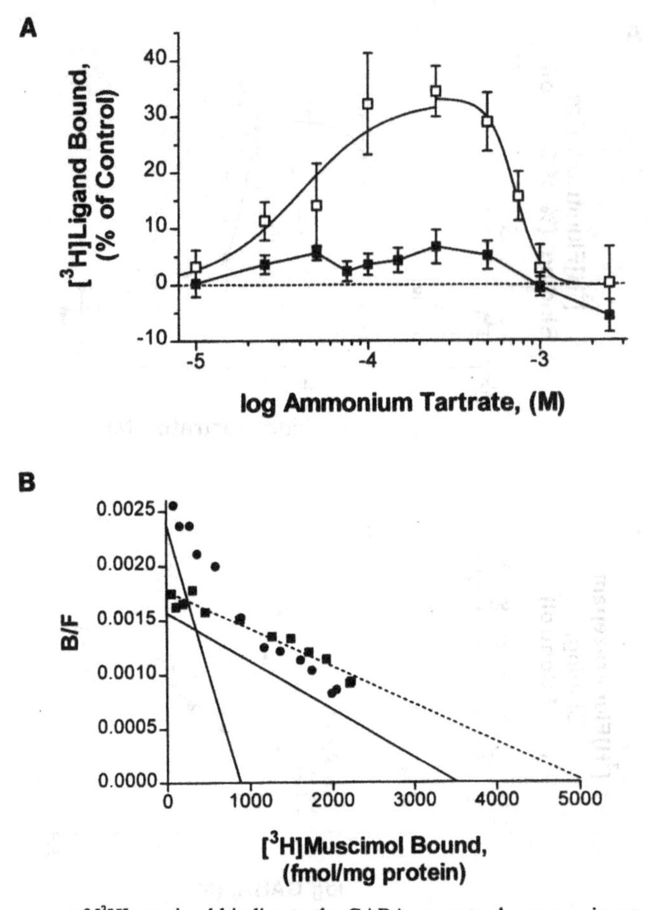

Figure 5. Enhancement of [^{3}H]muscimol binding to the $GABA_A$ receptor by ammonium tartrate (Panel A). Ammonium tartrate significantly increased the E_{max} of 500 nM [^{3}H]muscimol (□) binding above control levels (33%), with an EC_{50} = 40 μM. Increasing the ammonium tartrate concentration (500 μM to 2.5 mM) lowered the binding of 500 nM [^{3}H]muscimol to control levels (IC_{50} = 725 μM). In contrast, ammonium tartrate did not significantly modulate the binding of [^{3}H]SR 95-531 (■, E_{max} < 10%). Representative Scatchard-Rosenthal plots of the changes in [^{3}H]muscimol binding in the presence of 0 (●) and 500 μM (■) ammonium tartrate (Panel B). In the absence of ammonium tartrate, [^{3}H]muscimol bound to sites with high (K_d = 12 nM, B_{max} = 880 fmol/mg protein) and low affinities (K_d = 180 nM, B_{max} = 3400 fmol/mg protein). In the presence of 500 μM ammonium tartrate, the high affinity [^{3}H]muscimol binding site disappeared, with the remaining [^{3}H]muscimol binding displaying a K_d= 180 nM. The density of [^{3}H]muscimol binding to the remaining low affinity site was significantly increased by 47%, with the B_{max} = 5000 fmol/mg protein. From reference 10, with permission.

of GABA-enhanced [^{3}H]flunitrazepam binding to a maximum of 5-fold (500 μM ammonium tartrate, Figure 4B). Finally, there was a regional difference in the maximal efficacy of ammonium tartrate in enhancing [^{3}H]flunitrazepam binding to benzodiazepine receptors. The E_{max} for ammonium tartrate-induced enhancement of [^{3}H]flunitrazepam binding to benzodiazepine receptors in the cerebellum was 46% lower than that for the binding to the cortex or hippocampus.

Ammonium tartrate also increased the E_{max} of agonist ligand binding to the $GABA_A$ receptor (Figure 5A). Ammonium tartrate increased the binding E_{max} of the agonist

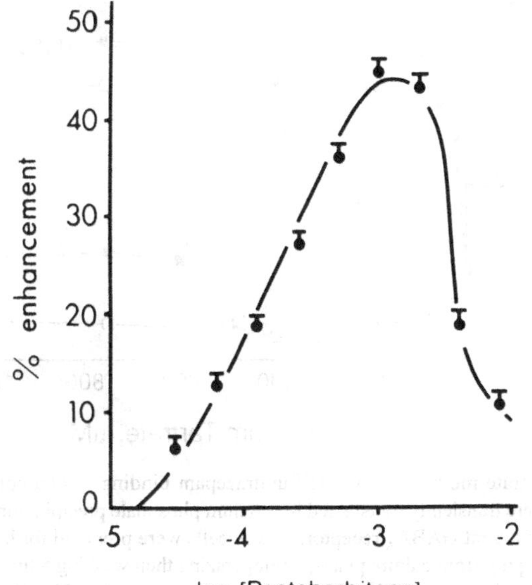

Figure 6. The effect of pentobarbital on [^{3}H]GABA (25 nM) binding to whole rat brain synaptosomes. From reference 16, with permission.

[^{3}H]muscimol (500 nM), but had no significant effect on the binding of the $GABA_A$ receptor antagonist [^{3}H]SR 95531 (Figure 5A). Saturation analysis of [^{3}H]muscimol binding in the presence of discrete concentrations of ammonium tartrate indicated that the high affinity component of [^{3}H]muscimol binding was lost, while the B_{max} for the low affinity [^{3}H]muscimol binding site increased 27% (Figure 5B). Further increasing the ammonium tartrate concentration to 2.5 mM not only resulted in the loss of the high affinity binding site, but also decreased the B_{max} for the low affinity binding site by 20%.

The ability of ammonium salts and benzodiazepine receptor ligands in combination to modulate [^{3}H]muscimol binding was also investigated. Ammonium tartrate further increased ability of both flunitrazepam to enhance (E_{max} = 90%), and DMCM (a β-carboline inverse agonist) to inhibit (I_{max} = 37%) [^{3}H]muscimol binding. Reciprocally, flunitrazepam (10 μM) increased the maximal enhancement of 500 nM [^{3}H]muscimol binding by ammonium tartrate by 97%. In contrast, DMCM reduced the EC_{50} for ammonium tartrate enhancement of [^{3}H]muscimol binding by 57%. Ro 15-1788 had no significant effect on ammonium tartrate's enhancement of [^{3}H]muscimol binding. Finally, ammonium tartrate was significantly more potent (189%) in enhancing [^{3}H]muscimol binding to $GABA_A$ receptors in the cerebellum than in the cortex or hippocampus.

IS NH_4^+ AN ENDOGENOUS BARBITURATE?

Many of the effects of NH_4^+ on radioligand binding to the $GABA_A$ receptor and GABA-gated Cl^- currents resemble those induced by barbiturates. Barbiturates increase benzodiazepine binding to its receptor by enhancing its affinity 2.6 fold[11,12]. Moreover, barbiturates increase the B_{max} of [^{3}H]muscimol binding 58%[13], and cause the loss of high

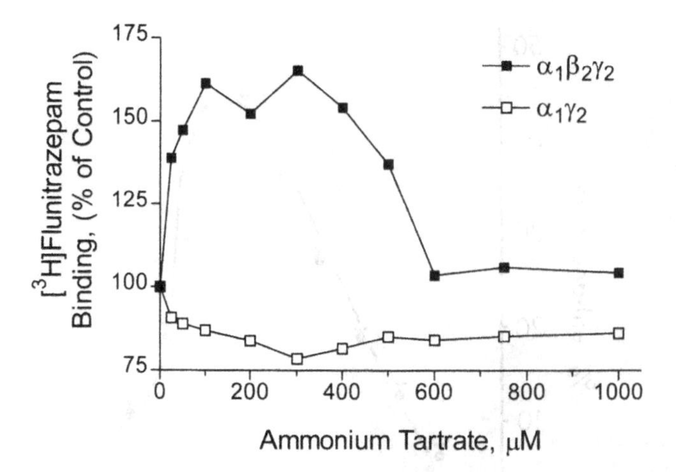

Figure 7. Ammonium tartrate modulation of [^{3}H]flunitrazepam binding to two constructs of the $GABA_A$ receptor. HEK-293 cells were transiently transfected by calcium phosphate precipitation with cDNAs encoding α_1, β_2 and/or γ_2 subunits of the rat $GABA_A$ receptor. These cells were prepared for binding assays within 48 hrs after transfection by scraping from culture plates, homogenizing then washing 5 times. Ammonium tartrate enhanced [^{3}H]flunitrazepam binding to the $\alpha_1\beta_2\gamma_2$ construct approximately 155% (■). This enhancment of [^{3}H]flunitrazepam binding by NH_4^+ is lost in cells expressing the $\alpha_1\gamma_2$ construct (□).

affinity binding sites[14,15]. Interestingly, pentobarbital has been reported to have a biphasic action on the binding of [^{3}H]GABA to the $GABA_A$ receptor, initially enhancing ligand binding by about 30%, then reducing ligand binding to control levels (Figure 6)[16]. In addition, there are significant regional differences in NH_4^+ modulation of ligand binding to the $GABA_A$ receptor (which is composed of α, β, and γ subunits)[17]. Heterogeneity in the subunit configuration of the $GABA_A$ receptor may account for these differences. Studies of recombinant $GABA_A$ receptors indicate that barbiturates require the β subunit to positively modulate ligand binding to $GABA_A$ receptors[18]. Using human embryonic kidney (HEK) cells transiently transfected with $\alpha_1\beta_2\gamma_2$ or $\alpha_1\gamma_2$ constructs of the GABAA receptor, we found that NH_4^+ modulation of ligand binding to the benzodiazepine receptor also requires the presence of the β subunit (Figure 7). The maximal enhancement of [^{3}H]flunitrazepam binding by NH_4^+ observed in cells expressing $\alpha_1\beta_2\gamma_2$ constructs (whose pharmacology and relative abundance most resembles that of the native $GABA_A$ receptor)[19] is approximately 2.5-fold greater than that observed in homogenates of cerebral cortex (Figure 7). In contrast, NH_4^+ had no effect on [^{3}H]flunitrazepam binding to HEK cells expressing $\alpha_1\gamma_2$ subunits. This suggests that both NH_4^+ and barbiturate-induced modulation of $GABA_A$ receptor function is dependent on the presence of a β subunit.

These data indicate several similarities between the effects of barbiturates and NH_4^+ on ligand binding to the $GABA_A$ receptor complex, there are nonetheless some important differences. Barbiturates enhance GABA-gated Cl^- currents 7-10 fold[20] , while NH_4^+ enhances these currents by 120%[9]. Unlike barbiturates, NH_4^+cannot directly induce Cl currents, but modestly increases the amplitude of pentobarbital-induced currents (112.5%)[9]. Finally, while NH_4^+ is less potent in enhancing agonist binding to benzodiazepine receptors in the cerebellum, barbiturates are less efficacious in increasing [^{3}H]diazepam binding to cerebellar benzodiazepine receptors[21]. Thus, it is still not clear whether NH_4^+ has a unique binding site on the $GABA_A$ receptor complex, or if it shares a site with barbiturates.

CONCLUSIONS

The data presented from both electrophysiological and neurochemical studies clearly indicate that pathophysiologically relevant concentrations of NH_4^+ (100 μM-1 mM) directly enhance GABA-ergic neurotransmission. The magnitude of the enhancement of GABAergic neurotransmission by NH_4^+ is not of the same magnitude as that induced by barbiturates or neurosteroids, but is very similar to that induced by benzodiazepine receptor agonists. The relatively limited magnitude of GABAergic enhancement by NH_4^+ may account for many of the neurological manifestations of early stages of hepatic encephalopathy, including confusion, depression, incoordination, analytical slowing, drowsiness, lethargy, and ataxia, but alone may be insufficient to cause coma. Instead, the direct actions of NH_4^+ on the GABA receptor may act synergistically with the other mechanisms by which GABAergic neurotransmission is increased in hepatic failure[21] to contribute to the development of coma. While the data clearly indicate that benzodiazepine receptor antagonists would be ineffective in ameliorating a purely hyperammonemic encephalopathy[9,10], it may be possible that other agents, such as the excitatory barbiturates (+)-MPPB or CHEB[12], or the neurosteroid antagonist pregnenolone sulfate[23], may be highly effective in selectively reversing the increase in GABAergic neurotransmission that accompanies hyperammonemic states. Studies of the effects of such agents on the manifestations of hepatic encephalopathy in animal models may pave the way for the development of new therapeutic modalities for the treatment of hepatic encephalopathy in man.

REFERENCES

1. G. Gabuzda, G.B Phillips, and C.S. Davidson, Reversible toxic manifestations in patients with cirrhsis of the liver given cation-exchange resins, *New Engl. J. Med.* 246:124 (1952).
2. H.D. Lux, E. Loracher, and E. Neher, The action of ammonium on postsynaptic inhibition of cat spinal motoneurons, Exp. Brain Res., 11:431 (1970).
3. W. Raabe and R.J. Gumnit, Disinhibition in cat motor cortex by ammonia, *J. Neurophysiol.* 38:347 (1975).
4. H.D. Lux, Ammonium and chloride extrusion: Hyperpolarizing synaptic inhibition in spinal motoneurons, *Science* 173:555 (1971).
5. B. E. Alger and R.A. Nicoll, Ammonia does not selectively block IPSPs in rat hippocampal pyramidal cells, *J. Neurophysiol.* 49:1381 (1983).
6. J.F. Iles and J.J.B. Jack, Ammonia: assessment of its action on postsynaptic inhibition as a cause of convulsions, *Brain* 103:555 (1983).
7. D.B. Flannery, Y.E. Hsia, and B. Wolf, Current status of hyperammonemia syndromes, *Hepatol.* 2: 495 (1982).
8. F. Vergara, F. Plum, and T.E. Duffy, α-Ketoglutaramate: increased concentrations in the cerebrospinal fluid of patients in hepatic coma, *Science* 183:81 (1974).
9. K. Takahashi, H. Kameda, M. Kataoka, K. Sanjou, N. Harata, and N. Akaike, Ammonia potentiates $GABA_A$ response in dissociated rat cortical neurons, *Neurosci. Lett.* 151:51 (1993).
10. J-H. Ha and A.S. Basile, Modulation of ligand binding to components of the $GABA_A$ receptor complex by ammonia: implications for the pathogenesis of hyperammonemic syndromes, *Brain Res.* 720:35 (1996).

11. P. Skolnick, V. Moncada, and J.L. Barker, Pentobarbital: dual actions to increase brai benzodiazepine receptor affinity, *Science* 211:1448 (1981).
12. F. Leeb-Lundberg, A. Snowman, and R.W. Olsen, Barbiturate receptor sites are coupled to benzodiazepine receptors, *Proc. Natl. Acad. Sci.* 77:7568 (1980).
13. J.A. Peters, E.F. Kirkness, H. Callachan, J.L. Lambert, and A.J. Turner, Modulation of the $GABA_A$ receptor by depressant barbiturates and pregnane steroids, *Br. J. Pharmacol.* 94:1257 (1988).
14. R.W. Olsen and A.M. Snowman, Chloride-dependent enhancement by barbiturates of γ-aminobutyric acid receptor binding, *J. Neurosci.* 12:1812 (1982).
15. U. Quast and O. Brenner, Modulation of [^{3}H]muscimol binding in rat cerebellar and cerebral cortical membranes by picrotoxin, pentobarbitone, and etomidate, *J. Neurochem.* 41:418 (1983).
16. R. Olsen and A. Tobin, Molecular biology of $GABA_A$ receptors, *FASEB J.* 4:1469 (1990).
17. M. Willow and G.A.R. Johnston, Dual action of pentobarbitone on GABA binding: role of binding site integrity. *J. Neurochem.* 37:1291 (1981).
18. B.D. Harris, G. Wong, E.J. Moody, and P. Skolnick, Different subunit requirements for volatile and nonvolatile anesthetics at γ-aminobutyric acid type A receptors, *Mol. Pharmacol.* 47:363 (1995).
19. H. Mohler, P. Malherbe, A. Draguhn, E. Sigel, J.M. Sequier, E. Persohn, and J.G. Richards, $GABA_A$ receptor subunits: functional expression and gene localization, in: *GABA and Benzodiazepine Receptor Subtypes,* G. Biggio and E. Costa, eds., Raven Press, New York, (1990).
20. N. Akaike, K. Hattori, N. Inomata, and Y. Oomura, γ-Aminobutyric and pentobarbitone-gated chloride currents in internally perfused frog sensory neurons, *J. Physiol.* 360:367 (1985).
21. P. Skolnick, K.C. Rice, J.L. Barker, and S.M. Paul, Interaction of barbiturates with benzodiazepine receptors in the central nervous system, *Brain Res.* 233:143 (1982
22. A.S. Basile, E.A. Jones, and P. Skolnick, The pathogenesis of hepatic encephalopathy: evidence for the involvement of benzodiazepine receptor ligands, *Pharmacol. Rev.* 43:27 (1991).
23. M.D. Majewska and R.D. Schwartz, Pregnenolone-sulfate: an endogenous antagonist of the γ-aminobutyric acid receptor complex in brain? *Brain Res.* 404:355 (1987).

THE PERIPHERAL BENZODIAZEPINE RECEPTOR AND NEUROSTEROIDS IN HEPATIC ENCEPHALOPATHY

Michael D. Norenberg, Yossef Itzhak and Alex S. Bender

Veterans Affairs Medical Center
Departments of Pathology and Biochemistry & Molecular Biology
University of Miami School of Medicine
Miami, FL 33101

INTRODUCTION

Hepatic encephalopathy (HE) represents one of the most common events in terminal liver failure. Acute HE (fulminant hepatic failure, FHF) presents with the abrupt onset of delirium, seizures, and coma, and has a mortality rate of about 90%. The principal cause of death in FHF is brain edema associated with increased intracranial pressure. Chronic HE, sometimes referred to as portal-systemic encephalopathy, most often occurs in the setting of cirrhosis and is characterized by change in personality, altered mood and behavior, diminished intellectual capacity, abnormal muscle tone and tremor (asterixis), stupor and coma. For reviews, see (Rothstein and Herlong, 1989; Lockwood. 1992).

While the mechanism responsible for HE remains controversial (see below), numerous studies have clearly shown that astrocytes and ammonia are critically involved. It is the intent of this article to briefly review the role of astrocytes, with particular emphasis on new data implicating the peripheral benzodiazepine receptor and associated neurosteroids in the pathogenesis of this disorder.

ASTROCYTES IN HE

Astrocytes are the most numerous cells in the central nervous system (CNS). Their cytoplasmic processes fill much of the interstices of the CNS and are intimately positioned at such critical sites such as around the synaptic complex and at the node of Ranvier. These dynamic cells have critical metabolic supportive functions involved in the maintenance and regulation of the extracellular microenvironment. They are involved in K^+ buffering and in the homeostasis of other ions including H^+ and Ca^{2+} (Walz, 1989; Ransom and Sontheimer, 1992; Kimelberg, et al., 1993), osmoregulation (Walz, 1989), development and regulation of the blood-brain barrier (Janzer and Raff, 1987; Risau and Wolburg, 1990), provision of nutrients and neurotransmitter precursors to neurons (Westergaard, et al., 1995), detoxification of ammonia, drugs and hormones (Norenberg, 1983; Abramovitz, et al., 1988), metabolism of CO_2 (Anderson, et al., 1984), free radical scavenging (Makar, et al., 1994), metal sequestration (Sawada, et al., 1994), uptake and release of neurotransmitters and neuromodulators (Schousboe, 1981), inflammatory/immune responses (Hertz, et al., 1990), and neurotrophism (Rudge, 1993; Rutishauser, 1993). Increasing evidence strongly indicates that astrocytes significantly influence neuronal excitability and neurotransmission (Nedergaard, 1994; Parpura, et al., 1994; Keyser and Pellmar, 1994; Mennerick and Zorumski, 1994). In view of these critical CNS functions, it is reasonable to assume that dysfunction of these cells would result in major neurological deficits.

The notion that astrocytes are critically involved in the pathogenesis of HE derives largely from pathological findings. The studies of Adams and Foley (1953), Norenberg (1981) and Martin et al. (1987) clearly show the consistent presence of abnormal astrocytes (Alzheimer type II change) in chronic HE. Moreover, there is a positive correlation between the severity of HE and the degree of Alzheimer type II astrocytosis. Almost all animal models of HE show the same astroglial change (Norenberg, 1981). In fulminant hepatic failure, astroglial swelling dominates the microscopic picture in human disease (Kato, et al., 1992) as well as in the majority of experimental animal studies (Norenberg, 1977; Voorhies, et al., 1983; Traber, et al., 1987; Swain, et al., 1991). Considering the important role for ammonia in HE, it should be noted that glutamine synthetase, the principal enzyme involved in ammonia metabolism is principally located in astrocytes (Norenberg, 1979), and that humans and animals with hyperammonemia, as well as ammonia-treated cultured astrocytes show Alzheimer type II changes. Furthermore, there is growing evidence of abnormalities in glutamatergic neuro-transmission in HE (Rao, et al., 1992; Szerb and Butterworth, 1992) where astrocytes are likely play a key role (Bender and Norenberg, 1996; Norenberg. 1996). Lastly, astrocytes may also be involved in the benzodiazepine/GABA hypothesis via the peripheral benzo-diazepine receptor, a concept that will be developed in this article.

While the significance of the astrocyte response in HE is still not clear, we have strongly advocated the view that HE represents a primary "gliopathy" in which a disturbance in critical astrocytic functions (such as neurotransmitter uptake and ion homeostasis) can result in neuronal dysfunction that lead to CNS derangements (Norenberg, et al., 1992).

MECHANISTIC CONSIDERATIONS

The pathogenetic mechanisms involved in HE are still unknown. Two views currently dominate: 1) the toxin/ammonia hypothesis, and 2) abnormal GABAergic neurotransmission related to the presence of endogenous benzodiazepines (BZDs).

To date, ammonia is the candidate that can best explain the clinical, pathological and neurochemical features of HE (Norenberg, 1981; Cooper and Plum, 1987; Record, 1991; Butterworth, 1991). Ammonia has many effects on the CNS (Cooper and Plum, 1987; Raabe, 1989; Szerb and Butterworth, 1992). The mechanisms of ammonia toxicity, however, are poorly understood. Views have ranged from altered bioenergetics, neuronal electro-physiological effects, changes in intracellular pH, and inhibition of various enzymes (Norenberg, 1981; Cooper and Plum, 1987). Ammonia also exerts many effects on astrocytes including decreases in glial fibrillary acidic protein (GFAP) and GFAP mRNA, which are consistent with the loss of GFAP observed in humans with HE (Sobel, et al., 1981). It decreases the cAMP response to β-adrenergic agonists, Ca^{2+} influx, protein phosphorylation, glycogen levels, and GABA uptake. It also causes cell swelling and alterations in energy and amino acid metabolism (Murthy and Hertz, 1987; Hertz, et al., 1987; Fitzpatrick, et al., 1988) (for review, see Norenberg, 1995).

The second major pathogenetic view deals with the role of heightened GABAergic neurotransmission in HE (Jones and Schafer, 1986; Basile, et al., 1991). Proponents of this view suggest that elevated GABA levels, hypersensitivity of the $GABA_A$ receptor, or excessive allosteric modulators of the $GABA_A$ receptor (e.g., benzodiazepines, BZDs) are significant factors in HE. Since GABA is the major inhibitory neurotransmitter in brain (Macdonald and Olsen, 1994), this seems like a plausible point of view. The $GABA_A$ receptor contains a modulatory binding site for BZDs ("central" BZD receptors) which exert their anxiolytic/ sedative effects by increasing $GABA_A$ receptor-mediated chloride currents (Olsen and Tobin, 1990). The rank order potency of BZDs for this binding site is clonazepam > diazepam > Ro5-4864. While the GABA/BZD hypothesis is controversial (Butterworth, 1992), it nonetheless has substantial support and represents a major point of interest among investigators at the present time.

PERIPHERAL BENZODIAZEPINE RECEPTORS

One aspect of the GABA/BZD hypothesis that has so far been little explored is the potential involvement of the "peripheral-type" benzodiazepine receptor (PBR), so named because it is found in many peripheral tissues. PBRs are found in especially high levels in steroidogenic organs such as adrenal cortex, testes, and ovary. In the CNS they are chiefly confined to glial cells (McCarthy and Harden, 1981; Schoemaker, et al., 1982; Bender and Hertz, 1985; Itzhak, et al., 1993) and have been found in high concentration in the choroid plexus, pineal, and ependymal cells (Benavides, et al., 1983; Schoemaker, et al., 1983; Moynagh, et al., 1991). While astrocytes clearly have PBRs, microglia appear to possess these receptors as well (Myers, et al., 1991; Stephenson, et al., 1995; Park, et al., 1996).

In contrast to the central BZD receptor that is present on the plasma membrane as part of the neuronal $GABA_A$ receptor complex, the PBR is primarily located on the outer mitochondrial membrane (Anholt, et al., 1986), although it has also been found in other subcellular components (O'Beirne, et al., 1990). The PBR has a different rank order of binding affinities from the central BZD receptor: PK 11195 (not a BZD but an isoquinoline carboximide) > Ro5-4864 > diazepam >> clonazepam (Parola, et al., 1993). Diazepam binding inhibitor (DBI) binds equally to both the central and peripheral receptors (Guidotti, et al., 1983). The PBR has distinct binding domains. Using the photoaffinity ligand PK 14105, the "PK" binding site has been identified as an 18 kDa protein (Garnier, et al., 1994; Antkiewicz Michaluk, et al., 1988). This site appears to be associated with two other proteins of 32 and 30 kDa size which have been identified as the voltage-dependent anion channel (VDAC; mitochondrial porin) and the adenine nucleotide carrier, respectively (McEnery, et al., 1992). It is unclear if BZDs bind to the same protein as PK 11195 or to other related proteins (Sprengel, et al., 1989; Garnier, et al., 1994). The isoquinoline/PK binding site gene has been cloned (Sprengel, et al., 1989).

The PBR has been implicated in cellular proliferation, inhibition of neurite outgrowth, inhibition of mitochondrial respiratory control, monocyte chemotaxis, immune function, enhancement of protooncogene expression, lipid metabolism, calcium homeostasis, and intermediate metabolism (Verma and Snyder, 1989; Parola, et al., 1993). However, the best studied function of the PBR is the regulation of steroid biosynthesis (Krueger and

Papadopoulos, 1992; Papadopoulos and Brown, 1995). The PBR serves as the rate limiting step in steroid synthesis since it is required for the transfer of cholesterol from the outer to the inner mitochondrial membrane (Krueger and Papadopoulos, 1990). Cholesterol is subsequently converted to pregnenolone, the parent compound for all neurosteroids, by the action of cytochrome P450scc (Mukhin, et al., 1989).

NEUROSTEROIDS

The capability of brain for *de novo* synthesis of steroids was described in the pioneering studies of Baulieu (1991) who showed that dehydroepiandrosterone (DHEA) and pregnenolone, as well as their sulfate and fatty acid esters, occurred in brain at levels that were independent of peripheral (i.e., adrenal or gonadal) sources. Such brain-derived steroids are referred to as neurosteroids. The brain can further oxidize pregnenolone to progesterone. The subsequent reduction of progesterone to tetrahydroprogesterone (THP; allopregnanolone; 3α-OH-5α-pregnan-20-one) via 5α-reductase and 3α-hydroxysteroid oxidoreductase has been shown in brain, brain slices and retina, as well as in mixed cultures of neurons and glia (Purdy, et al., 1991; Mellon and Deschepper, 1993; Korneyev, et al., 1993; Guarneri, et al., 1994) (Fig. 1). Tetrahydrodeoxycorticosterone (THDOC; 5α-pregnan-3α-21-diol-20-one) has not yet been definitively shown to be synthesized in brain. However, a recent report documents its synthesis in retina (Guarneri, et al., 1994). CNS contains significant amounts of steroid precursors such as cholesterol and its sulfate, and it clearly has the enzymatic machinery similar to steroidogenic tissues required for the synthesis of most neuroactive steroids. For reviews see (Baulieu, 1991; Lambert, et al., 1995).

Neurosteroids, particularly THP, alter neuronal excitability and have potent CNS depressant effects. Intravenous administration of THP produces anesthetic effects in mice (Mok, et al., 1991); intraventricular and intraperitoneal administration produces anxiolytic effects in rats (Bitran, et al., 1991) and mice (Wieland, et al., 1991); while intraperitoneal administration to mice has potent anticonvulsant activity (Belelli, et al., 1989). In contrast to the well known genomic effects of steroids, neurosteroid effects are mediated through direct actions on membrane receptors and channels. The 3α-reduced neurosteroids, THP and THDOC, are the most potent positive modulators of $GABA_A$ receptor known (Majewska, et al., 1986; Harrison, et al., 1987; Lambert, et al., 1987), resulting in enhanced GABA-mediated chloride currents.

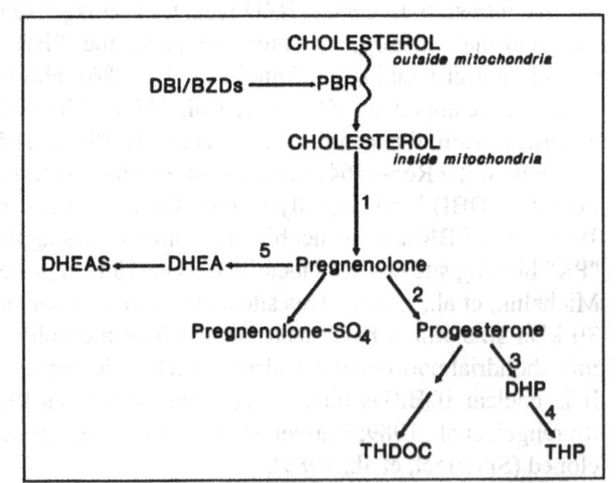

Figure 1. Pathways of neurosteroid synthesis. Numbers refer to biosynthetic enzymes. 1, cytochrome P450scc; 2, 3β-hydroxysteroid dehydrogenase; 3, 5α-reductase; 4, 3α-hydroxysteroid oxidoreductase; 5, 17α-hydroxylase-17-20-desmolase.

Specific steroid binding sites have been identified on the $GABA_A$ receptor which appear to be distinct from the BZD and barbiturate binding sites (Turner, et al., 1989). While pregnenolone, the parent molecule for neurosteroids is thought to be inactive at the $GABA_A$ receptor (Gee, 1988), its sulfated derivative, pregnenolone sulfate (PS), has potent effects on the $GABA_A$ receptor (Majewska, 1992). The binding of PS to brain membrane preparations indicates the existence of 3 binding sites associated with $GABA_A$ receptor: high affinity (5-500 nM); moderate affinity (20 μM); and low affinity (200-300 μM) (Majewska, et al., 1990). The high affinity binding sites (nM) correspond to sites that positively modulate the $GABA_A$ receptor, whereas the lower affinity sites (μM) mediate the negative modulatory effect of PS (Gee, 1988; Paul and Purdy, 1992). Indeed, several studies have demonstrated that nanomolar concentrations (levels of THP found in brain), are sufficient to activate the $GABA_A$ receptor (Gee, 1988). Certain neurosteroids, such as DHEA and its sulfated analogue DHEAS, have negative modulatory effects, but only at micromolar concentrations (Gee, 1988; Paul and Purdy, 1992). The physiological relevance of the antagonistic action of DHEA, DHEAS and PS on the $GABA_A$ receptor is unclear as relatively high concentrations are required for this effect.

While the focus of neurosteroid action has been on the neuronal $GABA_A$ receptor, there are data suggesting that neurosteroids may act directly on glia as well. DHEA and DHEAS increase astrocyte differentiation and decrease astrocyte proliferation in culture (Bologa, et al., 1987) and inhibit gliosis *in vivo* (Garcia-Estrada, et al., 1993). Gonadal hormones have potent effects on astrocytes by influencing their shape, intermediate filament content and distribution (see Garcia-Segura, et al., 1994; Jung-Testas, et al., 1992; Garcia-Estrada, et al., 1993, and references therein).

Most of the neurosteroids appear to be synthesized in glial cells following stimulation by DBI or other agonists of the PBR. It should be emphasized that DBI is an agonist of the PBR, in contrast to its action at the central BZD receptor where it appears to act as an inverse agonist. While it was originally believed that oligodendrocytes were the principal source of neurosteroids (Hu, et al., 1987; Jung-Testas, et al., 1989), there has been increasing evidence that astrocytes are also involved in their synthesis. Neurosteroid synthesis has been described in cultured astrocytes (Romeo, et al., 1992), and in C6 glia after treatment with DBI (Robel, et al., 1991; Papadopoulos, et al., 1992; Guarneri, et al., 1992; Korneyev, et al., 1993). In astrocyte cultures, Mellon and Descheppers (Mellon and Deschepper, 1993) definitively showed cytochrome P450scc and P450scc mRNA, which are required for the conversion of cholesterol to pregnenolone. Astrocytes also possess 5α-reductase most of the 3α-hydroxysteroid dehydrogenase (Krieger and Scott, 1989; Melcangi, et al., 1994), and have been shown to make abundant quantities of THP (Krieger and Scott, 1989; Kabbadj, et al., 1993). Figure 2 depicts glial-neuronal interactions mediated by neurosteroids that are generated by the action of BZDs on the PBR.

THE PBR IN HE/HYPERAMMONEMIA

Since prior studies had focused on the characterization of PBRs in whole membrane preparations and peripheral organs, we then focused our studies on characteristics of PBRs in cultured astrocytes. Saturation and competition binding experiments were performed in homogenate preparations of cultured astrocytes using tritium-labeled Ro5-4864 and PK 11195 (Itzhak, et al., 1993). Results indicated that Ro5-4864 and PK 11195 labeled one common binding site, while PK 11195 labeled an additional site that was less susceptible to binding by Ro5-4864. Subcellular fractionation studies indicated, however, that the binding of both PK

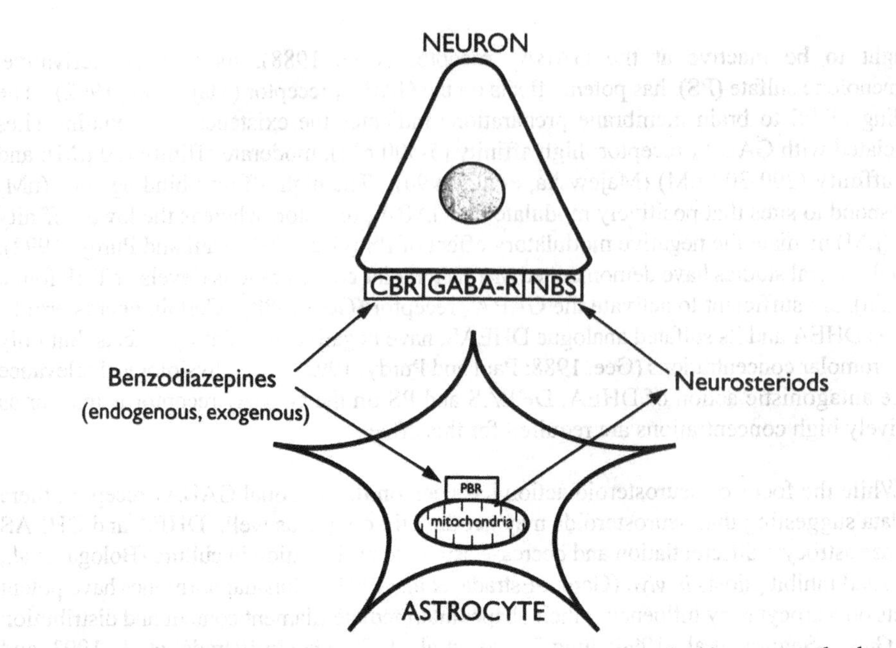

Figure 2. Glial-neuronal interactions mediated by neurosteroids that are synthesized in astrocytes by the action of BZDs on the PBR. Activation of the glial PBR may thus lead to increased $GABA_A$ergic activity. CBR, central benzodiazepine receptor; GABA-R, GABA receptor; NSB, neurosteroid binding site.

11195 and Ro5-4864 was associated primarily with the mitochondrial fraction of astrocytes. This study indicated the existence of non-overlapping PBR binding sites in astrocytes and thus suggests the existence of PBR receptor subtypes.

We had previously observed that ammonia (2-5 mM) caused an increase in the affinity of Ro5-4864 (Ducis, et al., 1988; Ducis, et al., 1989). Since Ro5-4864 and PK 11195 labeled non-overlapping binding sites (Itzhak, et al., 1993), we therefore examined the effect of ammonia on the binding parameters of [^{3}H]PK 11195 (Itzhak and Norenberg, 1994b). Cells treated with 2, 5 and 10 mM ammonium chloride for 24 h ammonia showed a 25, 48 and 44% increase in the Bmax of [^{3}H]PK 11195, respectively. These results demonstrate that ammonia causes upregulation of PK 11195 binding sites, while the same treatment causes primarily an increase in the affinity of Ro5-4864 to the PBR receptors. Using a cDNA probe of the PBR based on the sequence of Sprengel et al. (1989), Northern blot analysis showed that ammonia (5 mM) resulted in a 40% increase in PBR mRNA in cultured astrocytes, which is in good agreement with our binding data (unpublished observations).

Increased numbers of PBR receptors have been found in human postmortem tissue from encephalopathic patients (Lavoie, et al., 1990), and in portacaval-shunted rats (Giguere, et al., 1992). We have investigated whether the administration of ammonium acetate or the hepatotoxin, thioacetamide (TAA), to mice could also modulate PBRs in brain (Itzhak, et al., 1995). Treatment for 3 days with ammonium acetate or TAA showed a 34-55% increase in both the affinity and number of [^{3}H]Ro5-4864 binding sites (Table 1). Similarly, an 85% increase in the affinity and 38-46% increase in the number of [^{3}H]PK 11195 binding sites were observed in the ammonia- and TAA-treated animals as compared to control.

Table 1. Effect of 3-day treatment with thioacetamide (100 mg/kg) and ammonium acetate (5 mmol/kg) on PBRs in mouse brain

	[^{3}H]Ro5-4864		[^{3}H]PK 11195	
	Kd	Bmax	Kd	Bmax
Control	5.1±0.4	241±19	2.5±0.2	435±38
TAA	2.4±0.2 (-53%)*	322±23 (+34%)*	1.4±0.1(-44%) *	602±72 (+38%)*
NH_4 acetate	2.3±0.3 (-55%)*	351±38 (+45%)*	1.5±0.1(-40%)*	638±55 (+46%)*

Results represent the mean ± S.E.M of 3 experiments. Kd, dissociation constant in nM. Bmax, maximal number of binding sites in fmol/mg protein. *p<0.02. (From Itzhak, et al., 1995, with permission).

PK 11195 is an antagonist of the PBR. We reasoned that if the PBR was upregulated in hyperammonemia, blockage of this receptor might exert a protective effect in hyperammonemic states. We therefore examined the effect of PK 11195 in hyperammonemia (Itzhak and Norenberg, 1994a). Administration of ammonium acetate (8-15 mmol/kg, i.p.) to Swiss Webster mice resulted in a dose-dependent increase in mortality. Pretreatment with the "central" benzodiazepine receptor agonist clonazepam, or the "central" antagonist Ro15-1788 (flumazenil) (7 mg/kg each, i.p.) had no significant effect on the lethal response to 10 mmol/kg ammonium acetate. However, pretreatment with the putative antagonist of the PBR, PK 11195 (10 mg/kg, i.p.), reduced animal mortality from 50% to 10% (see Fig. 3).

We had speculated that the generation of positive modulators of the $GABA_A$ receptor derived from pregnenolone might have a causal role in HE, while negative modulators might be beneficial. To test this idea, we examined the effect of pregnenolone sulfate, an agent with negative modulatory effects on the $GABA_A$ receptor. Pregnenolone sulfate (PS; 20 mg/kg, i.p.) reduced animal mortality from 50 to 25% (Fig. 3). This dose of PS gives rise to approximately 1 μM of PS in brain, which is within the range required for the negative modulatory effect on the $GABA_A$ receptor.

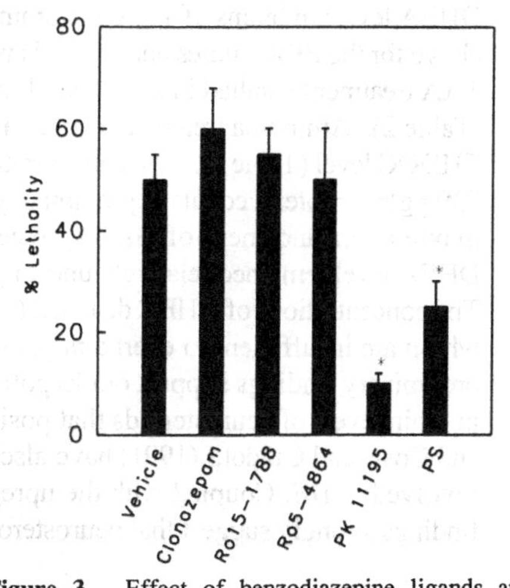

Figure 3. Effect of benzodiazepine ligands and pregnenolone sulfate (PS) on ammonia-induced toxicity. (Modified from Itzhak and Norenberg, 1994a, with permission).

NEUROSTEROIDS IN HE/HYPERAMMONEMIA

The above studies implicated the PBR in the pathogenesis of HE. Since the principal function of the PBR appears to be the generation of neurosteroids, we next investigated whether neurosteroids were also involved in HE (Itzhak, et al., 1995). Pregnenolone (the parent compound of neurosteroids) levels were determined in brain extracts from hyperammonemic mice, and mice treated with TAA by RIA. As shown in Fig. 4, brain pregnenolone levels from ammonia- and TAA-treated mice were elevated by 81 and 70%, respectively. The levels obtained in the membrane preparation, 50 pg/mg protein, correspond to ~15 nM. We also determined the total concentration of pregnenolone in whole brain homogenates (i.e., without centrifugation) of control, TAA and ammonium acetate-treated mice. Under these conditions, a higher concentration (50-60 nM) of pregnenolone was detected. Blood levels of pregnenolone were not elevated.

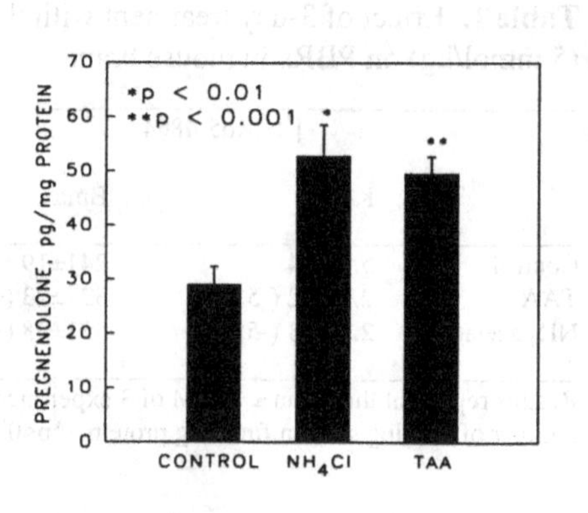

Figure 4. Pregnenolone levels in brain of mice treated with ammonium acetate and in TAA-treated animals with liver failure.

Since pregnenolone synthesis is dependent on the integrity of the PBR, we investigated the effect of DBI, an endogenous ligand of the PBR, on the rate of pregnenolone synthesis in the P-2 (mitochondrial) fraction obtained from hyperammonemic animals and animals treated with TAA (Itzhak, et al., 1995). DBI (5-10 nM) caused a 45-50% increase in pregnenolone synthesis. These findings suggest that brain is the source of the elevated neurosteroids found in hyperammonemia/HE.

To extend these pregnenolone studies, we have recently measured THP, THDOC, and DHEA levels in brains of TAA and ammonia-treated mice. Animals were treated as described above for the PBR studies and steroids were analyzed by HPLC/RIA. The results indicate that TAA treatment resulted in a marked (4- and 2-fold) increase in THDOC and THP, respectively (Table 2). Ammonia treatment caused a marked rise in THP but had only a minimal effect on THDOC level (Table 2). The concentration of THP detected in the brain of TAA-treated mice, 939 pg/mg protein, equals approximately 295 nM, a concentration which is known to produce maximal enhancement of $GABA_A$ receptor function (Lambert, et al., 1995). By contrast, DHEA level remained relatively unchanged following treatment with either TAA or ammonia. The concentrations of DHEA detected (117-125 pg/mg protein) equal approximately 35-38 nM which are insufficient to exert a negative modulatory effect on the $GABA_A$ receptor. These preliminary findings support our hypothesis that HE is associated primarily with an increase in brain levels of neurosteroids that positively modulate the $GABA_A$ receptor. Zaman (1990) and Costa and Guidotti (1991) have also suggested the possibility that neurosteroids may be involved in HE. Coupled with the upregulation of PBRs observed in the same animals, our findings strongly suggest that neurosteroid elevation is caused by an upregulation of the PBR.

Table 2. Neurosteroids in brain extracts of control, thioacetamide and ammonium acetate treated mice (pg/mg protein)

	THDOC	THP	DHEA
Control	50	451	117
TAA	217 (434%)	939 (208%)	125 (107%)
NH_4Ac	58 (116%)	636 (141%)	121 (103%)

Since cultured astrocytes exposed to ammonia results in an increase in PBR binding sites (Itzhak and Norenberg, 1994b) (see above), we examined whether this receptor upregulation was associated with an increase in the production of pregnenolone (Norenberg, et al., 1995).

We determined the basal and DBI-stimulated levels of pregnenolone in control and ammonia-treated cultured astrocytes. Following 24 h exposure to 5 mM ammonium chloride, cell membranes were incubated with mevalonolactone (10 mM) and DBI (10 μM) for 15 min at 37°C, steroids subsequently extracted with n-hexane, and pregnenolone levels were determined by RIA. Results presented in Fig. 5 indicate that DBI alone resulted in an 86% increase in pregnenolone synthesis; however, when added to ammonia-treated cells, DBI caused a 193% increase in pregnenolone synthesis. These findings, coupled with the ammonia-induced PBR upregulation, further supports a correlation between the elevated production of pregnenolone and the increase in PBR binding sites.

If neurosteroids are indeed involved in HE, we investigated whether the administration of THP and THDOC to mice can produce HE-like symptoms and histopathology. THP and THDOC solutions (20 mg/kg, each) were prepared in DMSO: β-cylodextrin (45%): water (1:2:1) (vehicle). The dose of THP used was calculated to achieve a brain level approximating that observed in animal models of HE (200-300 nM, based on results presented in Table 2) that is within the pathophysiological relevant concentrations known to have a maximal effect on the $GABA_A$ receptor (Lambert, et al., 1995). For comparison, we also examined the effect of TAA (100 mg/kg) which was prepared in the same vehicle. Control animals received vehicle only (0.1 ml/10 g). All drug solutions were administered for 3 consecutive days. Stage of encephalopathy was graded by the criteria of Gammal et al. (1990) and the results are summarized in Table 3. Our findings demonstrate that THP produces potent sedative effects in mice, and following the third injection, 2 out of 4 animals were in coma that lasted 2-3 h. The sedative effects of THP are long lasting since 24 h after the administration of the third injection animals remained in stage 3 encephalopathy. THDOC was found to be less potent, and the maximal stage observed was 3 in 2 out of the 4 animals tested. The most pronounced effects produced by TAA were observed 24 h after the administration of the third TAA injection. The maximal stage recorded was 3. The delayed response to TAA, as opposed to THP, is due to the fact that TAA first has to produce liver toxicity, which then leads to HE. THP, however, has immediate direct effects on $GABA_A$ receptor.

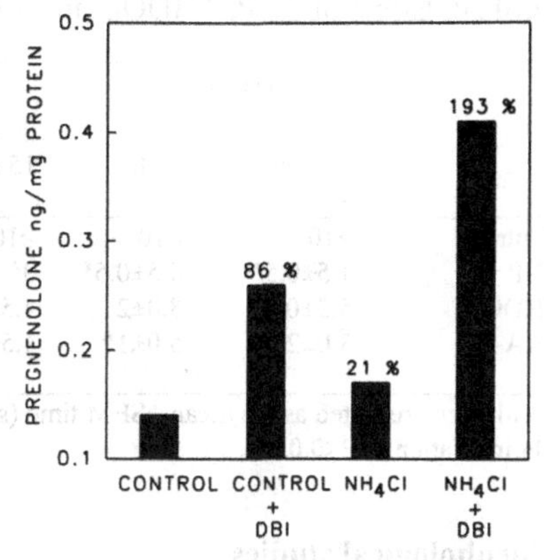

Figure 5. Pregnenolone levels in cultured astrocytes treated with ammonia and DBI..

Table 3. Effect of THP, THDOC and TAA on animal behavior

	Day 1		Day 2		Day 3	
	15 min	24 h	15 min	24 h	15 min	24 h
Control	0	0	0	0	0	0
THP	2-3	1	4	1	4-5	3
THDOC	1	0	2	0	2-3	1
TAA	0	1	1	3	3	3

Behavior was scored on a 5-stage scale, 15 min and 24 h after daily drug administration: 0 = normal behavior (moving about the cage, sniffing and rearing); 1 = lethargy; 2 = mild ataxia; 3 = lack of spontaneous activity, but normal righting reflex; 4 = loss of righting reflex; 5 = coma. N=4 for each condition.

In addition to animal behavior, motor coordination was also examined by measuring the time that animals stayed on a metal bar (50 cm long x 0.9 cm diameter) without falling (normal mice were able to maintain balance for more than 10 sec). Results presented in Table 4 show once again that THP is a much more potent CNS depressant than THDOC. The highest impairment of motor coordination produced by TAA was evident 24 h after the third injection of TAA. Taken together, the results observed suggest that THP produces CNS depressant effects similar to the outcome of exposure to the hepatotoxin, TAA. In a previous study (Itzhak and Norenberg, 1994a), we injected pregnenolone sulfate (20 mg/kg), a negative modulator of the $GABA_A$ receptor, and no behavioral changes were observed.

Table 4. Effect of THP, THDOC and TAA on motor coordination

	Day 1		Day 2		Day 3	
	15 min	24 h	15 min	24 h	15 min	24 h
Control	>10	>10	>10	>10	>10	>10
THP	1.5±0.5*	4.5±0.5*	0*	3.2±0.3*	0*	1.5±0.5*
THDOC	5.5±0.5*	8.0±2	4.5±1*	6.5±1	3.5±0.5	5.5±0.5*
TAA	8.0±2	5.0±1*	4.5±0.5*	2.5±0.5*	3.0±1*	1.5±0.5*

Results are presented as the mean ±SEM time (seconds) spent on a bar, 15 min and 24 h after daily drug administration. *P<0.05.

Morphological studies

Brains of mice treated with neurosteroids were fixed by immersion in 10% formaldehyde and processed routinely for hematoxylin and eosin staining. As shown in Fig. 6, 3-day treatment with THP resulted in Alzheimer type II-like changes in astrocytes, characterized by enlarged pale nuclei, and chromatin margination. Increased numbers of astrocytes were apparent as evidenced by the frequency of paired and triplet nuclei. The changes were seen throughout the CNS including cerebral cortex, basal ganglia, thalamus, brainstem and cerebellum (Bergmann glia). They were particularly striking in the basal forebrain, and striatum and less evident in the white matter. No changes were observed in neurons or other cellular elements. These histological findings, which constitute the classic changes observed in human and experimental HE, correlated with the level of encephalopathy (Tables 3 and 4). THDOC showed similar changes but were of lesser magnitude than THP. These results show that neurosteroids are capable of inducing alterations in brain that correspond with changes described in patients with HE.

BZDs AND ASTROCYTE SWELLING

Astrocyte swelling is the dominant morphologic change in acute HE. The importance of astrocyte swelling lies in its mass effect resulting in increased intracranial pressure and in a reduction in cerebral blood flow by compression of the cerebral microvasculature. Another important effect of swelling is its impact on glial function.

The factors responsible for glial swelling are poorly understood. Swelling correlates well with levels of ammonia (Swain, et al., 1992; Ganz, et al., 1989), and cell culture studies have

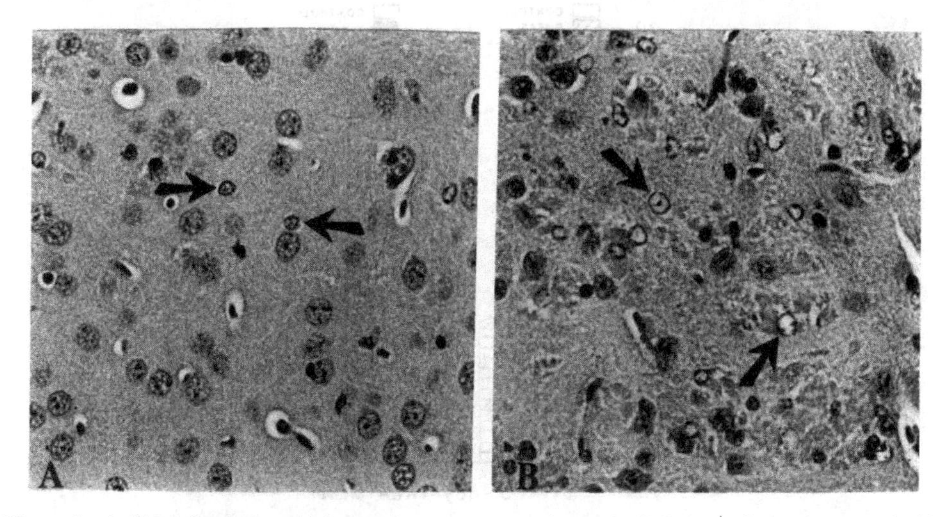

Figure 6. A. Normal striatum with inconspicuous astrocytes (arrows). B Striatum from mice treated with THP showing numerous Alzheimer type II-like astrocytes (arrows), characterized by enlarged pale nuclei and marginated chromatin. (H and E, x300).

shown that 3-day treatment with ammonia results in glial swelling (Norenberg, et al., 1991). More recently, we have found that co-treatment of cells with ammonia and glutamate caused a rise in cell volume as early as one hour (unpublished observations). The mechanism for ammonia-induced glial swelling is not known, although recent studies have suggested that the generation of glutamine during the ammonia detoxification process may generate excessive intracellular osmoles leading to the influx of water and cell swelling (Takahashi, et al., 1991).

We have investigated the possibility that BZDs and neurosteroids may also be involved in influencing glial cell volume (Norenberg and Bender, 1994). Our studies indicated that the PBR agonist Ro5-4864 (10 μM) enhanced the ammonia-induced swelling in cultured astrocytes by 20%, while the PBR antagonist PK 11195 (10 μM) attenuated such swelling by 23% (Fig. 7). These findings suggest that BZDs exacerbate ammonia-induced astroglial swelling which may contribute to the morbidity of acute HE.

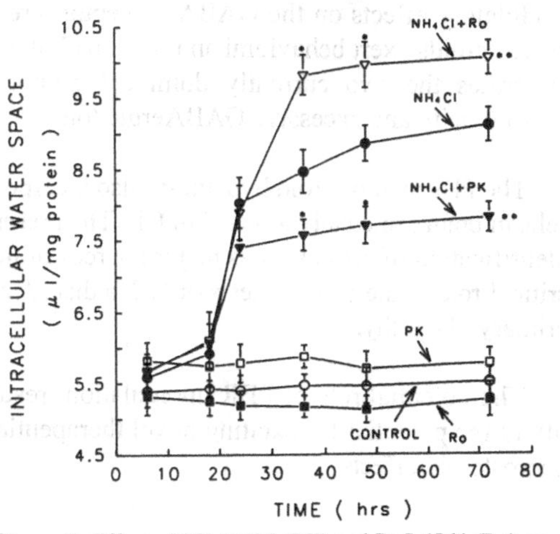

Figure 7. Effect of PK 11195 (PK) and Ro5-4864 (Ro) on ammonia-induced astrocyte swelling. (Modified from Norenberg and Bender, 1994, with permission).

We have also examined the effects of various neurosteroids on cell volume and on ammonia-induced astrocyte swelling. Three day treatment with neurosteroids at 1-10 μM slightly increased cell swelling. However, ammonia-induced swelling was potentiated by 60% (Fig. 8).

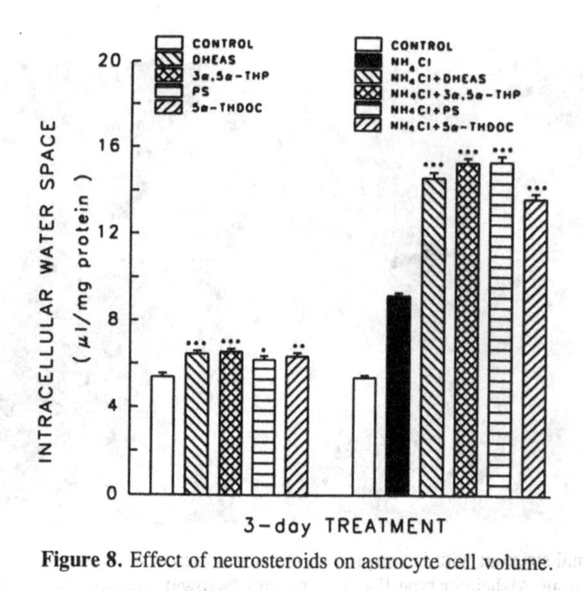

Figure 8. Effect of neurosteroids on astrocyte cell volume.

SUMMARY

Ammonia and astrocytes are inextricably involved in the mechanism of HE. We propose that ammonia, by upregulating the astrocytic peripheral benzodiazepine receptor, results in the production of neurosteroids that exert a positive modulatory effect on the $GABA_A$ receptor which contributes to the neuroinhibition and neurologic dysfunction associated with hepatic encephalopathy. In support for this hypothesis, we, and others, have shown: 1) that the PBR is upregulated in animal models of hyperammonemia/HE as well as in ammonia-treated astrocyte cultures; 2) that PK 11195, a specific blocker of the PBR, ameliorates ammonia toxicity *in vivo*; 3) that the synthesis of pregnenolone, the parent compound for all neurosteroids, is increased in ammonia-treated astrocyte cultures and in *in vivo* models of HE; 4) that levels of THP and THDOC, pregnenolone-derived neurosteroids with positive modulatory effects on the $GABA_A$ receptor, are elevated in animal models of HE; and 5) neurosteroids exert behavioral and neuropathologic changes similar to HE. This hypothesis integrates the two currently dominant pathogenetic views of HE, namely, ammonia neurotoxicity and excessive GABAergic tone.

The PBR/neurosteroid hypothesis also incorporates the pathogenetic role of astrocytes, the cells in brain principally affected in HE. The presence of the PBR on astrocytes as well as the identification of astrocytes as major sources of neurosteroids serves again to highlight their critical role in the pathogenesis of HE, a disorder which we have viewed for some time as a primary gliopathy.

The potential role of PBR upregulation resulting in increased neurosteroid production offers the potential for exciting novel therapeutic approaches to HE through modulation of neurosteroid effects.

Acknowledgments

The authors are grateful to Dr. Roy Dombro for his assistance and advice in the conduct of our studies; to Linnell Baker and Ana Roig-Cantisano for technical support, and to Dr. Jocelyn Bruce for her critical review of the manuscript.

REFERENCES

Abramovitz, M., Homma, H., Ishigaki, S., Tansey, F., Cammer, W., and Listowsky, I., 1988, Characterization and localization of glutathione-S-transferases in rat brain and binding of hormones, neurotransmitters, and drugs, *J. Neurochem.* 50:50.

Adams, R.D., and Foley, J.M., 1953, The neurological disorder associated with liver disease, *Assoc. Res. Nerv. Ment. Dis. Proc.* 32:198.

Anderson, R.E., Engstrom, F.L., and Woodbury, D.M., 1984, Localization of carbonic anhydrase in the cerebellum of normal and audiogenic seizure mice, *Ann. N. Y. Acad. Sci.* 429:502.

Anholt, R.R.H., Pedersen, P.L., DeSouza, E.B., and Snyder, S.H., 1986, The peripheral-type benzodiazepine receptor: localization to the mitochondrial outer membrane, *J. Biol. Chem.* 261:576.

Antkiewicz Michaluk, L., Mukhin, A.G., Guidotti, A., and Krueger, K.E., 1988, Purification and characterization of a protein associated with peripheral-type benzodiazepine binding sites, *J. Biol. Chem.* 263:17317.

Basile, A.S., Jones, E.A., and Skolnick, P., 1991, The pathogenesis and treatment of hepatic encephalopathy: evidence for the involvement of benzodiazepine receptor ligands, *Pharmacol. Rev.* 43:27.

Baulieu, E.E. ,1991, Neurosteroids: a new function in the brain, *Biol. Cell.* 71:3.

Belelli, D., Bolger, M.B., and Gee, K.W., 1989, Anticonvulsant profile of the progesterone metabolite 5-α-pregnan-3-α-ol-20-one, *Eur . J. Pharmacol.* 166:325.

Benavides, J., Quarteronet, D., Imbault, F., Malgouris, C., Uzan, A., Renault, C., Dubroeucq, M.C., Gueremy, C., and Le Fur, G., 1983, Labelling of "peripheral-type" benzodiazepine binding sites in the rat brain by using [^{3}H]PK 11195, an isoquinoline carboxamide derivative: kinetic studies and autoradiographic localization, *J. Neurochem.* 41:1744.

Bender, A.S., and Hertz, L., 1985, Binding of (^{3}H) Ro5-4864 in primary cultures of astrocytes, *Brain Res.* 341:41.

Bender, A.S., and Norenberg, M.D., 1996, Effects of ammonia on L-glutamate uptake in cultured astrocytes, *Neurochem. Res.* 21:567.

Bitran, D., Hilvers, R.J., and Kellog, C.K., 1991, Anxiolytic effects of 3 α-hydroxy-5α[β]-pregnan-20-one: endogenous metabolites of progesterone that are active at the GABA-A receptor, *Brain Res.* 561:157.

Bologa, L., Sharma, J., and Roberts, E., 1987, Dehydroepiandrosterone and its sulfated derivative reduce neuronal death and enhance astrocytic differentiation in brain cell cultures, *J. Neurosci. Res.* 17: 274.

Butterworth, R.F., 1991, Pathophysiology of hepatic encephalopathy; the ammonia hypothesis revisited, in: *Progress in Hepatic Encephalopathy and Metabolic Nitrogen Exchange,* F. Bengtsson, B. Jeppsson, T. Almdal, and H. Vilstrup, eds., CRC Press, Boca Raton.

Butterworth, R.F., 1992, Pathogenesis and treatment of portal-systemic encephalopathy: an update, *Dig. Dis. Sci.* 37:321.

Cooper, A.J.L., and Plum, F., 1987, Biochemistry and physiology of brain ammonia, *Physiol. Rev.* 67:440.

Costa, E., and Guidotti, A., 1991, Diazepam binding inhibitor (DBI): a peptide with multiple biological actions, *Life Sci.* 49:325.

Ducis, I., Norenberg, L.O.B., and Norenberg, M.D., 1988, Effect of ammonia on the benzodiazepine receptor in cultured astrocytes, *Soc. Neurosci. Abst.* 14:1082.

Ducis, I., Norenberg, L.O.B., and Norenberg, M.D., 1989, Effect of ammonium chloride on the astrocyte benzodiazepine receptor, *Brain Res.* 499:362.

Fitzpatrick, S.M., Cooper, A.J., and Hertz, L., 1988, Effects of ammonia and β-methylene-DL-aspartate on the oxidation of glucose and pyruvate by neurons and astrocytes in primary culture, *J. Neurochem.* 51:1197.

Gammal, S.H., Basile, A.S., Geller, D., Skolnick, P., and Jones, E.A., 1990, Reversal of the behavioral and electrophysiological abnormalities of an animal model of hepatic encephalopathy by benzodiazepine receptor ligands, *Hepatology*, 11:371.

Ganz, R., Swain, M., Traber, P., DalCanto, M., Butterworth, R.F., and Blei, A.T., 1989, Ammonia-induced swelling of rat cerebral cortical slices: implications for the pathogenesis of brain edema in acute hepatic failure, *Metab. Brain Dis.* 4:213.

Garcia-Estrada, J., Del Rio, J.A., Luquin, S., Soriano, E., and Garcia-Segura, L.M., 1993, Gonadal hormones down-regulate reactive gliosis and astrocyte proliferation after a penetrating brain injury, *Brain Res.* 628:271.

Garcia-Segura, L.M., Luquín, S., Párducz, A., and Naftolin, F., 1994, Gonadal hormone regulation of glial fibrillary acidic protein immunoreactivity and glial ultrastructure in the rat neuroendocrine hypothalamus, *Glia*, 10:59.

Garnier, M., Dimchev, A.B., Boujrad, N., Price, J.M., Musto, N.A., and Papadopoulos, V., 1994, *In vitro* reconstitution of a functional peripheral-type benzodiazepine receptor from mouse Leydig tumor cells, *Mol. Pharmacol.* 45:201.

Gee, K.W., 1988, Steroid modulation of the GABA/benzodiazepine receptor-linked chloride ionophore, *Molec. Neurobiol.* 313:291.

Giguere, J.F., Hamel, E., and Butterworth, R.F., 1992, Increased densities of binding sites for the 'peripheral-type' benzodiazepine receptor ligand [^{3}H]PK 11195 in rat brain following portacaval anastomosis, *Brain Res.* 585:295.

Guarneri, P., Guarneri, R., Cascio, C., Pavasant, P., Piccoli, F., and Papadopoulos, V., 1994, Neurosteroidogenesis in rat retinas, *J. Neurochem.* 63:86.

Guarneri, P., Papadopoulos, V., Pan, B., and Costa, E., 1992, Regulation of pregnenolone synthesis in C6-2B glioma cells by 4'-chlorodiazepam, *Proc. Natl. Acad. Sci. U. S. A.* 89:5118.

Guidotti, A., Forchetti, C.M., Corda, M.G., Konkel, D., Bennett, C.D., and Costa, E., 1983, Isolation and characterization and purification to homogeneity of an endogenous polypeptide with agonistic action on benzodiazepine receptors, *Proc. Natl. Acad. Sci. U. S. A.* 80:3531.

Harrison, N.L., Majewska, M.D., Harrington, J.W., and Barker, J.L., 1987, Structure activity relationships for steroid interaction with the gamma-aminobutyric acidA receptor complex, *J. Pharmacol. Exp. Ther.* 241:346.

Hertz, L., McFarlin, D., and Waksman, B., 1990, Astrocytes: auxiliary cells for immune responses in the central nervous system, *Immunol. Today*, 11:265.

Hertz, L., Murthy, C.R.K., Lai, J.C.K., Fitzpatrick, S.M., and Cooper, A.J.L., 1987, Some metabolic effects of ammonia on astrocytes and neurons in primary culture, *Neurochem. Pathol.* 6:97.

Hu, Z.Y., Bourreau, E., Jung-Testas, I., Robel, P., and Baulieu, E.-E., 1987, Neurosteroids: oligodendrocyte mitochondria convert cholesterol to pregnenolone, *Proc. Natl. Acad. Sci. U. S. A.* 84:8215.

Itzhak, Y., Baker, L., and Norenberg, M.D., 1993, Characterization of the peripheral-type benzodiazepine receptor in cultured astrocytes: evidence for multiplicity, *Glia*, 9:211.

Itzhak, Y., and Norenberg, M.D., 1994a, Attenuation of ammonia toxicity in mice by PK 11195 and pregnenolone sulfate, *Neurosci. Lett.* 182:251.

Itzhak, Y., and Norenberg, M.D., 1994b, Ammonia-induced upregulation of peripheral-type benzodiazepine receptors in cultured astrocytes labeled with [^{3}H]PK 11195, *Neurosci. Lett.* 177:35.

Itzhak, Y., Roig-Cantisano, A., Dombro, R.S., and Norenberg, M.D., 1995, Acute liver failure and hyperammonemia increase peripheral-type benzodiazepine receptor binding and pregnenolone synthesis in mouse brain, *Brain Res.* 705: 345.

Janzer, R.C., and Raff, M.C., 1987, Astrocytes induce blood-brain barrier properties in endothelial cells, *Nature*, 325: 253.

Jones, E.A., and Schafer, D.F., 1986, Hepatic encephalopathy: a neurochemical disorder, *Prog. Liver Dis.* 8: 525.

Jung-Testas, I., Hu, Z.Y., Baulieu, E.E., and Robel, P., 1989, Neurosteroids: biosynthesis of pregnenolone and progesterone in primary cultures of rat glial cells, *Endocrinology*, 125:2083.

Jung-Testas, I., Renoir, M., Bugnard, H., Greene, G.L., and Baulieu, E.-E., 1992, Demonstration of steroid hormone receptors and steroid action in primary cultures of rat glial cells, *J. Steroid Biochem. Mol. Biol.* 41:621.

Kabbadj, K., El-Etr, M., Baulieu, E.-E., and Robel, P., 1993, Pregnenolone metabolism in rodent embryonic neurons and astrocytes, *Glia*, 7:170.

Kato, M., Hughes, R.D., Keays, R.T., and Williams, R., 1992, Electron microscopic study of brain capillaries in cerebral edema from fulminant hepatic failure, *Hepatology*, 15:1060.

Keyser, D.O., and Pellmar, T.C., 1994, Synaptic transmission in the hippocampus: critical role for glial cells, *Glia*, 10:237.

Kimelberg, H.K., Jalonen, T., and Walz, W., 1993, Regulation of the brain microenvironment: transmitters and ions, in: *Astrocytes: Pharmacology and Function*, S. Murphy, ed., Academic Press, San Diego.

Korneyev, A., Guidotti, A., and Costa, E., 1993, Regional and interspecies differences in brain progesterone metabolism, *J. Neurochem.* 61:2041.

Korneyev, A., Pan, B.S., Polo, A., Romeo, E., Guidotti, A., and Costa, E., 1993, Stimulation of brain pregnenolone synthesis by mitochondrial diazepam binding inhibitor receptor ligands in vivo, *J. Neurochem.* 61:1515.

Krieger, N.R., and Scott, R.G., 1989, Nonneuronal localization for steroid converting enzyme: 3α-hydroxysteroid oxidoreducatase in olfactory tubercle of rat brain, *J. Neurochem.* 52:1866.

Krueger, K.E., and Papadopoulos, V., 1990, Peripheral-type benzodiazepine receptors mediate translocation of cholesterol from outer to inner mitochondrial membranes in adrenocortical cells, *J. Biol. Chem.* 265:15015.

Krueger, K.E., and Papadopoulos, V., 1992, Mitochondrial benzodiazepine receptors and the regulation of steroid biosynthesis, *Annu. Rev. Pharmacol. Toxicol.* 32:211.

Lambert, J.J., Belelli, D., Hill-Venning, C., and Peters, J.A., 1995, Neurosteroids and $GABA_A$ receptor function, *Trends Pharmacol. Sci.* 16:295.

Lambert, J.J., Peters, J.A., and Cotrell, G.A., 1987, Actions of synthetic and endogenous steroids on the $GABA_A$ receptor, *Trends Pharmacol. Sci.* 8:224.

Lavoie, J., Layrargues, G.P., and Butterworth, R.F., 1990, Increased densities of peripheral-type benzodiazepine receptors in brain autopsy samples from cirrhotic patients with hepatic encephalopathy, *Hepatology*, 11:874.

Lockwood, A.H., 1992, *Hepatic Encephalopathy,* Butterworth-Heinemann, Boston.

Macdonald, R.L., and Olsen, R.W., 1994, $GABA_A$ receptor channels, *Annu. Rev. Neurosci.* 17:569.

Majewska, M.D., 1992, Neurosteroids: endogenous bimodal modulators of the $GABA_A$ receptor: mechanism of action and physiological significance, *Prog. Neurobiol.* 38:379.

Majewska, M.D., Demirgoren, S., and London, E.D., 1990, Binding of pregnenolone sulfate to rat brain membranes suggests multiple sites of steroid action action at the GABA-A receptor, *Eur. J. Pharmacol.* 189:307.

Majewska, M.D., Harrison, N.L., Schwartz, R.D., Barker, J.L., and Paul, S.M., 1986, Steroid hormone metabolites are barbiturate-like modulators of the GABA receptor, *Science*, 232:1004.

Makar, T.K., Nedergaard, M., Preuss, A., Gelbard, A.S., Perumal, A.S., and Cooper, A.J., 1994, Vitamin E, ascorbate, glutathione, glutathione disulfide, and enzymes of glutathione metabolism in cultures of chick astrocytes and neurons: evidence that astrocytes play an important role in antioxidative processes in the brain, *J. Neurochem.* 62:45.

Martin, H., Voss, K., Hufnagl, P., Wack, R., and Wassilew, G., 1987, Morphometric and densitometric investigations of protoplasmic astrocytes and neurons in human hepatic encephalopathy, *Exp. Pathol.* 32:241.

McCarthy, K.D., and Harden, T.K., 1981, Identification of two benzodiazepine binding sites on cells cultured from rat cerebral cortex, *J. Pharmacol. Exp. Ther.* 216:183.

McEnery, M.W., Snowman, A.M., Trifiletti, R.R., and Snyder, S.H., 1992, Isolation of the mitochondrial benzodiazepine receptor: association with the voltage-dependent anion channel and the adenine nucleotide carrier, *Proc. Natl. Acad. Sci. U. S. A.* 89:3170.

Melcangi, R.C., Celotti, F., and Martini, L., 1994, Progesterone 5-α-reduction in neuronal and in different types of glial cell cultures: type 1 and 2 astrocytes and oligodendrocytes, *Brain Res.* 639: 202.

Mellon, S.H., and Deschepper, C.F., 1993, Neurosteroid biosynthesis: genes for adrenal steroidogenic enzymes are expressed in the brain, *Brain Res.* 629:283.

Mennerick, S., and Zorumski, C.F., 1994, Glial contributions to excitatory neurotransmission in cultured hippocampal cells, *Nature*, 368:59.

Mok, W.M., Herschkowitz, S., and Krieger, N.R., 1991, In vivo studies identify 5α-pregnan-3α-ol-20-one as an active anesthetic agent, *J. Neurochem.* 57:1296.

Moynagh, P.N., Bailey, C.J., Boyce, S.J., and Williams, D.C., 1991, Immunological studies on the rat peripheral-type benzodiazepine acceptor, *Biochem. J.* 275:419.

Mukhin, A.G., Papadopoulos, V., Costa, E., and Krueger, K.E., 1989, Mitochondrial benzodiazepine receptors regulate steroid biosynthesis, *Proc. Natl. Acad. Sci. U. S. A.* 86:9813.

Murthy, C.R., and Hertz, L., 1987, Acute effect of ammonia on branched-chain amino acid oxidation and incorporation into proteins in astrocytes and in neurons in primary cultures, *J. Neurochem.* 49:735.

Myers, R., Manjil, L.G., Cullen, B.M., Price, G.W., Franckowiak, R.S., and Cremer, J.E., 1991, Macrophage and astrocyte populations in relation to (^{3}H)PK 11195 binding following a local ischemic lesion, *J. Cereb. Blood Flow Metab.* 11:314.

Nedergaard, M., 1994, Direct signaling from astrocytes to neurons in cultures of mammalian brain cells, *Science*, 263:1768.

Norenberg, M.D., 1977, A light and electron microscopic study of experimental portal-systemic (ammonia) encephalopathy, *Lab. Invest.* 36:618.

Norenberg, M.D., 1979, The distribution of glutamine synthetase in the rat central nervous system, *J. Histochem. Cytochem.* 27:756.

Norenberg, M.D., 1981, The astrocyte in liver disease, in: *Advances in Cellular Neurobiology, Vol. 2,* S. Fedoroff and L. Hertz, eds., Academic Press, New York.

Norenberg, M.D., 1983, Immunohistochemistry of glutamine synthetase, in: *Glutamine, Glutamate, and GABA in the Central Nervous System,* L. Hertz, E. Kvamme, E.G. McGeer, and A. Schousboe, eds., Alan R. Liss, New York.

Norenberg, M.D., 1995, Hepatic encephalopathy, in: *Neuroglia,* H. Kettenmann and B.R. Ransom, eds., Oxford, New York.

Norenberg, M.D. Astrocytic-ammonia interactions in hepatic encephalopathy. *Semin. Liver Dis.* (In press).

Norenberg, M.D., Baker, L., Norenberg, L.-O.B., Blicharska, J., Bruce-Gregorios, J.H., and Neary, J.T., 1991, Ammonia-induced astrocyte swelling in primary culture, *Neurochem. Res.* 16:833.

Norenberg, M.D., and Bender, A.S., 1994, Astrocyte swelling in liver failure: role of glutamine and benzodiazepines, *Acta Neurochir.* 60 (Suppl):24.

Norenberg, M.D., Neary, J.T., Bender, A.S., and Dombro, R.S., 1992, Hepatic encephalopathy: a disorder in glial-neuronal communication, in: *Neuronal-Astrocytic Interactions. Implications for Normal and Pathological CNS Function,* A.C.H. Yu, L. Hertz, M.D. Norenberg, E. Sykova, and S.G. Waxman, eds., Elsevier, Amsterdam.

Norenberg, M.D., Roig-Cantisano, A., and Itzhak, Y., 1995, Peripheral benzodiazepine receptors and pregnenolone synthesis in models of hepatic encephalopathy and in ammonia-treated astrocytes, *J. Neurochem.* 64 (Suppl):56.

O'Beirne, G.B., Woods, M.J., and Williams, D.C., 1990, Two subcellular locations for peripheral-type benzodiazepine acceptors in rat liver, *Eur. J. Biochem.* 188:131.

Olsen, R.W., and Tobin, A.J., 1990, Molecular biology of $GABA_A$ receptors, *FASEB J.* 4:1469.

Papadopoulos, V., and Brown, A.S., 1995, Role of the peripheral-type benzodiazepine receptor and the polypeptide diazepam binding inhibitor in steroidogenesis, *J. Steroid Biochem. Mol. Biol.* 53:103.

Papadopoulos, V., Guarneri, P., Krueger, K.E., Guidotti, A., and Costa, E., 1992, Pregnenolone biosynthesis in C6-2B glioma cell mitochondria: regulation by a mitochondrial diazepam binding inhibitor receptor, *Proc. Natl. Acad. Sci. U. S. A.* 89:5113.

Park, C.H., Carboni, E., Wood, P.L., and Gee, K.W., 1996, Characterization of peripheral benzodiazepine type sites in a cultured murine BV-2 microglial cell line, *Glia,* 16:65.

Parola, A.L., Yamamura, H.I., and Laird, H.E.I., 1993, Peripheral-type benzodiazepine receptors, *Life Sci.* 52:1329.

Parpura, V., Basarsky, T.A., Liu, F., Jeftinija, K., Jeftinija, S., and Haydon, P.G., 1994, Glutamate-mediated astrocyte-neuron signalling, *Nature,* 369:744.

Paul, S.M., and Purdy, R.H., 1992, Neuroactive steroids, *FASEB J.* 6:2311.

Purdy, R.H., Morrow, A.L., Moore, P.H., and Paul, S.M., 1991, Stress-induced elevation of gamma-aminobutyric acid type A receptor-active steroids in rat brain, *Proc. Natl. Acad. Sci. U. S. A.* 88: 4553.

Raabe, W.A., 1989, Neurophysiology of ammonia intoxication, in: *Hepatic Encephalopathy: Physiology and Treatment,* R.F. Butterworth and G. Pomier Layrargues, eds., Humana Press, Clifton, New Jersey.

Ransom, B.R., and Sontheimer, H., 1992, The neurophysiology of glial cells, *J. Clin. Neurophysiol.* 9:224.

Rao, V.L.R., Murthy, C.R.K., and Butterworth, R.F. ,1992, Glutamatergic synaptic dysfunction in hyperammonemic syndromes, *Metab. Brain Dis.* 7:1.

Record, C.O., 1991, Neurochemistry of hepatic encephalopathy, *Gut,* 32:1261.

Risau, W., and Wolburg, H., 1990, Development of the blood-brain barrier, *Trends Neurosci.* 13:174.

Robel, P., Jung-Testas, I., Hu, Z.Y., Akwa, Y., Sananes, N., Kabbadj, K., Eychenne, B., Sancho, M.J., Kang, K.I., Zucman Morfin, R., and Baulieu, E.E., 1991, Neurosteroids: biosynthesis and metabolism in cultured rodent glia and neurons, in: *Neurosteroids and Brain Function,* E. Costa and S.M. Paul, eds., Thieme Med Pub, New York.

Romeo, E., Auta, J., Kozikowski, A.P., Ma, D., Papadopoulos, V., Puia, G., Costa, E., and Guidotti, A. 1992, 2-Aryl-3-indoleacetamides (FGIN-1): a new class of potent and specific ligands for the mitochondrial DBI receptor (MDR), *J. Pharmacol. Exp. Ther.* 262:971.

Rothstein, J.D., and Herlong, H.F., 1989, Neurologic manifestations of hepatic disease, *Neurol. Clin.* 7:563.

Rudge, J.S. ,1993, Astrocyte-derived neurotrophic factors, in: *Astrocytes. Pharmacology and Function,* S. Murphy, ed., Academic Press, San Diego.

Rutishauser, U., 1993, Adhesion molecules of the nervous system, *Curr. Opin. Neurobiol.* 3:709.

Sawada, J., Kikuchi, Y., Shibutani, M., Mitsumori, K., Inoue, K., and Kasahara, T., 1994, Induction of metallothionein in astrocytes by cytokines and heavy metals, *Biol. Signals,* 3:157.

Schoemaker, H., Boles, R.G., Horst, D., and Yamamura, H.I., 1983, Specific high-affinity binding sites for [^{3}H]Ro5-4864 in rat brain and kidney, *J. Pharmacol. Exp. Ther.* 225:61.

Schoemaker, H., Morelli, M., Deshmukh, P., and Yamamura, H.I., 1982, [^{3}H]Ro5-4864 benzodiazepine binding in the kainate lesioned striatum and Huntington's diseased basal ganglia, *Brain Res.* 248: 396.

Schousboe, A., 1981, Transport and metabolism of glutamate and GABA in neurons and glial cells, *Int. Rev. Neurobiol.* 22:1.

Sobel, R.A., DeArmond, S.J., Forno, L.S., and Eng, L.F., 1981, Glial fibrillary acidic protein in hepatic encephalopathy. An immunohistochemical study, *J. Neuropathol. Exp. Neurol.* 40:625.

Sprengel, R., Werner, P., Seeburg, P.H., Mukhin, A.G., Santi, M.R., Grayson, D.R., Guidotti, A., and Krueger, K.E. , 1989, Molecular cloning and expression of cDNA encoding a peripheral-type benzodiazepine receptor, *J. Biol. Chem.* 264:20415.

Stephenson, D.T., Schober, D.A., Smalstig, E.B., Mincy, R.E., Gehlert, D.R., and Clemens, J.A., 1995, Peripheral benzodiazepine receptors are colocalized with activated microglia following transient global forebrain ischemia in the rat, *J. Neurosci.* 15:5263.

Swain, M., Butterworth, R.F., and Blei, A.T., 1992, Ammonia and related amino acids in the pathogenesis of brain edema in acute ischemic liver failure in rats, *Hepatology*, 15:449.

Swain, M.S., Blei, A.T., Butterworth, R.F., and Kraig, R.P., 1991, Intracellular pH rises and astrocytes swell after portacaval anastomosis in rats, *Am. J. Physiol. Regul. Integr. Comp. Physiol.* 261:R1491.

Szerb, J.C., and Butterworth, R.F., 1992, Effect of ammonium ions on synaptic transmission in the mammalian central nervous system, *Prog. Neurobiol.* 39:135.

Takahashi, H., Koehler, R.C., Brusilow, S.W., and Traystman, R.J., 1991, Inhibition of brain glutamine accumulation prevents cerebral edema in hyperammonemic rats, *Am. J. Physiol. Heart Circ. Physiol.* 261:H825.

Traber, P.G., DalCanto, M., Ganger, D., and Blei, A.T., 1987, Electron microscopic evaluation of brain edema in rabbits with galactosamine-induced fulminant hepatic failure: ultrastructure and integrity of the blood-brain barrier, *Hepatology*, 7:1272.

Turner, M.M., Ransom, R.W., Yang, J.S., and Olsen, R.W., 1989, Steroid anaesthetics and naturally occurring analogs modulate the gamma-aminobutyric acid receptor complex at a site distinct from barbiturates, *J. Pharmacol. Exp. Ther.* 248:960.

Verma, A., and Snyder, S.H., 1989, Peripheral type benzodiazepine receptors, *Annu. Rev. Pharmacol. Toxicol.* 29:307.

Voorhies, T.M., Ehrlich, M.E., Duffy, T.E., Petito, C.K., and Plum, F., 1983, Acute hyperammonemia in the young primate. Physiologic and neuropathological correlates, *Pediatric Res.*, 17:970.

Walz, W., 1989, Role of glial cells in the regulation of the brain ion microenvironment, *Prog. Neurobiol.* 33: 309.

Westergaard, N., Sonnewald, U., and Schousboe, A., 1995, Metabolic trafficking between neurons and astrocytes: the glutamate glutamine cycle revisited, *Dev. Neurosci.* 17:203.

Wieland, S., Lan, N.C., Mirasedeghi, S., and Gee, K.W., 1991, Anxiolytic activity of the progesterone metabolite 5α-pregnan-3α-ol-20-one, *Brain Res.* 565:263.

Zaman, S.H., 1990, Endogenous steroids and pathogenesis of hepatic encephalopathy [letter], *Lancet.* 336: 573.

ORNITHINE AMINOTRANSFERASE AS A THERAPEUTIC TARGET IN HYPERAMMONEMIAS

Nikolaus Seiler

Groupe de Recherche en Thérapeutique Anticancéreuse,URA, CNRS 1529
Institut de Recherche Contre le Cancer, Faculté de Médecine, Université de Rennes 1, 2, av. du Pr. Léon Bernard, F-35043 RENNES Cedex, France

1. INTRODUCTION

L-Ornithine:2-oxoacid aminotransferase (OAT) is a mitochondrial matrix enzyme, present in most tissues (1). It catalyses the transfer of the terminal (δ) amino group of L-ornithine (2,5-diamino-pentanoic acid) (Orn) to 2-oxoglutarate, producing glutamic acid semialdehyde and glutamic acid (2). It has been suggested many years ago that OAT competes with L-ornithine carbamoyltransferase (OCT) for the intramitochondrially available Orn, and thus decreases the rate of urea formation via the urea cycle (3). In favor of this suggestion are protective effects of large doses of Orn and arginine (Arg) in acute ammonia intoxication (4,5). Administration of these amino acids is assumed to enhance mitochondrial Orn concentrations and thus increase due to the improved substrate availability the rate of both reactions, citrullin (Cit) formation and transamination. Inhibition of OAT and the consequent increase of Orn concentrations in liver appeared to be a potential alternative to the administration of Orn .

In 1988 the racemic mixture of 5-(fluoromethyl)ornithine (5FMOrn; 5-fluoro-2.5-diaminohexanoic acid) (Fig. 1), the first selective inactivator of OAT, was synthesized (6). It became possible to observe *in vivo* metabolic and physiologic consequences of the near-complete inactivation of OAT in the vertebrate organism. Transamination turned out to be the major catabolic pathway of Orn in all tissues. In the absence of active OAT the mammalian organism appears unable to eliminate Orn at a sufficient rate, and its massive accumulation in organs and tissues is observed (6,7). Since even long-term administration of 5FMOrn did not produce toxic effects (8) it seemed logical to ask whether acute or chronic inactivation of OAT would be of therapeutic use, in particular as a method to enhance the detoxifica-

Advances in Cirrhosis, Hyperammonemia, and Hepatic Encephalopathy
Edited by Felipo and Grisolía, Plenum Press, New York, 1997

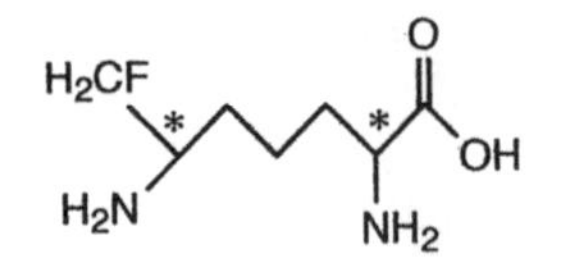

5-(Fluoromethyl)ornithine

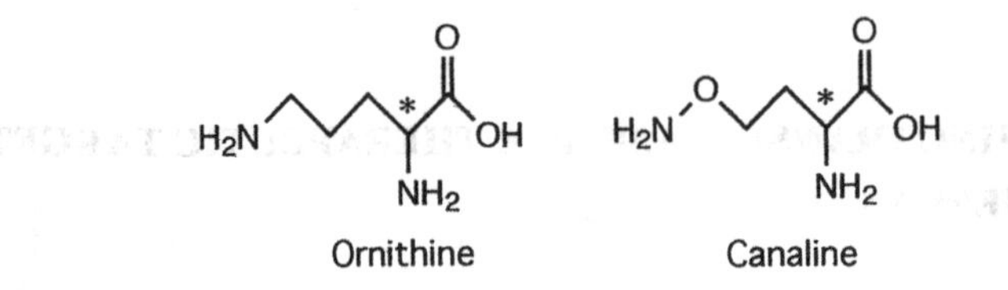

Fig. 1. Structural formulae of 5-(fluoromethyl)ornithine, ornithine and canaline. The asterisks indicate asymmetric centers .

tion of excessive ammonia in diseases with elevated blood and tissue ammonia concentrations.

In the present review ammonia (NH_3) and ammonium (NH_4^+), the protonated form of NH_3, is used synonymously, keeping in mind, however, that at (physiological) pH 7.4, 1.7% of NH_3 is in equilibrium with 98.3 % of its protonated form (9).

2. BIOCHEMICAL ASPECTS OF ORNITHINE METABOLISM

Orn and the inhibitory neurotransmitter, 4-aminobutyric acid (GABA), have certain features in common: They are not incorporated into polypeptides and their major catabolic pathways are initiated by the transfer of the ω-amino groups to 2-oxoglutarate. These reactions are catalyzed by similar pyridoxal phosphate-dependent aminotransferases. Both amino acids are present in all tissues of the vertebrate organism, though at different concentrations: In accordance with its neurotransmitter function GABA is highest in brain (10), whereas the highest Orn concentration is found in liver (8,11), in agreement with its role in urea formation. Owing to its well established physiological function all aspects of GABA metabolism have been extensively studied (12), and several inhibitors of 4-aminobutyrate:2-oxoglutarate aminotransferase (GABA-T) were synthesized. One of these became an antiepileptic drug (13). In contrast, Orn was nearly entirely neglected during the last decades. Hence, disregarding its function as substrate of the urea cycle, our knowledge of physiological and pharmacological aspects of Orn is incomplete.

In liver Orn is at the crossing of three major metabolic pathways (Fig. 2):

(a) Catalyzed by OCT, Orn reacts with carbamoyl phosphate to form Cit. The final product of the urea cyle, Arg, is hydrolyzed by arginase to form Orn and urea. Cit formation occurs nearly exclusively in liver. In most other organs OCT activity is low or absent. However, most tissues contain arginase. In muscle Orn is mainly formed by transfer of the amidino group of arginine to glycine (11) (Fig. 2).

(b) Orn is decarboxylated by ornithine decarboxylase (ODC) to form putrescine (1,4-butanediamine). This reaction is the initial, highly regulated step of polyamine formation. The transformation of putrescine to spermidine, and the formation of spermine from spermidine is catalyzed by specific synthases, and requires decarboxylated S-adenosyl-L-methionine as substrate. The latter is formed by decarboxylation of S-adenosyl-L-methionine. The enzyme that catalyzes this reaction (S-adenosyl-L-methionine decarboxylase), and ODC are inducible enzymes. In many instances they limitate the rate of polyamine formation (14,15).

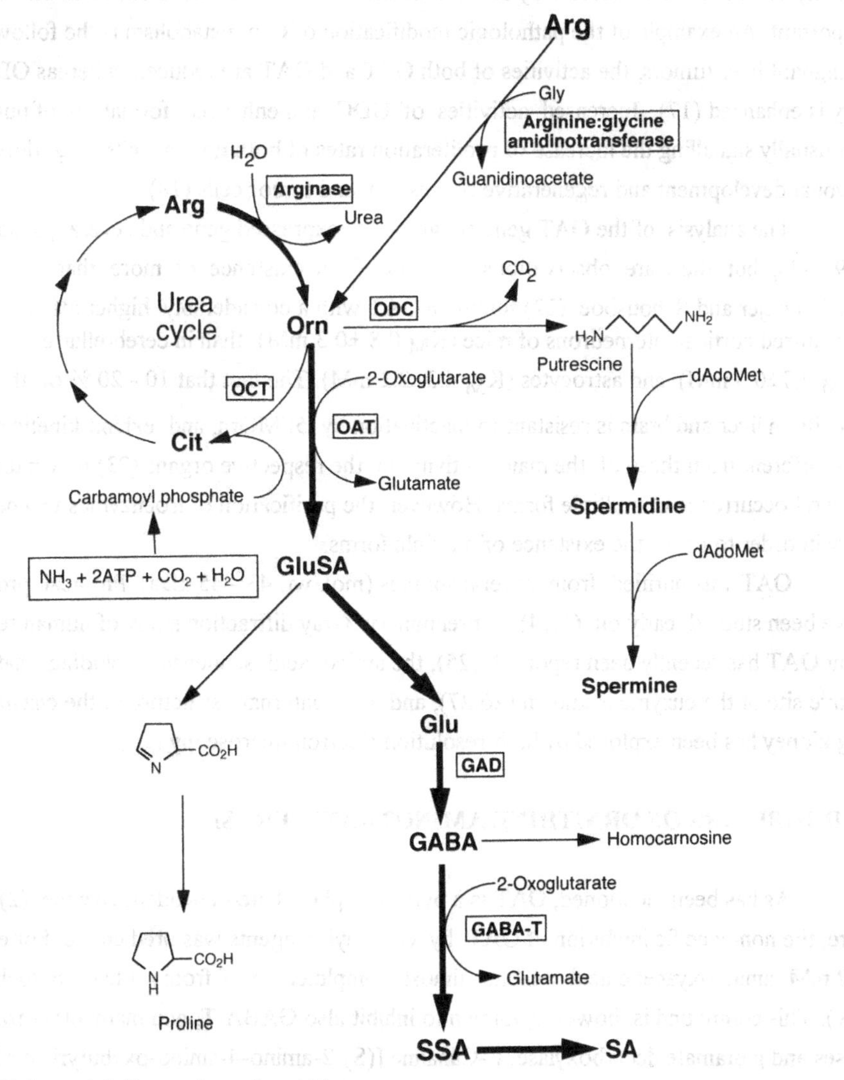

Fig. 2. Major metabolic reactions of ornithine.
Abbreviations: *Enzymes* : OAT ornithine : 2-oxoglutarate aminotransferase; OCT ornithine : carbamoyl-transferase; ODC ornithine decarboxylase; GAD glutamic acid decarboxylase; GABA-T 4-aminobutyric acid : 2-oxo-acid aminotransferase. *Metabolites*: Arg arginine; Cit citrulline; Gly glycine; Glu glutamic acid; GluSA glutamic acid semialdehyde; GABA 4-aminobutyric acid; dAdoMet decarboxylated S-adenosylmethionine

(c) The OAT-catalyzed reaction of Orn with 2-oxoglutarate occurs in all tissues, predominantly in liver. Products of the reaction are glutamic acid and glutamic acid semialdehyde. The latter is mainly transformed to glutamic acid, but it is also a precursor of proline, which may be formed via Δ^1-pyrroline 5-carboxylic acid (11,16) (Fig. 2).

From the organ distribution of the enzymes involved in Orn metabolism it is evident that its role as precursor of putrescine is general, whereas its function within the urea cycle is nearly exclusive for liver. The relative rates of the three reactions of Orn, decarboxylation, carbamoylation and transamination, change with physiologic and pathologic conditions. The activity of liver OAT is affected by several factors among which hormones and diet are most important. An example of the pathologic modification of Orn metabolism is the following: In malignant liver tumors, the activities of both OCT and OAT are reduced, whereas ODC activity is enhanced (17). Increased activities of ODC and enhanced formation of putrescine are usually signalling the increase of proliferation rates of both normal cells, (e.g. during embryonal development and regenerative processes), and tumor cells (18).

The analysis of the OAT gene suggests one expressed gene and several pseudogenes (19 - 21), but there are observations in favor of the existence of more than one form of OAT: Drejer and Schousboe (22) found an OAT with a considerably higher affinity for Orn in cultured cortical interneurons of mice (K_M 0.8 ±0.3 mM) than in cerebrellar granule cells (K_M 4.7±0.9 mM) and astrocytes (K_M 4.3±2.2 mM). The fact that 10 - 20 % of the OAT activity in liver and brain is resistant to inactivation by 5FMOrn, and exhibit kinetic properties different from those of the major activity in the respective organs (23) may indicate the general occurrence of multiple forms. However, the purification of isoenzymes will be necessary in order to prove the existence of multiple forms.

OAT was purified from several sources (mol. wt. 43 - 45 kDa). Physical properties have been studied early on (2,24). A preliminary X-ray diffraction study of human recombinant OAT has recently been reported (25), the amino acid sequence, including that of the active site of the enzyme is known (26,27), and the quaternary structure of the enzyme from pig kidney has been explored by high-resolution electron microscopy (28).

3. INHIBITORS OF ORNITHINE AMINOTRANSFERASE

As has been mentioned, OAT is a pyridoxal phosphate-dependent enzyme (2), therefore, the non-specific inhibition of OAT by carbonyl reagents was predictable. For example 0.2 mM aminooxyacetic acid inhibits almost completely OAT from rat liver mitochondria (29). This compound is, however, known to inhibit also GABA-T, and many other transaminases and glutamate decarboxylase. L-Canaline [(S)-2-amino-4-amino-oxybutyric acid] (Fig. 1) also reacts as a pyridoxal phosphate scavenger (30). Owing to its close structural relationship with Orn it is nevertheless a rather potent and selective inhibitor of OAT (31) . Inactivation by canaline is not restricted to the natural S-enantiomer, however, the inactivation rate by the R-enantiomer is considerably slower (32). Although selective *in vitro,* L-canaline is not well suited for *in vivo* studies. It appears to be rapidly metabolized. Consequently high doses are required, and inhibition is relatively short lasting (7,32).

Based on the fact that the key step of Orn transamination is the abstraction of the pro-S hydrogen atom at C5 (33), the synthesis of an enzyme-activated irreversible inhibitor of OAT was conceived. Enzyme-activated irreversible inhibitors (mechanism based inactivators) are relatively unreactive molecules which require structural similarity to the natural substrate, in order to allow competition for binding within the active site of the enzyme. Moreover, they have to react within the active site in a manner similar to the natural substrate, in order to become transformed into a reactive molecule which is capable to inactivate the enzyme (34,35). Owing to these requirements, enzyme-activated irreversible inhibitors are usually selective. The close relationship between GABA-T and OAT is documented by the fact that most enzyme-activated irreversible inhibitors of GABA-T (4-amino-5-hexynoic acid; 4-amino-5,6-heptadienoic acid; 5-amino-1,3-cyclohexadienyl carboxylic acid (Gabaculine)) are potent inactivators of OAT, both *in vitro* and *in vivo* (36 - 38). Since 3-aminopropionic acid and 4-aminobutyric acid with fluoromethyl- or difluoromethyl-groups attached to their terminal carbon atoms had been identified as potent inactivators of GABA-T (39) the structural analog of Orn with a fluoromethyl group at C5 (6-fluoro-2,5-diaminohexanoic acid , 5-(fluoromethyl)ornithine, 5FMOrn) (Fig. 1) was synthesized in the form of a racemic mixture, which contained the four enantiomers in equal amounts. This compound turned out to be a higly selective and potent inactivator of OAT, both *in vitro* and *in vivo* (6). It does not inactivate GABA-T or any other enzyme for which Orn is a substrate. Among the four enantiomers of 5FMOrn only one, namely (2S,5S)-5-fluoro-2,5-diaminohexanoic acid, reacts with of OAT (32). The three other enantiomers do not compete effectively with the active isomer, nor do they exert any measurable pharmacologic or toxic effects in rodents at the doses which were active in acute and chronic experiments. The key observations made with the racemate were confirmed by the selective synthesis of the active enantiomer of 5FMOrn, and its pharmacologic evaluation (40). All observations with 5FMOrn reported in this chapter have been obtained with the racemate, but there is no doubt that one can expect to obtain very similar results by using (2S,5S)-5-fluoro-2,5-diaminohexanoic acid, the active enantiomer, at 25% of the dose of the racemate.

4. BIOCHEMICAL EFFECTS OF ORNITHINE AMINOTRANSFERASE INHIBITION BY 5-(FLUOROMETHYL)ORNITHINE

In agreement with the properties of an enzyme-activated irreversible inhibitor (mechanism-based inhibitor) 5FMOrn inactivates OAT *in vitro* in a concentration- and time-dependent manner (Fig 3). The inactivation rate is reduced in the presence of Orn, indicating competition for binding within the active site of the enzyme. The reaction mechanism of 5FMOrn has not been fully clarified. The spectral changes of OAT during reaction with 5FMOrn are similar to those observed during reaction with Orn: The maximum of the pyridoxal band at 420 nm disappears, and concomitantly the pyridoxamine band at 330 nm increases. In a second step a slow shift of the absorption maximum from 330 nm to 458 nm was observed. The chromophore corresponding to this band was not removed by extensive dialysis. Based on these findings a reaction scheme was formulated (32). 5FMOrn forms within the active site of OAT a Schiff-base with pyridoxal phosphate The release of F^- causes the formation of a reactive intermediate, which after rearrangement binds irreversibly to Lys^{292}, the same Lys residue in the active site of the enzyme, to which pyridoxal phosphate is normally attached . The chromophore with the maximum at 458 nm is the result of the slow hydrolysis of an imino group of the inactivation complex; it is not essential for the inactivation of the enzyme.

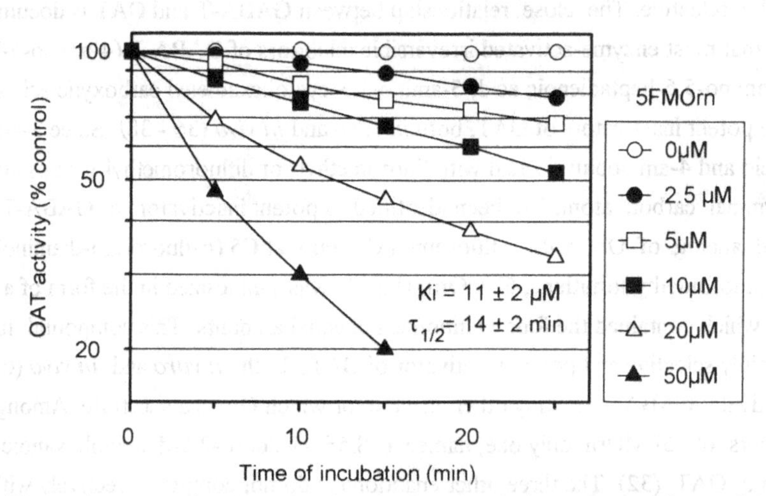

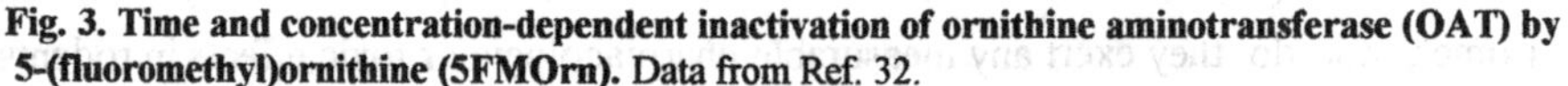
Fig. 3. Time and concentration-dependent inactivation of ornithine aminotransferase (OAT) by 5-(fluoromethyl)ornithine (5FMOrn). Data from Ref. 32.

If administered to mice the compound causes a dose- and time-dependent decrease of OAT activity in all tissues. Table 1 summarizes data on OAT activity and Orn concentrations in liver and brain of mice 16 h (the time of maximal Orn concentrations) after a single intraperitoneal dose of 5FMOrn. A dose of 25 $mg \cdot kg^{-1}$ produced maximal (80 - 90%) inactivation between 16 and 24 h. The compound is also orally active and can be conveniently administered with the drinking fluid. The extent of OAT inhibition is organ dependent.

It has already been mentioned that a certain fraction of OAT activity present in most tissues is refractory to inactivation by 5FMOrn, but this residual activity is competitively inhibited by 5FMOrn. Canaline, gabaculine, amino-oxy acetic acid and 4-amino-5-hexynoic acid are inhibitors of the 5FMOrn-refractory OAT (23). The fact that tissue Orn concentrations increase with increasing doses of 5FMOrn, even when maximal inactivation of OAT has been achieved (6) is due to the competitive inhibition of the 5FMOrn-refractory OAT. During the time of maximal OAT inactivation, Orn concentrations increase dramatically in all organs, including the brain, but decline after partial recovery of the enzyme, as is shown for liver in Fig. 4. The time-concentration changes of Orn after a single dose of 5FMOrn are typical for the inhibition of enzymes which are present in large excess. Their activity is made

Table 1. Ornithine aminotransferase (OAT) activity and ornithine (Orn) concentration in liver and brain of mice16 h after a single intraperitoneal dose of 5-fluoromethylornithine (5FMOrn)

5FMOrn	Liver		Brain	
i.p. dose	OAT activity	Orn	OAT activity	Orn
$\mu mol \cdot kg^{-1}$	$\mu mol \cdot g^{-1} \cdot h^{-1}$	$\mu mol \cdot g^{-1}$	$\mu mol \cdot g^{-1} \cdot h^{-1}$	$nmol \cdot g^{-1}$
0	171±2	0.3±0.08	22.4±0.3	18±6
4.2	86±10*	0.6±0.2	10.4±0.8*	51±18*
10.5	62±7*	1.1±0.3*	7.5±0.4*	145±36*
21.0	28±7*	1.5±0.5*	6.9±0.4*	208±78*
31.5	30±11*	4±2*	5.7±0.7*	262±86*
42.0	31±2*	4±2*	5.2±0.4*	351±127*
84.0	16±3*	11±3*	4.8±0.3*	659±84*

Mean value ± S.D. (n = 3); The asterisks indicate a statistically significant difference (p < 0.01 between control and treated mice; (multiple range and multiple F-tests).Data from ref. 51.

rate limiting only when inhibition is near-complete, since even a fraction of the physiologically available enzyme activity is sufficient to control normal steady state levels of the substrate. Long-term administration of 5FMOrn causes a gradual increase of Orn in all organs to reach a new stady state level after about 4 or 5 days of treatment (Table 2). The dramatic accumulation of Orn in all tissues indicates that the cells of the vertebrate organism have the ca-

Table 2. Ornithine concentration in organs of mice after oral administration of daily 40 $mg \cdot kg^{-1}$ of 5-fluoromethylornithine (5FMOrn) (mean values ± S.D.; $nmol \cdot g^{-1}$ of tissue)

Tissue	Days of treatment with 5FMOrn 0	1	4	13
Liver	689±21	2300±230	6200±960	7170±2670
Kidney	41±12	450±130	1367±215	922±62
Spleen	62±12	246±43	318±8	281±60
Lung	158±23	268±47	342±85	345±50
Skeletal muscle	50±21	215±26	472±136	432±53
Eye	88±26	648±49	1067±167	855±217
Brain:				
Hemispheres	31±9	679±57	1065±105	1249±136
Brainstem	18±2	1027±250	1725±268	1783±129
Medulla	20±3	1239±289	1625±340	1530±151
Cerebellum	25±6	972±162	1659±164	1221±296

Female C57BL mice (n = 4) received a solution of 0.036% of 5FMOrn in tap water as drinking fluid. The average fluid intake corresponded to a daily drug intake of about 40 $mg \cdot kg^{-1}$ (168 $\mu mol \cdot kg^{-1}$). Data from ref. 8.

pacity to store Orn and that transamination is the major catabolic pathway. In the absence of active OAT the cells of the vertebrate organism lack the ability to remove excessive Orn by an alternative mechanisms (e.g. by release) at a rate sufficiently high to avoid Orn accumulation .

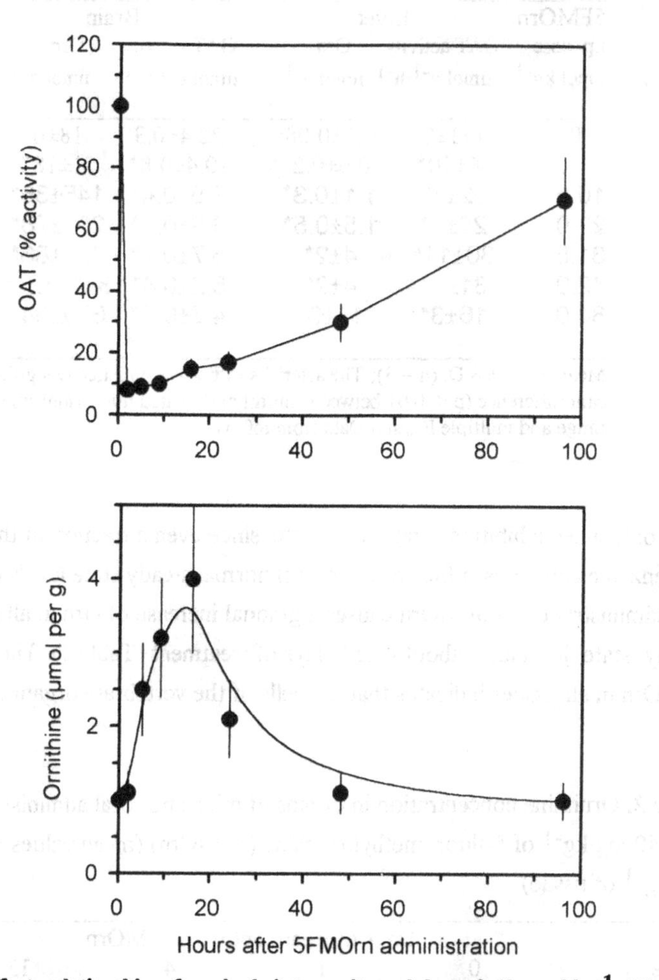

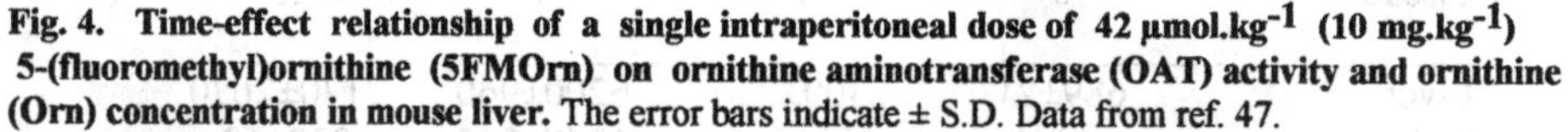
Fig. 4. Time-effect relationship of a single intraperitoneal dose of 42 µmol.kg^{-1} (10 mg.kg^{-1}) 5-(fluoromethyl)ornithine (5FMOrn) on ornithine aminotransferase (OAT) activity and ornithine (Orn) concentration in mouse liver. The error bars indicate ± S.D. Data from ref. 47.

Even after long-term administration of 5FMOrn brain GABA concentrations were unaffected, demonstrating the lack of an effect of the drug on GABA-T. However, in brain carnosine and homocarnosine, and in skeletal muscle anserine concentrations decreased significantly after chronic dosing of 5FMOrn (8). One potential explanation for this finding, the substitution of histidine by Orn in these dipeptides, could not be substantiated. Thus the biochemical basis and the physiological significance of the effect of 5FMOrn administration on formation and metabolism of the histidine-dipeptides is still unclear.

5. ORNITHINE, GYRATE ATROPHY OF THE CHOROID AND RETINA, AND 5-(FLUOROMETHYL)ORNITHINE

Owing to the selectivity and potency of 5FMOrn as an inhibitor of OAT it was expected that the compound would be useful to establish an animal model of hereditary OAT deficiency. However, even the chronic administration of 5FMOrn to adult mice at daily intraperitoneal doses of 10-20 mg/kg, or by oral administration (with the drinking fluid) at an average daily dose of 40 mg/kg did not produce any apparent toxic effects or behavioral changes (8). Specific attention was paid to the visual system since it appears to be general consensus that the elevated Orn concentration in the eye is a major pathogenetic factor in gyrate atrophy of the choroid and retina. This assumption was based, among others, on the observation that visual function in children with hereditary OAT deficiency improved following reduction of plasma Orn by diet (41), and injections of Orn into the eye of adult rats produced retina degeneration (42). The latter approach is, however, inappropriate. The observed effects can be explained by the fact that the transamination of each molecule of Orn produces two molecules of glutamate, a well known excitotoxic amino acid (43). Glutamate formation from Orn does not occur in the absence of OAT activity. This may explain the lack of any effect of elevated intraocular Orn concentrations on the retina of adult mice in the presence of 5FMOrn (8).

The above mentioned effects of chronic elevation of Orn concentrations on carnosine, homocarnosine and anserine metabolism (8) demonstrate that our knowledge of the biochemical consequences of chronically elevated Orn concentrations in the vertebrate organism is insufficient. 5FMOrn is a tool that may allow us to explore metabolic aspects of chronic OAT deficiency which have hitherto not been considered as potential pathogenetic factors of hereditary OAT deficiencies. It is interesting to note in this context that in newborn mice with hereditary OAT deficiency a paradoxical hypoornithinemia and retinal degeneration was observed (44), suggesting the importance of developmental events in retinal degeneration.

6. DETOXIFICATION OF AMMONIA BY INACTIVATION OF ORNITHINE AMINOTRANSFERASE

A logical consequence of the long-term blockade of OAT is the channelling of Orn into the remaining pathways. From the metabolic scheme (Fig. 2) the enhanced formation of putrescine was predicted. This could indeed be observed. In brain, which is a nearly closed system with regard to polyamine metabolism, the increase of Orn concentrations caused only a marginal increase of polyamine concentrations, but instead, polyamine turnover and elimination rates were enhanced (45) - a consequence of the homeostatic regulation of polyamine metabolism.

Therapeutic applications of enhanced polyamine formation are presumably tissue regeneration and repair, because these processes require an increased access to polyamines (8). Enhancement of liver regeneration in the presence of excessive amounts of Orn plays presumably a role in the protective effect of 5FMOrn in thioacetamide (TAA)-induced encephalopathy (46) (see below). Disregarding this aspect in the present review the enhancement of polyamine formation will not be considered further.

6.1. PROTECTION AGAINST ACUTE AMMONIA INTOXICATION

In addition to a generally enhanced putrescine formation, in liver the enhanced formation of Cit is to be expected from the selective elevation of Orn concentrations (Fig. 2). In agreement with this expectation a single dose of 20 $mg \cdot kg^{-1}$ 5FMOrn to normal mice caused an increase of liver Cit concentrations from 43 to 190 $nmol \cdot g^{-1}$, and the urinary excretion of this amino acid was more than doubled (46). This observation indicates that under physiological conditions liver OCT is not saturated with Orn, and that urea formation can be enhanced by the increase of intramitochondrial Orn concentrations, even though the increase of urea concentration in blood and liver was marginal. (Since Orn is a matrix enzyme, elevation of Orn concentrations due to OAT inhibition occur first intramitochondrially).

Urinary orotic acid excretion by healthy mice was not significantly reduced by 5FMOrn administration, indicating that under physiological conditions the intramitochondrially formed carbamoyl phosphate was not an important source for orotic acid formation. If, however, excessive orotic acid formation was induced in mice by administration of an ammonium salt, pretreatment with 5FMOrn nearly completely normalized the excessive urinary orotic acid excretion (47). The exorbitant increase of urinary orotic acid in hyperammonemic states is a consequence of excessive carbamoyl phosphate formation, and a functional (not absolute) deficiency of Orn or Arg (48). The above mentioned observations clearly demonstrate that a functional deficiency of Orn can be compensated by preventing its catabolism. Excessive carbamoyl phosphate formation in hyperammonemic states is a consequence of the activation of carbamoyl phosphate synthetase, presumably by acetylglutamate (49), and the enhancement of the synthesis rate due to saturation of the enzyme by its substrate ammonia. In addition, ammonia appears to have a direct stimulatory effect on Cit formation in a model system containing OAT, OCT, glutamate dehydrogenase, and carbamoyl phosphate (50).

More impressive than the effects on biochemical parameters appears the protection by 5FMOrn against lethal intoxication with ammonium salts. In Tab. 3 the dose - effect relationship for intraperitoneal 5FMOrn doses between 0.5 $mg \cdot kg^{-1}$ and 20 $mg \cdot kg^{-1}$ (given 16 h before intoxication with ammonium acetate) are shown. Pretreatment with 10 $mg \cdot kg^{-1}$ of the drug before administration of a lethal dose (13 $mmol \cdot kg^{-1}$) of ammonium acetate is sufficient to protect during more than ten hours 90% of the animals from death (51). The oral administration of the drug is nearly as efficient as its injection.

Protection by 5FMOrn is not a direct effect of the drug. It is most probably correlated with the liver Orn concentration. If ammonium salts are given at times when tissue Orn

Tab. 3. Protection of mice against a lethal dose of ammonium acetate by pretreatment with 5-(fluoromethyl)ornithine (5FMOrn)

5FMOrn i.p.dose $\mu mol \cdot kg^{-1}$	Percent animals With loss of righting reflex	With tonic seizure	Surviving
0	100	100	0
2.1	100	80	20
4.2	90	50*	50*
10.5	80	50*	60*
21.0	70	50*	70*
31.5	70	20*	80*
42.0	50*	10*	90*
84.0	60*	10*	90*

Each treatment group consisted of 10 female CD1 mice. 5FMOrn was administered 16 h before the intraperitoneal injection of 13 $mmol \cdot kg^{-1}$ ammonium acetate. The asterisks indicate a statistically significant difference ($p < 0.05$) between the control and a treated group (Fischer's exact probability test). Data from ref. 51.

concentrations are submaximal, the protective effect is diminished concomitantly, and no significant protection against ammonia intoxication is achieved within the first hour after 5FMOrn administration, i.e. at the time of highest drug concentration in tissues.

The K_M for Orn of rat liver OCT is reported to be 0.4 mM at pH 7.7 (52) and 1.82 mM at pH 7.5 (53); the K_M for carbamoyl phosphate is very low (22 - 26 μM) (52 - 53). The total Orn concentration in mouse liver is around 0.3 mM; 16 h after the administration of 10 $mg \cdot kg^{-1}$ (42 $\mu mol.kg^{-1}$) 5FMOrn it increased to about 40 mM (Table 1). The effective intramitochondrial Orn concentration is not known, but it is evident that at 40 mM Orn the OCT is saturated with its substrate. Hence a further increase of liver Orn concentration by higher doses of 5FMOrn does neither improve the rate of Cit formation nor the protection against ammonia intoxication.

6.2. Enhancement of the Protective Effect of 5-(Fluoromethyl)ornithine Against Acute Ammonia Intoxication

Starting forty years ago with the work of Greenstein and his colleagues (4) until present, amino acids and other compounds expected to enhance urea formation, and to improve detoxification of ammonia by other pathways, were tested in animal models of acute ammonia intoxication, and clinically in patients, mostly with liver cirrhosis (Table 4).

Some of the compounds found earlier to be efficient in antagonizing acute ammonia intoxication, were tested together with 5FMOrn in CD1 mice, with the aim to identify synergistically acting drug combinations. The most conspicuous results are summarized in Table

5. In order to achieve a protective effect by injections of Orn and Arg against a subcutaneous dose of 13 mmol·kg^{-1} ammonium acetate, 10 mmol·kg^{-1} of the amino acids have to be injected. Citrullin was more effective, but the protection by amino acids and the compounds shown in Table 5 lasts only 1 to 2 h. Pretreatment with 5 µmol·kg^{-1} 5FMOrn, a partially protective dose against intoxication with 13mmol·kg^{-1} ammonium acetate enhanced the protective effect of all other drugs, except that of N-acetyl-L-glutamate. With one exception, namely the combined treatment with 5FMOrn and Arg, the drug combinations prevented the enhancement of brain ammonia concentration more efficiently than the individual drugs (54).

Table 4. Amino acids and other compounds suggested as protective agents aga inst intoxication with ammonium salts, or as treatments of hyperammonemic states

Compound	Experimental model	Ref. No.
Ornithine	Ammonia intoxication	5
Arginine	Ammonia intoxication	4, 95
Citrulline	Ammonia intoxication	5, 96
N-Acetylglutamate	Ammonia intoxication	97
N-Carbamylglutamate	Ammonia intoxication	49, 97, 98
α-Methylglutamate	Ammonia intoxication	99
Branched-chain amino acids	Exercise-induced hyperammonemia	100
L-Carnitine	Ammonia intoxication	56, 59
MK 801	Ammonia toxicity	101
Ornithine/branched chain amino acids	Treatment of portal systemic encephalopathy	69
Ornithine or Arginine/ N-carbamylglutamate	Ammonia intoxication	102
Ornithine/aspartate	Ammonia intoxication	102, 103
	Clinical trial in liver cirrhosis	104
Ornithine/benzoate	Ammonia intoxication	102
	Treatment of inborn errors of urea synthesis	105

Alone, as well as in combination with a submaximal dose of 5FMOrn, none of the amino acids and drugs were effectively protecting against death, if the intraperitoneal dose of ammonium acetate was elevated to 15 mmol·kg^{-1} (Table 5). Even pretreatment with a maximal dose of 5FMOrn, and administration of the amino acids at 5 or 10 mmol·kg^{-1} did not protect against this elevated dose of ammonium acetate. However, 5FMOrn showed significant protective effects in combination with carnitine, acetylcarnitine and MK-801, (Table 5), i.e. with those compounds, which do not act by improvement of the saturation of urea cycle enzymes, but by different mechanisms.

In acute intoxications with high doses of ammonium salts protection against death by 5FMOrn and by substrates of urea cycle enzymes relies on the prevention of the accumul-

Table 5. Effect of treatment with 5-fluoromethylornithine in combination with amino acids and related compounds known to protect against acute ammonia intoxication. Comparison of effects after intoxication with 13 mmol·kg^{-1} and 15 mmol·kg^{-1} ammonium acetate

Amino acid or Drug	Dose	Ammonium acetate 13 mmol.kg^{-1}	15 mmol.kg^{-1}
	mmol.kg^{-1}	Percent surviving animals	
A. Single drug treatment (no pretreatment with 5FMorn)			
None	-	0	0
L-Ornithine	10	90	10
L-Arginine	10	90	0
L-Citrulline	0.75	40	0
	5	100	0
N-Acetyl-L-glutamate	5	10	0
L-Carnitine	15	10	0
L-Acetylcarnitine	15	30	0
MK 801	0.006	80	0
B. Pretreatment with 5 μmol.kg^{-1} 5FMOrn, a submaximally protecting dose.			
None	-	40	0
L-Ornithine	10	100	0
L-Arginine	10	90-100	0
L-Citrulline	0.75	80*	0
N-Acetyl-L-glutamate	5	20	0
L-Carnitine	15	60*	0
L-Acetylcarnitine	15	100*	0
C. Pretreatment with 100 μmol.kg^{-1} 5FMOrn, a maximally protecting dose.			
None	-	90-100	0
L-Ornithine	10	90-100	20
L-Arginine	10	90-100	0
L-Citrulline	5	100	0
N-Acetyl-L-glutamate	5	90-100	0
L-Carnitine	15	90-100	60*
L-Acetylcarnitine	15	90-100	60*
MK 801	0.006	90-100	60*

Each treatment group consisted of 10 female CD1 mice (20 ± 2 g). Pretreatment with 5FMOrn (intraperitoneal injection) was 15 h before the subcutaneous administration of the drugs. One hour after drug administration ammonium acetate was given by intraperioneal injection.The asterisks indicate a statistically significant difference ($p<0.05$) between groups treated with a single drug and the combination of the drug with 5FMOrn. (Fischer's exact probability test). Data from Ref. 54.

ation of a lethal concentration of ammonia in the brain. This is indicated by the results shown in Table 6. Neither Cit nor glutamine was significantly affected by the pretreatment with 5FMOrn, but brain ammonia concentration was considerably below that found in non-treated mice.

Table 6 . Accumulation of ammonia in blood and brain of mice 10 min after the administration of 8 mmol·kg^{-1} ammonium acetate. Effects of pretreatment with 100 μmol·kg^{-1} 5-(fluoromethyl)ornithine 16 h before ammonium acetate administration

Treatment	Blood Ammonia μmol·ml^{-1}	Brain Ammonia μmol·g^{-1}	Ornithine nmol·g^{-1}	Citrulline nmol·g^{-1}	Glutamine μmol·g^{-1}
None	0.17±0.05	1.1±0.1	19±3	13±3	6.3±0.6
5FMOrn	0.14±0.04	1.21±0.03	703±85	16±5	6.0±0.8
NH_4^+	1.8±0.5	7±2	40±22	19±5	11±3
5FMOrn + NH_4^+	0.9±0.2*	3.3±0.9*	960±400	16±4	11±2

5FMOrn and ammonium acetate (NH_4^+) were administered by intraperitoneal injections. The asterisks indicate statistically significant differences (p = 0.05) between ammonium acetate-treated groups due to treatment with 5FMOrn. (Multiple range anad multiple F-tests). Data from Ref. 51.

After a dose of 13 mmol·kg^{-1} ammonium acetate the removal of ammonia from the circulation by saturation of the urea cycle with the appropriate substrates is sufficiently fast and avoids the accumulation of lethal concentrations in brain. However, the maximum rate of urea formation after 15 mmol·kg^{-1} is obviously insufficient to counteract the accumulation of lethal brain ammonia concentrations. Death of the intoxicated mice could be prevented only by activating other, independent supportive mechanisms. The observed synergistic effects of 5FMOrn with carnitine, acetylcarnitine and blockers of the N-methyl-D-aspartate (NMDA) receptors, of which MK801 is an example, could become of practical importance in the therapy of hyperammonemic states. Unfortunately our knowledge of the mechanisms underlying the protective effects of these compounds is insufficient. The blockade of central NMDA receptors is, of course, the obvious basis of the effects of MK 801 and related NMDA receptor blockers. However, in view of the ubiquity of NMDA receptors in the vertebrate brain a more detailed mapping of the involved neuronal systems will be necessary in order to allow us to talk about specific mechanisms. It appears that NMDA antagonists do not exert an anticonvulsant effect but selectively prevent a lethal effect of ammonia, presumably respiratory arrest. While mice intoxicated with a lethal dose of ammonium acetate usually die after the first tonic convulsion, pretreatment with three different NMDA antagonists, including MK 801, prevented death, but the animals exhibited series of tonic hind limb extensions (51).

It has been repeatedly shown that carnitine and acetylcarnitine administration lowers the amount of ammonia accumulating in the brain in acutely intoxicated experimental animals (54 - 56). For the mode of action of carnitine and acetylcarnitine in ammonia intoxication no firmly established explanation exists at present. From the high doses required, metabolic effects are likely. Thus it has been proposed that the carnitine-induced intramitochondrial generation of reducing equivalents would overcome the ammonia-induced blocking of the maleate-aspartate shuttle, leading to increased ATP production, and owing to an increase in acetylCoA levels the formation of N-acetyl-L-glutamate would be enhanced (57 - 59). N-Acetyl-L-glutamate is considered to be the physiological regulator of carbamoyl phosphate synthase (60). The experiments of Ratnakumari et al. (61) with chronically hyperammonemic sparse-fur mice are in support of an improvement of the state of energy metabolism in brain and liver. In agreement with previous results (62) they found as the most important effect of L-carnitine administration enhanced ATP and CoA pools in these mice. Matsuoka et al. (56) also point out the importance of the amelioration of brain energy metabolism. They also believe that cholinergic effects of acetylcarnitine (63,64) could contribute in addition to the protective effects. Felipo et al. (65) found that the exposure of neuronal cultures to L-carnitine increases the affinity of glutamate for the quisqualate receptors and prevents glutamate neurotoxicity by preventing excessive Ca^{2+} influx.

6.3. Effects of 5-(Fluoromethyl)ornithine in animal models of chronically elevated ammonia

Two animal models of chronically elevated blood and tissue ammonia concentrations were used to study effects of 5FMOrn:

(a) Rats with portacaval anastomoses (66)

(b) Mice with a hereditary abnormal ornithine carbamoyltransferase (67).

Administration of 5FMOrn at concentrations which were effective in protecting mice against acute intoxication with ammonia reduced OAT activity equally well in the liver of shunted and sham operated rats, and liver Orn concentrations were increased to the same extent. However, the treatment had no significant effect on ammonia detoxification and urea formation in rats with portacaval anastomoses. Likewise, a series of other pathological symptoms of portacaval shunting (plasma and brain amino acid patterns, plasma enzyme activities, locomotor behavior, etc.) were not significantly shifted toward normal values by treatment with 5FMOrn. These observations leave us with the following tentative explanation: Owing to the shunt, the blood flow through the liver is reduced to such an extent that the capacity of the apparently normal, though "small" liver is sufficient to form urea from the ammonia present in the fraction of blood which perfuses the liver from collaterals. The presence of an excessive amount of Orn in the shunted liver is, as in normal liver, of no importance for urea formation, since there is no functional deficit of Orn. This idea is supported by the fact that the ammonia content of the liver of shunted rats was not significantly different from that of sham operated animals. In contrast, in normal mice intoxicated with an ammonium salt, the liver ammonia concentration was enhanced proportionately with the blood concentration, irrespective of pretreatment with 5FMOrn (47).

It is known that in human cirrhotic liver the specific activities of urea cycle enzymes are reduced (68). Nevertheless, Herlong et al. (69) observed an improvement of the clinical grade of encephalopathy by infusion of ornithine salts of branched chain oxoacids. In portacaval shunted rats infusion of ornithine aspartate did not improve the clinical grade of encephalopathy, even though plasma and brain ammonia concentrations were reduced by 35% due to the treatment (70).

Mice with X-chromosome sparse-fur (spf) mutation have an abnormal form of liver OCT (71). Both, in spf mice and in human hereditary OCT deficiency (72), ammonia detoxification via urea formation is impaired. Therefore, plasma and tissue ammonia levels are chronically elevated, and massive amounts of orotic acid are excreted. OCT of spf mice has a different pH - sensitivity, and its affinity for Orn has been reported to be 0.6 mM, compared with 0.2 mM for the normal enzyme (71). Human OCT deficiencies are heterogenous. Based on their enzyme kinetics and immunological properties, at least five groups of mutations were distinguished. Among these two were similar to spf and sparse-fur with abnormal skin and hair (spf-ash) mouse mutants (72). The similarity of the kinetic properties of OCT in spf mutant mice and the human hereditary disease, and the similarity of the major metabolic aberrations - chronic elevation of ammonia in plasma and tissues, and excessive urinary excretion of orotic acid - make spf mice an interesting model for therapy experiments.

Administration of 5FMOrn with the drinking fluid (20 mg/100 ml; daily drug consumption 1.3-1.6 mg per mouse) caused a decrease of urinary orotic acid concentration from about 3000 $nmol \cdot mg^{-1}$ creatinine to 140-150 $nmol \cdot mg^{-1}$ creatinine (Fig. 5). These values are only insignificantly higher than those observed in untreated normal males (120 ± 50 $nmol \cdot mg^{-1}$ creatinine) (67). Likewise, plasma and tissue amonia concentrations were reduced by this treatment close to normal values (Fig. 6). Once again it was observed that neither urinary orotic acid excretion, nor ammonia concentration of normal male controls was diminished to a significant extent by administration of 5FMOrn. The amelioration of hyperammonemia by 5FMOrn is also documented by the reduction of the pathologically high blood glutamine levels to control values, the increase of citrulline concentration (which is far below normal values in spf mice) and the general normalization of the abnormal amino acid pattern in blood (Fig. 7). During and shortly after the treatment period of the animals gained weight and appeared less jittery, although their locomotor and exploratory behavior was not significantly changed (67). Administration of high doses of Orn was also able to reduce pathological manifestations of spf mice (73), but the effect was less impressive than in the case of 5FMOrn administrations.

The effect of 5FMOrn on orotic acid excretion by spf mice was, as expected, reversible. Surprisingly, however, low urinary orotic acid concentrations were still observed 5 days after termination of drug administration (Fig. 5), although after single doses of the drug normal tissue Orn concentrations are observed already at about 48 h, i.e. at a time when OAT was only recovered by about 30 % (Fig. 4). A satisfactory explanation for the long-lasting effect of 5FMOrn on orotic acid excretions by spf mice is presently not available.

With regard to the availability of Orn within the mitochondria, there is a principal difference between exogenously administered Orn and the enhancement of Orn concentrations by inactivation of OAT. This difference may contribute to the long-lasting effect of 5FMOrn in spf mice and is, therefore, briefly discussed. If OAT is inactivated, the increase of Orn oc-

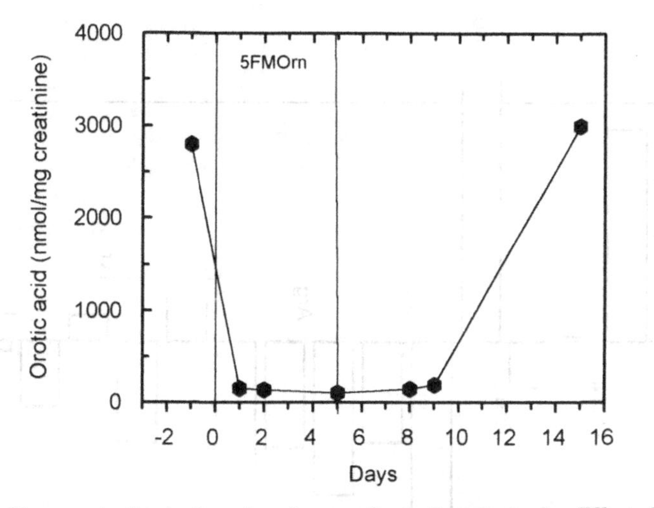

Fig. 5. Orotic acid concentration in the urine of sparse-fur (spf) mutant mice. Effect of oral administration of 5-(fluoromethyl)ornithine (5FMOrn) on urinary orotic acid concentration. The vertical lines indicate the period of 5FMOrn administration (20 mg 5FMOrn per 100 ml tap water; daily drug consumption 1.3 - 1.6 mg). Mean values of 8 animals. Data from ref. 67.

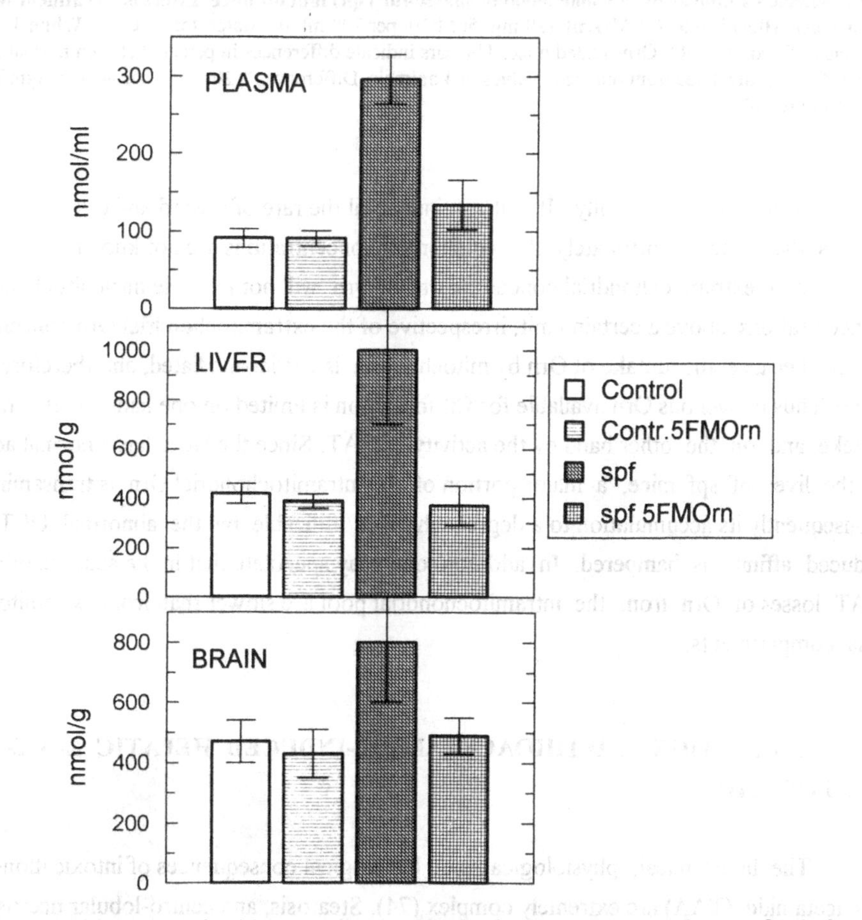

Fig.6. Ammonia concentration in plasma, liver and brain of normal controls and sparse-fur (spf) mutant mice before and after treatment with 5-(fluoromethyl)-ornithine (5FMOrn). The mice received a solution of 5FMOrn as drinking fluid (20 mg/100 ml tap water) for 4 days. The error bars indicate ±S.D. (n = 4). Data from ref. 67.

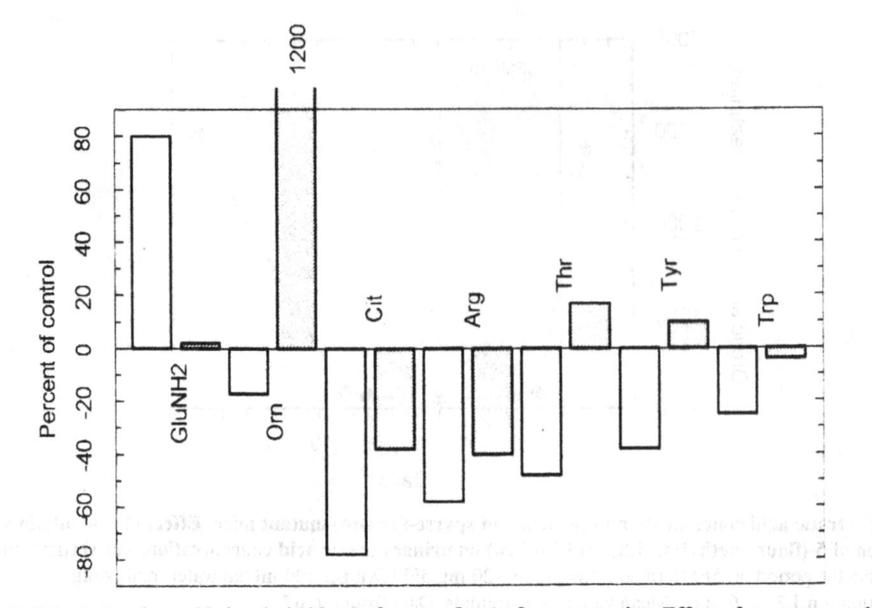

Fig.7. Selected amino acids in whole blood of sparse-fur (spf) mutant mice. Effect of treatment with 5-(fluoromethyl)ornithine (5FMOrn) (20 mg 5FMOrn per 100 ml tap water for 4 days). White bars: no treatment; filled bars: 5FMOrn-treated mice. The bars indicate differences in percent between normal males and spf mice, calculated from the mean values of 4 animals. Differences > 20 % are considered significant. Data from ref. 67.

curs first intramitochondrially. It will continue until the rate of inward and outward flow of Orn is the same. Unfortunately the equilibrium concentrations are not known. In contrast, elevation of extramitochondrial concentrations of Orn will not increase intramitochondrial concentrations above a certain limit, irrespective of the extramitochondrial Orn concentration, because the uptake of Orn by mitochondria is carrier-mediated, and therefore saturable. Thus exogenous Orn available for Cit formation is limited on one hand by the rate of uptake, and on the other hand by the activity of OAT. Since the latter has a normal activity in the liver of spf mice, a major portion of the intramitochondrial Orn is transaminated. Consequently its accumulation to a degree which is utilizable by the abnormal OCT with reduced affinity is hampered. In addition one may speculate that in the absence of active OAT losses of Orn from the intramitochondrial pool are slower than from extramitochondrial compartments.

7. OAT INHIBITION AND THIOACETAMIDE-INDUCED HEPATIC ENCEPHALOPATHY

The biochemical, physiological, and histological consequences of intoxications with thioacetamide (TAA) are extremely complex (74). Steatosis, and centro-lobular necrosis, fibrosis, cirrhosis and haematoma are chronic lesions of the liver, and two different modes of cell death, apoptosis and necrosis, are induced (75). In spite of the ill defined processes that lead to the development of the symptoms, intoxications with TAA were nevertheless widely used as a model of hepatic encephalopathy. Mostly in rats, a variety of biochemical, physiological, pharmacological, and behavioral apects of this syndrome were studied (76 - 85). The model was also used to test drugs (86 - 87).

After administration of single intraperitoneal doses of 600 mg·kg^{-1} TAA, 90 - 100 % of male CD1 mice died within 48 h. The toxicity of TAA turned out to be very much dependent on strain and body weight of the mice, therefore, only CD1 mice with a narrow body weight range were used. Administration of a single dose of 20 mg·kg^{-1} of 5FMOrn either shortly before or after TAA administration protected about 90 % of the animals from death during the first 24 h, but the mice died subsequently. However, if the first dose of 5FMOrn was given within the period between 30 min before and 30 min after TAA administration, and a second dose 24 h after TAA, a higly significant protective effect was achieved (Fig. 8) (88). In this model, as well as in a less acute mouse model, in which 100 mg.kg^{-1} doses of TAA were given repeatedly at 24 h intervals, treatment with 5FMOrn diminished all pathological symptoms of the intoxication: Liver haemorrhage was less important, plasma enzyme levels (LDH, GOT) were reduced, pathologic amino acid patterns in blood, liver and brain were shifted towards normal values (46,88), and the TAA-induced reduction of locomotor and exploratory activity was enhanced close to normal behavior. In an *in vivo* liver function test the rate of $^{14}CO_2$-respiration after injection of D-[1-^{14}C]-galactose increased from 45-61 % to 86-91% of control, if TAA-intoxicated mice were treated with 5FMOrn (46). This, together with the mentioned reduction of liver haemorrhage suggested that the amelioration of the symptoms was due to a less damaged liver.

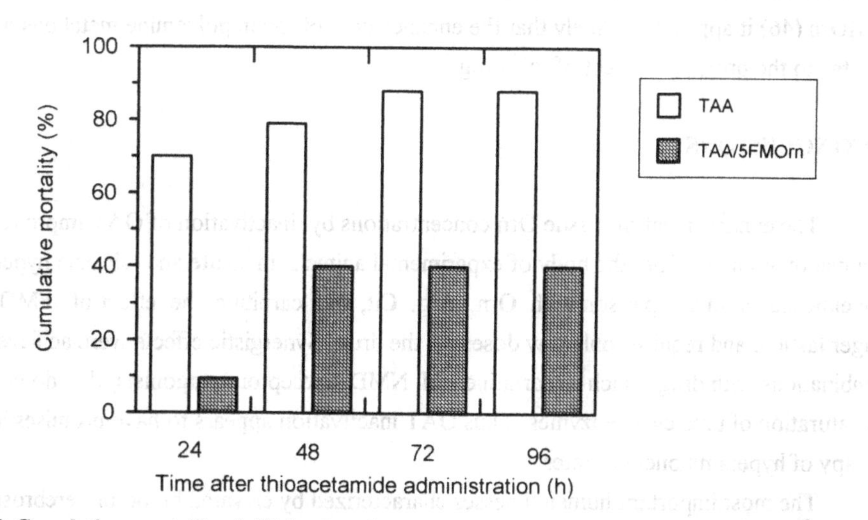

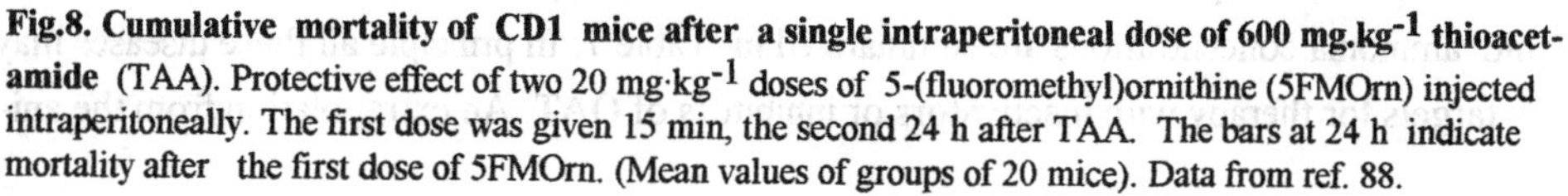
Fig.8. Cumulative mortality of CD1 mice after a single intraperitoneal dose of 600 mg.kg^{-1} thioacetamide (TAA). Protective effect of two 20 mg·kg^{-1} doses of 5-(fluoromethyl)ornithine (5FMOrn) injected intraperitoneally. The first dose was given 15 min, the second 24 h after TAA. The bars at 24 h indicate mortality after the first dose of 5FMOrn. (Mean values of groups of 20 mice). Data from ref. 88.

The protection by 5FMOrn of TAA-induced liver damage is not well understood. In the acute model (600 mg·kg^{-1} TAA) the time between intoxication with a lethal dose of TAA, the gradual deterioration of liver function, and the development of symptoms of encephalopathy, ending with death, is for most mice less than 24 h. Maximal Orn concentrations in brain and liver after 5FMOrn administration are observed around 16 h (Fig. 4). Protective effects of 5FMOrn were restricted to a short period from about 30 min before, until 30 min after TAA administration (88). Especially the fact that pretreatment with 5FMOrn several h before administration of TAA was ineffective, and that a second dose of the drug 24 h after intoxication was necessary, seems to indicate that highly elevated Orn concentrations were required for effective protection between about 10 and 18 h of the development of the syndrome, and for the period between 24 and 48 h after TAA administration.

About 6 h after TAA administration, ODC activity (89), and putrescine concentrations (90,91) start to increase and are maximal between about 10 h and 24 h in the intoxicated liver. The increase of spermidine and spermine concentrations (91), the enhancement of RNA metabolism (89,92,93) and the initiation of DNA synthesis and mitosis of hepatocytes (94) are events that follow 24 to 48 h after TAA administration. These changes are indications of regenerative processes. One may, therefore, consider the enhancement of putrescine concentrations as the initial step of a cascade of events that are induced to antagonize the pathological process initiated by TAA, and to restore normal liver function.

As was discussed in a previous section the enhancement of Orn favors the formation of putrescine and of polyamines. Thus in TAA-induced hepatic encephalopathy the support of regenerative processes by an increase of the rate of putrescine formation in liver due to the improvement of Orn availability is currently the best explanation for the protective effect of 5FMOrn. Even though CNS effects of TAA intoxication are considerably ameliorated by 5FMOrn (46) it appears not likely that the enhancement of brain polyamine metabolism contributes to the protective effect of this drug.

8. CONCLUSIONS

The enhancement of tissue Orn concentrations by inactivation of OAT improved the removal of ammonia from the body of experimental animals in acute and chronic hyperammonemic states. In comparison with Orn, Arg, Cit, and carnitine the effect of 5FMOrn is longer lasting, and requires only low doses of the drug. Synergistic effects were achieved by combinations with drugs, such as carnitine and NMDA receptor antagonists, that do not act via saturation of urea cycle enzymes. Thus OAT inactivation appears to have promises in the therapy of hyperammonemic states.

The most important human illnesses characterized by elevated blood or cerebrospinal fluid ammonia concentrations are summarized in Table 7. In principle all these diseases may be targets for therapy with inactivators or inhibitors of OAT. An extrapolation from the animal models to human illnesses is, however, difficult. In view of the fact that spf mice have a very similar abnormality as was described for some human OCT deficiencies (namely an OCT with a low affinity for Orn), and in view of the profound recuperation of the major pathological manifestations of spf mice by low oral doses of 5FMOrn, it appears likely that the administration of 5FMOrn would have comparable effects in the analogous human hereditary OCT deficiencies.

Table 7. Human illnesses and therapeutic interventions which are associated with elevated blood or cerebrospinal fluid ammonia concentrations *

Hepatic encephalopathy (106,107)	Systemic carnitine deficiency (122)
Fulminant hepatic failure (108)	Hyperornithinemia, hyperammonemia, homocitrullinemia syndrome (123)
Alzheimer's disease (109 - 111)	Nonketotic hyperglycinemia (124)
Urinary tract (bladder) infections (112,113)	Progressive neuronal degeneration of childhood (Alper syndrome) (125)
Congestive heart failure (114)	Ureterosigmoidostomy (126 - 128)
Pulmonary emphysema (115)	Complications of hemodialysis (129)
Shock (116)	Valproate therapy (130 - 132)
IgD multiple melanomas (117)	
Hereditary deficiencies of urea cycle enzymes (118,119)	
Reye's syndrome (120,121)	

* Reference No in parenthesis

Since a certain capacity of the liver to form urea is a prerequisite for the efficacy of the method, those diseases which do not imply a severely impaired liver function may be the most favourable targets for OAT inhibitors. Among these Alzheimer's disease is the most frequent disease and deserves, therefore, especial consideration. Reduction of brain ammonia concentrations in Alzheimer patients is expected to diminish cognitive deficits and to reduce the progression rate of the disease by reducing ammonia-induced excitotoxic mechanisms (133)

Protection against lethal TAA intoxications by 5FMOrn suggests the activation of regenerative processes in the liver due to the elevated Orn concentrations. In view of this possibility it may be of interest to examine the therapeutic potentials of OAT inactivation in liver cirrhosis, even though in rats with portacaval anastomosis this approach was not successful as a method to enhance the removal of ammonia.

The development of 5FMOrn as a potential drug is still at an early stage. However, the chemical synthesis of the active enantiomer of 5FMOrn has been solved (40), and the most important characteristics of the compound are known, and appear favourable. Moreover, OAT - inactivation is not only a new therapeutic target, but has, in contrast to most drugs, a clear mechanistic basis. Somewhat premature speculations concerning its major areas of potential applications may, therefore, be justified, the more so since in these therapeutic areas new appoaches are urgently needed.

REFERENCES

1. Herzfeld,A. and Knox,W.E. 1968, The properties, developmental formation and estrogen induction of ornithine aminotransferase in rat tissues. J. Biol. Chem. **243**: 3327-3332.
2. Peraino,C., Bunville, L.G. and Tahmisian,T.N. 1969, Chemical, physical and morphological properties of ornithine aminotransferase from rat liver. J. Biol. Chem. **244**: 2241-2249.
3. McGivan,J.D. , Bradford,N.M. and Beavis,A.D. 1977, Factors affecting the activity of ornithine aminotransferase in isolated rat liver mitochondria. Biochem.J. **162**: 147-156.
4. Greenstein,J.P., Winnitz,M., Gullino,P. and Birnbaum,S.M. 1955, The prevention of ammonia toxicity by L-arginine and related compounds. Arch. Biochem. Biophys. **59**: 302-303.
5. Greenstein,J.P., Winitz,M., Gullino, P., Birnbaum, S.M. and Otey,M.C. 1956, Studies on the metabolism of amino acids and related compounds in vivo. III. Prevention of ammonia toxicity by arginine and related compounds. Arch. Biochem. Biophys. **64**: 342-354.
6. Daune,G., Gerhart, F. and Seiler, N. Biochem. J. 1988, 5-Fluoromethylornithine, an irreversible and specific inhibitor of L-ornithine : 2-oxo-acid aminotransferase. Biochem. J. **253**: 481-488.
7. Seiler,N. and Daune-Anglard ,G. 1993, Endogenous ornithine in search for CNS functions and therapeutic applications. Metab. Brain Dis. **8**: 151-179.
8. Daune-Anglard,G., Bonaventure,N. and Seiler,N.,1993, Some biochemical and pathophysiological aspects of long-term elevation of brain ornithine concentrations. Pharmacol. & Toxicol. **73**: 29-34.
9. Cooper,A.J.L. and Plum, F. 1987, Biochemistry and physiology of brain ammonia. Physiol. Rev. **67**: 440-519
10. Perry,T.L. 1982, Cerebral amino acid pools. In *Handbook of Neurochemistry* (Lajtha, A. Ed.) 2nd. ed, Plenum Press, New York, vol. 1; pp 151-188.
11. Meister,A. 1965, *Biochemistry of the Amino Acids*, 2nd. ed. , Academic Press, New York, pp 108-113.
12. Seiler,N. and Lajtha,A. 1987, Functions of GABA in the vertebrate organism. In *Neurotrophic Activity of GABA During Development* .(Redburn,D.A.; Schousboe,A. Eds.), Alan Liss Inc. New York, pp 1-56.
13. Grant,S.M. and Heel,R.C. 1991, Vigabatrin: A review of its pharmacodynamic and pharmacokinetic properties and therapeutic potential in epilepsy and disorders of motor control. Drugs **41**: 889-926.
14. Pegg,A.E. 1986, Recent advances in the biochemistry of polyamines in eukaryotes. Biochem. J. **234**: 249-262.
15. Seiler,N. and Heby,O. 1988, Regulation of cellular polyamines in mammals. Biochim.Biophys. Hung. **23**:1-36.

16. Shih, V.E. 1981, Regulation of ornithine metabolism. Enzyme **26**:254-258.

17. Weber,G., Queener,S.F. and Morris,H.P. (1972) Imbalance in ornithine metabolism in hepatomas of different growth rates as expressed in behavior of L-ornithine carbamoyl transferase activity. Cancer Res. **32**: 1933-1940.

18. Jänne,J., Pösö,H. and Raina,A., 1978, Polyamines in rapid growth and cancer. Biochim. Biophys. Acta **473**: 241-293.

19. Shull,J.D., Pennington,K.L., George,S.M. and Kilibarda,K.A. 1991, The ornithine aminotransferase-encoding gene family of rat: Cloning, characterization, and evolutionary relationships between a single expressed gene an three pseudogenes. Gene **104**: 203-209.

20. Shull,J.D., Pennington,K.L., Pitot,H.C., Boryca,V.S. and Schulte,B.L. 1992, Isolation and characterization of the rat gene encoding ornithine aminotransferase. Biochim. Biophys. Acta **1132**: 214-218.

21. Shull,J.D., Esumi,N., Colwell,A.S., Pennington,K.L. and Jendoubi,M. 1995, Sequence of the promoter region of the mouse gene encoding ornithine aminotransferase. Gene **162**: 275-277.

22. Drejer,J. and Schousboe,A. 1984, Ornithine-δ-aminotransferase exhibits different kinetic properties in astrocytes, cerebral cortical neurones and cerebellar granule cells in primary culture. J. Neurochem. **42**: 1194-1197.

23. Daune,G. and Seiler,N. 1988, Interrelationsships between ornithine, glutamate and GABA - III. An ornithine aminotransferase activity that is resistant to inactivation by 5-fluoromethylornithine. Neurochem. Int. **13**: 383-391.

24. Boernke, W.E., Stevens, F.J. and Peraino, C. 1981, Effects of self-association of ornithine aminotransferase on its physicochemical characteristics. Biochemistry **20**: 115-121.

25. Shen,B.W., Ramesh,V., Mueller,R., Hohenester,E., Hennig,M. and Jansinius,J.N. , 1994, Crystallization and preliminary x-ray diffraction studies on recombinant human ornithine aminotransferase. J. Mol. Biol. **243**: 128-130.

26. Mueckler,M.M. and Pitot,H.C. 1985, Sequence of the precursor to rat ornithine aminotransferase from a cDNA clone. J. Biol. Chem. **260**:12993-12997.

27. Simmaco,M., John,R.A., Barra,D. and Bossa,F. 1986, The primary structure of ornithine aminotransferase. Identification of active-site sequence and site of post-translational proteolysis. FEBS Lett. **199**: 39-42.

28. Lünsdorf,H.,Hecht,H.-J. and Tsai,H. 1994, High-resolution electron microscopic studies on the quaternary structure of ornithine aminotransferase from pig kidney. Eur. J. Biochem. **225**: 205-211.

29. Murphy,B.J. and Brosnan,M.E. 1976, Subcellular localization of ornithine decarboxylase in liver of control and growth-hormone-treated rats. Biochem. J. **157**: 33-39.

30. Kito,K., Sanada,Y. and Katunuma,N. 1978, Mode of inhibition of ornithine aminotransferase by L-canaline. J. Biochem. (Tokyo) **83**: 201-206.

31. Rosenthal,G.A. 1978, The biological and biochemical properties of L-canaline, a naturally occurring structural analogue of L-ornithine. Life Sci. **23**: 93-98.
32. Bolkenius,F.N., Knödgen,B. and Seiler,N. 1990, D,L-Canaline and 5-fluoromethyl-ornithine. Comparison of two inactivators of ornithine aminotransferase. Biochem. J. **268**: 409-414.
33. Williams,J.A.; Bridge,G.; Fowler,L.J.,John,R.A. 1982, The reaction of ornithine aminotransferase with ornithine. Biochem. J. **201**: 221-225.
34. Abeles,R.H. 1978, Suicide enzyme inactivators. In *Enzyme-Activated Irreversible Inhibitors* (Seiler,N., Jung,M.J. and Koch-Weser,J. Eds.) Elsevier/North Holland, Amsterdam., pp 1-12.
35. Rando,R.R. 1978, Principles of catalytic enzyme inhibition. In *Enzyme-Activated Irreversible Inhibitors.* (Seiler,N.;Jung,MJ.;Koch-Weser,J. Eds.) Elsevier:North Holland, Amsterdam pp.13-26.
36. Jung,M.J. and Seiler,N. 1978, Enzyme-activated irreversible inhibitors of L-ornithine:2-oxoacid aminotransferase. J. Biol. Chem.**253**: 7431-7439.
37. Jung,M.J., Heydt,J.G. and Casara,P. 1984, γ-AllenylGABA, a new inhibitor of 4-aminobutyrate aminotransferase. Comparison with other inhibitors of this enzyme. Biochem. Pharmac. **33**: 3717.-3720.
38. Daune,G. and Seiler,N. 1988, Interrelationships between ornithine, glutamate and GABA. II. Concequences of inhibition of GABA-T and ornithine aminotransferase in brain. Neurochem. Res.**13**: 69-75.
39. Bey,P., Jung,M.J., Gerhart,F., Schirlin,D., Van Dorsselaer,V. and Casara,P. 1981 omega-Fluoromethyl analogues of omega amino acids as irreversible inhibitors of 4-aminobutyrate:2-oxoglutarate aminotransferase. J. Neurochem. **37**: 1341-1344.
40. Ducep,J.B., Jund,K., Lesur,B., Sarhan,S., Schleimer,M., Zimmermann,P.R. and Seiler,N. 1996, Inhibition of ornithine aminotransferase: a new target for therapeutic intervention. In *Biomedical Frontiers of Fluorine Chemistry* (Ojima,I., McCarthy,J.R. and Welch,J.T. Eds.), ACS Books, American Chemical Society, Washington.
41. Kaiser-Kupfer,M.I., De Monasterio,F.M., Valle,D.L. Walser,M., and Brusilow S. 1980, Gyrate atrophy of the choroid and retina. Improved visual function following reduction of plasma ornithine by diet. Science **210**: 1128-1131.
42. Kuwabara,T., Ishikawa,Y. and Kaiser-Kupfer,M.I. 1980, Experimental model of gyrate atrophy in animals. Ophthalmology **88**: 331-334.
43. Garthwaite,G., Williams,G.D. and Garthwaite,J. 1992, Glutamate toxicity: An experimental and theoretical analysis. Eur. J. Neurosci. **4**: 353-360.
44. Wang,T., Lawler,A.M., Steel,G., Sipila,I., Milan,A.H., and Valle,D. (1995) Mice lacking ornithine-δ-aminotransferase have paradoxical neonatal hypoornithine-aemia and retinal degeneration. Nature Genet. **11**:185-190.
45. Seiler,N., Daune,G., Bolkenius,F.N. and Knödgen,B. 1989, Ornithine aminotransferase activity, tissue ornithine concentrations, and polyamine metabolism. Int. J. Biochem. **21**: 425-432.

46. Sarhan,S., Knödgen,B., Grauffel,C. and Seiler,N. 1993, Effects of inhibition of ornithine aminotransferase on thioacetamide-induced hepatógenic encephalopathy. Neurochem. Res. **18**: 539-549.
47. Seiler,N., Grauffel,C., Daune,G. and Gerhart,F. 1989, Ornithine aminotransferase activity, liver ornithine concentration and acute ammonia intoxication. Life Sci. **45**: 1009-1019.
48. Zieve,L. 1986, Conditional deficiencies of ornithine or arginine. J. Am. Coll. Nutr. **5**: 167-176.
49. Grisolia,S., Minana,M.D., Grau,E. and Felipo,V. 1994. Control of urea synthesis and ammonia detoxification. In *Cirrhosis, Hyperammonemia and Hepatic Encephalopathy* (Grisolia,S. and Felipo,V. eds.), Plenum Press, New York, pp. 1-12.
50. Matsuzawa,T., Kobayashi,T., Tashiro,K. and Kasahara,M. 1994, Changes in ornithine metabolic enzymes induced by dietary protein in small intestine and liver:intestine-liver relationship in ornithine supply to liver. J; Biochem. (Tokyo) **116**: 721-727.
51. Seiler,N., Sarhan,S., Knoedgen,B., Hornsperger,J.M. and Sablone,M. (1993) Enhanced endogenous ornithine concentrations protect against tonic seizures and coma in acute ammonia intoxication. Pharmacol.&Toxicol. **72**: 116-123.
52. Lusty,C.J., Jilka,R. and Nietsch,E.H. 1979, Ornithine transcarbamylase of rat liver. Kinetic, physical and chemical properties. J. Biol. Chem. **254**: 10030-10036.
53. Raijman, L. 1974, Citrullin synthesis in rat tissues and liver content of carbamoyl-phosphate and ornithine. Biochem. J. **138**: 225-223.
54. Sarhan,S., Knödgen,B. and Seiler,N. 1994, Protection against lethal ammonia intoxication: Synergism between endogenous ornithine and L-carnitine. Metab. Brain Dis. **9**: 67-79.
55. Matsuoka,M., Igisu,H., Kohryama,K. and Inoue,N. 1991, Suppression of neurotoxicity of ammonia by L-carnitine. Brain Res. **567**: 328-331.
56. Matsuoka,M. and Igisu,H. 1993, Comparison of the effects of L-carnitine, D-carnitine and acetyl-L-carnitine on the neurotoxicity of ammonia. Biochem. Pharmacol. **46**:159-164.
57. Costell,M., O'Connor,J.E., Miguez,H.P. and Grisolia,S. 1984, Effects of L-carnitine on urea synthesis following acute ammonia intoxication in mice. Biochem. Biophys. Res. Commun. **120**: 726-733.
58. O'Connor, J.E., Costell, M. and Grisolia,S. 1984, Protective effect of L-carnitine in hyperammonemia. FEBS Lett. **166**: 331-334.
59. O'Connor,J.E., Costell,M. and Grisolia,S. 1984, Prevention of ammonia toxicity by L-carnitine. Neurochem. Res. **9**: 563-570.
60. Meijer,A.J. and Hensgens,H.E.S.J. 1982, Ureogenesis. In: *Metabolic Compartmentation* (Sies,H. ed.) Academic Press, New York, pp. 259-286.
61. Ratnakumari,L., Qureshi,I. and Butterworth,R.F. 1993, Effect of L-carnitine on cerebral and hepatic energy metabolites in congenitally hyperammonemic sparse-fur mice and its role during benzoate therapy. Metabolism **42**:1039-1046.

62. Robinshaw,J.D. and Neely,J.R. 1985, Coenzyme A metabolism. Am. J. Physiol. **248:** E1-E9.

63. Janiri,L. and Tempesla,E.A. 1983, A pharmacological profile of the effects of carnitine and acetylcarnitine on the central nervous system. Int. J. Clin. Pharmacol. Res. **3**: 295-306.

64. Imperato,A. Romacci,M.T. and Angelucci,L. 1989, Acetylcarnitine enhances acetylcholine release in the striatum and hippocampus of awake freely moving rats. Neurosci. Lett. **107**: 251-255.

65. Felipo,V., Minana,M.D., Cabedo,H. and Grisolia,S. 1994,. L-carnitine increases the affinity of glutamate for quisqualate receptors and prevents glutamate neurotoxicity. Neurochem. Res. **19**: 373-377.

66. Therrien,G., Sarhan,S., Knödgen,B., Butterworth,R.F. and Seiler,N. 1994, Effects of ornithine aminotransferase inactivation by 5-fluoromethylornithine in rats following portacaval anastomosis. Metab. Brain Dis. **9:** 211-224.

67. Seiler,N., Grauffel,C., Daune-Anglard,G., Sarhan,S. and Knödgen,B. 1994, Decreased hyperammonemia and orotic aciduria due to inactivation of ornithine aminotransferase in mice with a hereditary abnormal ornithine carbamoyl-transferase. J. Inher. Metab. Dis. **17**: 691-703.

68. Khatra,B.S., Smith III, R.B., Millikan,W.J., Sewell, C.W., Warren,W.D. and Rudman, D. 1974, Activities of Krebs-Henseleit enzymes in normal and cirrhotic human liver. J. Lab. Clin. Med. **84**: 708-715.

69. Herlong,H.F., Maddrey,W.C. and Walser,M. 1980, The use of ornithine salts of branched chain ketoacids in portal systemic encephalopathy. Ann. Intern. Med. **93**: 545-550.

70. Vogels,B.A.P.M., Maas, M.A.W., deHaan, J.G., Jörning,G.G.A., Slotboom, J., and Bovee, W.M.M.J. 1993, The effect of ornithine-aspartate (OA) on encephalopathy due to portosystemic shunting and hyperammonemia. Abstr. No; 113/O, 8th Intern. Symposium on Ammonia, Rome, Italy.

71. DeMars,R., LeVan,S.L., Trend,B.L. and Russel, L.B. 1976, Abnormal carbamoyl-transferase in mice having the sparse-fur mutation. Proc. Natl. Acad. Sci USA **73**: 1693-1697.

72. Briand,P., Francois,B., Rabier,D. and Cathelineau,L. 1982, Ornithine transcarbamylase deficiencies in human males; kinetic and immunochemical classification. Biochim. Biophys. Acta **704**:100-106.

73. Nelson,J., Qureshi,I.A., Vasudevan,S. and Sarma, D.S.R. 1993, The effect of various inhibitors on the regulation of orotic acid excretion in sparse-fur mutant mice (spf/Y) deficient in ornithine transcarbamylase. Chem. Biol. Interact. **89**: 35-47.

74. Rappaport,A.M. 1979, Physioanatomical basis of toxic liver injury. In: Toxic Injury of the Liver. (Farber,E. and Fisher,M.M. eds.) pp. 1 - 57, Marcel Dekker, New York.

75. Ledda-Columbano,G.M., Coni,P., Curto,M., Giacomini,L., Faa,G., Oliverio,S., Piacentini,M. and Columbano,A. 1991, Induction of two different modes of cell death, apoptosis and necrosis, in rat liver after a single dose of thioacetamide. Am. J. Pathol. **139**: 1099-1109.

76. Albrecht,J., Hilgier,W. and Rafalowska,U. 1990, Activation of arginine metabolism to glutamate in rat brain synaptosomes in thioacetamide-induced hepatic encephalopathy: an adaptive response? J. Neurosci. Res. **25**: 125-130.

77. Albrecht,J., Hilgier,W., Januszewski,S., Kapuscinski,A. and Quack,G. 1994, Increase of the brain uptake index for L-ornithine in rats with hepatic encephalopathy. Neuroreport **5:** 671-673.

78. Peeling,J., Shoemaker,L., Gauthier,T., Benarroch,A., Sutherland,G.R. and Minuk, G.Y. 1993, Cerebral metabolic and histological effects of thioacetamide-induced liver failure. Am. J. Physiol. **265:** G572-G578.

79. Zimmermann,C., Ferenci,P., Pifl,C., Yurdaydin,C., Ebner,J., Lassmann,H., Roth, E. and Hörtnagl,H. 1989, Hepatic encephalopathy in thioacetamide-induced acute liver failure in rats: Characterization of an improved model and study of amino acid-erg neurotransmission. Hepatology **9:** 594-601.

80. Basile,A.S., Pannell,L., Jaouni,T., Gammal,S.H., Fales,H.M., Jones,E.A. and Skolnick,P. 1990, Brain concentrations of benzodiazepines are elevated in an animal model of hepatic encephalopathy. Proc. Natl. Acad. Sci. USA **87**: 5263-5267.

81. Gammal,S.H., Basile,A.S., Geller,D., Skolnick,P. and Jones,E.A. 1990, Reversal of behavioral and electrophysiological abnormalities of an animal model of hepatic encephalopathy by benzodiazepine receptor ligands. Hepatology **11**: 371-378.

82. Osada,J.H., Aylagas ,M.J., Miro-Obradors,M.J., Palacios-Alaiz,E. and Cascales, M. 1990, Effect of thioacetamide administration on rat brain phospholipid metabolism. Neurochem. Res. **15**: 927-931.

83. Püspök,A., Herneth,A., Steindl,P and Ferenci,P. 1993, Hepatic encephelopathy in rats with thioacetamide-induced acute liver failure is not mediated by endogenous benzodiazepines. Gastroenterology **105**: 851-857.

84. Hilgier,W., Zitting,A. and Albrecht,J. 1985, The brain octopamine and phenylethanolamine content in rats in thioacetamide-induced hepatogenic encephalopathy. Acta Neurol. Scand. **71**:195-198.

85. Wysmyk,U., Oja,S.S., Saransaari,P. and Albrecht,J. 1992, Enhanced GABA release in cerebral cortical slices derived from rats with thioacetamide-induced hepatic encephalopathy. Neurochem. Res. **17**:11878-1190.

86. Kretzschmar,M., Machnik,G., Mueller,A., Splinter,F.K., Zimmermann,T. and Klinger,W. 1991, Experimental treatment of thioacetamide-induced liver cirrhosis by metenolone acetate. A morphological and biochemical study. Exp. Pathol. **42**:37-46.

87. Krähenbühl,S. and Reiche,J. 1992, Adaptation of mitochondrial metabolism in liver cirrhosis. Different strategies to maintain a vital function. Scand. J. Gastroenterol. **27**: Suppl. **193**: 90-96.

88. Seiler,N., Sarhan,S. and Knödgen,B. 1992. Inhibition of ornithine aminotransferase by 5-fluoromethylornithine: Protection against acute thioacetamide intoxication by elevated tissue ornithine levels. Pharmacol.& Toxicol. **7:** 373-380.
89. Fausto,N. 1970, RNA and amine synthesis in the liver of rats given injections of thioacetamide. Cancer Res. **30:**1937-1942.
90. Raina,A. and Jänne,J. 1970, Polyamines and the accumulation of RNA in mammalian systems.Fed. Proc. **29**: 1568-1574.
91. Seiler,N., Bolkenius,F.N. and Knödgen,B. 1980, Acetylation of spermidine in polyamine catabolism. Biochim. Biophys. Acta **633**:181-190.
92. Steele,W.J., Okamura,N. and Busch,H. 1965, Effects of thioacetamide on the composition and biosynthesis of nucleolar and nuclear ribonucleic acid in rat liver. J. Biol. Chem. **240**:1742-1749.
93. Kizer,D.E., Shirley,B.C., Cox,B. and Howell,B.A. 1965, Effect of thioacetamide on adenylic acid deaminase activity and nuclear ribonucleic acid metabolism in rat liver. Cancer Res. **25**: 596-603.
94. Reddy,J., Chiga,M. and Svoboda,D. 1969, Initiation of the division cycle of rat hepatocytes following a single injection of thioacetamide. Lab. Invest. **20**: 405-411.
95. Gullino,P., Winitz,M., Birnbaum,S.M., Cornfield,J., Otey, C. and GreensteinJ.P. 1956, Studies on the metabolism of amino acids and related compounds in vivo. I. Toxicity of essential amino acids, individually and in mixtures, and the protective effect of L-arginine. Arch. Biochem. Biophys. **64**: 319-332.
96. Stephens,J.R. and Levy,R.H. 1994, Effects of valproate and citrulline on ammonium-induced encephalopathy. Epilepsia **35**: 164-171.
97. Chiosa,K., Nicolescu,V., Bonciocat,C. and Stancu,C. 1965, The protective action of N-acetyl and N-carbamoyl derivatives of glutamic and aspartic acids against ammonia intoxication. Biochem. Pharmacol. **14**: 1635-1643.
98. Grau,E., Felipo,V., Minana,M.D. and Grisolia,S. 1992, Treatment of hyperammonemia with carbamylglutamate in rats. Hepatology **15**: 446-448.
99. Lamar,Jr. C. 1970, Ammonia toxicity in rats: protection by alpha-methylglutamic acid. Toxicol. Appl. Pharmacol. **17**: 795-803.
100. MacLean,D.A. and Graham,T.E. 1993, Branched-chain amino acid supplementation augments plasma ammonia responses during exercise in humans. J. Appl. Physiol. **74**: 2711-2717.
101. Marcaida, G., Felipo,V., Hermengildo,C., Minana, M.D. and Grisolia,S. 1992, Acute ammonia toxicity is mediated by the NMDA type glutamate receptors. FEBS Lett. **296**: 67-68.
102. Zieve,L., Lyftogt,C. and Raphael,D. 1986, Ammonia toxicity: comparative protective effect of various arginine and ornithine derivatives, aspartate, benzoate and carbamyl glutamate. Metab. Brain Dis. **1**: 25-35.

103. Salvatore,F., Cimino,F., D'Ayello-Caracciola,M. and Cittadini,D. 1964, Mechanism of protection by L-ornithine - L-aspartate mixtures and by arginine in ammonia intoxication. Arch. Biochem. Biophys. **107**: 499-503.

104. Staedt,U., Leweling,H., Gladisch,R., Kortsik,C., Hagmueller,E. and Holm,E. 1993, Effect of ornithine aspartate on plasma ammonia and plasma amino acids in patients with cirrhosis. A double-blind, randomized study using a four-fold crossover design. J. Hepatol. **19**: 424-430.

105. Batshaw,M.L., Brusilow,S., Waber,L., Blom,W., Brubakk,A.M., and Burton,B.K. 1982, Treatment of inborn errors of urea synthesis. Activation of alternative pathways of waste nitrogen synthesis and excretion. N. Engl. J. Med. **306**: 1387-1392.

106. Plum,F. 1971, The CSF in hepatic encephalopathy Exp. Biol. Med. **4:**34-41.

107. Butterworth,R.F. 1992, Pathogenesis and treatment of portal-systemic encephalopathy: An update. Dig. Dis. Sci. **37**: 321-327..

108. Capocaccio,L. and Angelico,M. 1991, Fulminant hepatic failure. Clinical features, epidemiology, and current management. Dig. Dis. Sci. **36:** 775.

109. Fisman,M., Gordon,B., Felcki,V., Helmes,E., Appel,J. and Rabhern,K. 1986. Hyperammonemia in Alzheimer's disease. Am. J. Psychiatry , **142**: 71-73.

110. Branconnier,R.J., Dessain,E.C., McNiff,M.E. and Cole,J.O. 1986. Blood ammonia and Alzheimer's disease. Am. J. Psychiatry **143**: 1313.

111. Hoyer,S., Nitsch,R. and Oesterreich,K. 1990, Ammonia is endogenously generated in the brain in the presence of presumed and verified dementia of Alzheimer type. Neurosci Lett. **117**: 358-362.

112. Samtoy,B. and DeBeukelaer,M.M. 1980, Ammonia encephalopathy secondary to urinary tract infection with *Proteus mirabilis*. Pediatrics **65**:294-297.

113. Drayna,C.J., Titcomb,C.B., Varma,R.R. and Soergel,K.M. 1981, Hyperammonemic encephalopathy caused by infection in a neurogenic bladder. N. Eng. J. Med. **304**: 766-768.

114. Valero,A., Alroy,G., Eisenkraft,B. and Itskovitch,J. 1974, Ammonia metabolism in chronic obstructuve pulmonary disease with special reference to congestive right ventricular failure. Thorax **29**:703-709.

115. Dutton,R.J., Nicholas,W., Fisher,C.J. and Renzetti Jr.,A.D. 1959, Blood ammonia in a chronic pulmonary emphysema. N. Eng. J. Med. **261**:1369-1373.

116. Nelson,R.M. and Seligson,D. 1963, Studies on blood ammonia in normal and shock states. Surgery, **34**: 1-8.

117. Caminal,L., Castellanos,E., Mateos,V., Astudillo,A., Moreno,C. and Dieguez,M.A. 1993. Hyperammonemic encephalopathy as the presenting feature of IgD multiple myeloma. J. Intrn. Med. **233**: 277-279.

118. Brusilow,S.W. 1984, Arginine, an indispensable amino acid for patients with inborn errors of urea synthesis. J. Clin. Invest. **74**: 2144-2148.

119. Bachmann,C. and Colombo,J.P. 1980, Diagnostic value of orotic acid excretion in heritable disorders of the urea cycle and in hyperammonemia due to organic acidurias. Eur. J. Pediatr. **134**:109-113.
120. Huttenlocher,R.P., Schwartz,A.D. and Klatskin,G. 1969, Reye's syndrome: ammonia intoxication as a possible factor in the encephalopathy. Pediatrics **43:** 443-454.
121. Shannon,D.C., DeLong,R., Bercu,B., Glick,T., Herrin,J.T., Moylan,F.M.B. and Todres,I.D. 1975, Studies on the pathophysiology of Reye's syndrome: hypeammonemia in Reye's syndrome. Pediatrics, **56**: 999-1004.
122. Chapoy,P.R., Angelini,C., Brown,W.J., Stiff,J.E.; Shug,A.L. and Cederbaum,S.D. 1980, Systemic carnitine deficiency - a treatable inherited lipid-storage disease presenting as Reye's syndrome. N. Eng. J. Med. **303**: 1389-1394.
123. Gordon,B.A., Gatield,D.P. and Haust,D. 1987, The hyperornithinemia, hyperammonemia, homocitrullinemia syndrome: an ornithine transport defect remediable with ornithine supplements. Clin. Invest. Med. **10**:329-336.
124. Schiffmann,R., Boneh,A., Ergaz,Z. and Glick,B. 1992. Nonketotic hyperglycinemia presenting with pin-point pupils and hyperammonemia. Isr. J. Med. Sci. **28**: 91-93.
125. Wilson,D.C., McGibben,D., Hicks,E.M. and Allen,I.V. 1993, Progressive neuronal degeneration of childhood (Alpers syndrome) with hepatic cirrhosis. Eur. J. Pediatr. **152**: 260-262.
126. Mortensen,E., Lyng,G. and Juhl,E. 1972, Ammonia-induced coma after ureterosigmoidostomy. Lancet **1**:1024.
127. Edwards,R.H. 1984, Hyperammonemic encephalopathy related to ureterosigmoidostomy. Arch. Neurol. **41**: 1211-1212.
128. Van Laethem,J.L., Gay,F., Franck,N. and van Gossum,A. 1992, Hyperammonemic coma in a patient with ureterosigmoidostomy and normal liver function Dig. Dis. Sci. **37**: 1754-1756.
129. Canzanello,V.J., Rasmussen,R.T. and McGoldrick,M.D. 1983, Hyperammonemic encephalopathy during hemodialysis. Ann. Intern. Med. **99:**190-191.
130. Batshaw,M.L. and Brusilow,S.W. 1982, Valproate-induced hyperammonemia. Ann. Neurol.**11**: 319-321.
131. Zaret,B.S., Beckner,R.R., Marini,A.M., Wagle,W. and Passarelli,C. 1982, Sodium valproate-induced hyperammonemia without clinical hepatic dysfunction. Neurology **32:** 206-208.
132. Binek,J., Hany,A., Egloff,B. and Heer, M. 1991, Acute fatal hepatic failure under valproic acid therapy. Schweiz. M. Med. Wochenschr. **121**:228-233.
133. Seiler,N. 1993, Is ammonia a pathogenetic factor in Alzheimer's disease? Neurochem. Res. **18**: 235-245..

SPARSE–FUR (spf) MOUSE AS A MODEL OF HYPERAMMONEMIA: ALTERATIONS IN THE NEUROTRANSMITTER SYSTEMS

I.A. Qureshi and K.V. Rama Rao

Division of Medical Genetics, Hôpital Sainte–Justine
Montréal, Québec, H3T 1C5, Canada

INTRODUCTION

Literature on sparse–fur (spf) mutant mouse, as an animal model of congenital hyperammonemia has been reviewed earlier[1,4]. Our current estimates indicate that over one hundred full–fledged articles have been published on spf mice since 1976, when the X–linked hepatic ornithine transcarbamylase (OTC; E.C. 2.1.3.3.) deficiency associated with the sparse–fur mutation was described for the first time[5]. An allelic form, the spf^{ash} (abnormal skin and hair) mutation, having a somewhat different phenotype to spf mouse, was also shown to have a quantitative deficiency of the hepatic OTC[6]. These publications have covered various aspects of the expression of the spf gene, including the clinical pathology, neurochemical pathology, behavior, experimental carcinogenesis and pharmacogenetics. Moreover, the spf mouse is now established as an animal model to study the effects of transgenic and viral–mediated gene therapy[7,12]. As indicated in Figure. 1, this has brought in a dramatic increase in new research studies on the spf and spf^{ash} mice, a big majority of which were initiated from our laboratory. It can be said that the spf mouse is now established as the most appropriate model to study the pathology and therapy of chronic hyperammonemic encephalopathy, particularly of hereditary origin. In the following text, we shall briefly review the nature and expression of the spf mutation, at the hepatic and intestinal levels, and its similarity to the human OTC deficiency. Particular emphasis shall be given to the neurochemical pathology in the spf mouse, from the point of view of metabolic and neurotransmitter abnormalities.

INHERITED ABNORMALITY IN THE SPARSE–FUR MOUSE

Nature of the Mutation

The X–linked spf mutation arose spontaneously in the progeny of an irradiated male at Oak Ridge National Laboratories, where it was maintained on various genetic backgrounds[5]. The mice originally used in our laboratory, in the study of their suitability as animal models of congenital

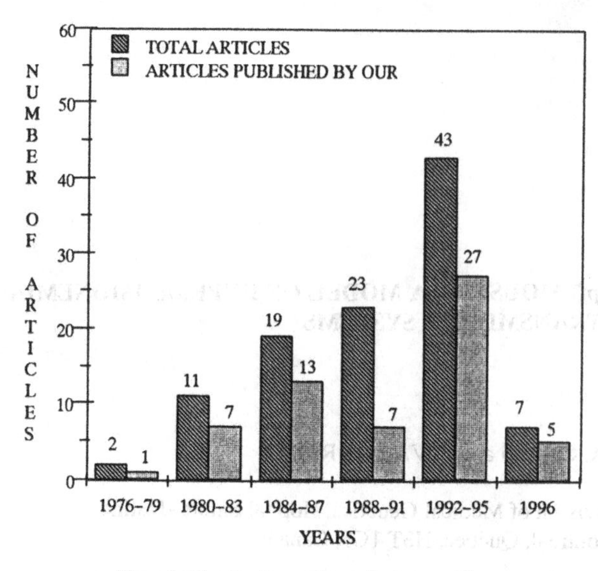

Figure 1. 20 years of research on spf mouse model.

hyperammonemia[13], were the progeny of +/Y males (22 A stock) and spf/+ female heterozygotes derived from SPFCP strains and bred at Oak Ridge. The characteristic phenotype of young spf/Y males born from the above stock was their small size, absent or relatively sparse fur and wrinkled skin. These traits were clearly discernible at 7 to 10 days. Hemizygous affected spf/Y males had an excitable hyper-reactive temperament. Furless males were frequently observed to be somnolent. The behavior of the heterozygous spf/+ females is not distinguishable from normal littermates, although a few show hyper-reactivity. Except for abnormal skin appearance, gross lesions in spf/Y males are not remarkable. Some hemizygous males have urinary bladder stones composed of orotic acid.

Various biochemical and enzymological studies had predicted that the spf mouse could have a single point mutation. Veres et al.,[14] have now verified a single base substitution in the complementary DNA for OTC from the spf mouse, by means of techniques for rapid mutation analysis. The OTC gene in the spf mouse contains a C to A transversion that alters a histidine residue to an aspargine residue.

Breeding of the Mutant OTC gene in spf Mice

To obtain viable affected males for breeding, it was necessary to transfer the spf gene to a suitable genetic background. Demars et al.,[5] transferred the spf gene to C57BL6J strain. In our laboratory, we have used CD-1 outbred albino males (Canadian Breeding Farms and Laboratories, St-Constant, Quebec) to transfer the gene by alternate matings of +/Y x spf/+ females and viable spf/Y males x +/+ females. Eighty percent of the new spf/Y males are now fully furred at weaning. The mortality has been reduced from 80% to 20% and the breeding capability of surviving males is normal.

Consequent to the transfer of the spf gene to the new genetic background, it has also been possible to generate viable spf/spf homozygous females. The spf/spf females are bred with +/Y males or spf/Y males to give spf/Y males that could be seperated from the female progeny by simple sexing[4].

HEPATIC AND INTESTINAL EXPRESSION OF MUTANT OTC IN spf MOUSE

The chemical lesions of the spf mouse are the important distinguishing features. Besides a decreased activity of hepatic and intestinal OTC (Table 1), there are significant increases in the urinary orotic acid excretion, serum ammonia and glutamine in spf/Y males and to a lesser extent in spf/+ females. In affected mice, orotate excretion is correlated to the decreased hepatic and intestinal OTC activity and increased serum ammonia and glutamine. The etiology of congenital hyperammonemias in spf mice may be linked to the structural mutation in the OTC molecule, to limit its capacity to catalyze the formation of citrulline from carbamyl phosphate and ornithine[15]. A recent study by Batshaw et al.,[7] using ^{15}N stable isotopes, has shown that the production of hepatic urea is also compromised in spf mice. Excess mitochondrial carbamyl phosphate volatilizes to ammonia or shifts into cytosol to form orotic acid by an induction of the pyrimidine pathway. Ammonia being a neurotoxin, is the cause of neurological symptoms associated with hyperammonemia. The spf^{ash} mouse has a somewhat different phenotype to that of spf mouse. The hepatic OTC activity is 5 to 10% of normal as compared to 13% in spf mice but the enzyme is kinetically normal. A comparison of spf and spf^{ash} strains[6] had shown that although the deficiency of hepatic OTC is comparable, the excretion of orotate is lower in the spf^{ash} mouse.

Studies conducted by several investigators have indicated that although the immunoreactive OTC protein levels increased, the translatable mRNA of the hepatic OTC gene in spf mice was only 26–58% of the normal expression (Table 1)[16,19].

SIMILARITY OF THE spf MOUSE TO HUMAN OTC DEFICIENCY

Primary Deficiency of the OTC enzyme

The human deficiency of OTC, the second enzyme of the urea cycle, was first described, in 1962[20]. Evidence for its X-linked dominant inheritance was presented in 1973[21]. Affected male hemizygote infants generally die in the first few weeks after birth, due to acute hyperammonemic

Table 1. Percent residual activity and mrna abundance of hepatic and intestinal ornithine transcarbamylase (otc) in the congenitally hyperammonemic spf–mouse

Liver	Intestine	pH	Reference
12	14–38	7.5	Qureshi et al., (1979 & 1985)[13,23]
10–20+	N.D	7.5	Gushiken et al.,(1985)[79]
11	11	7.5	Malo et al., (1986)[80]
10	N.D	7.5	Ohtake et al., (1987)[17]
10	N.D	7.5	Ratnakumari et al., (1992)[33]
4.5	N.D	7.5	Selier et al., (1994)[81]
20	N.D	7.5	Robinson et al., (1995)[55]
22	N.D	7.6	Demars et al., (1976)[5]
10	N.D	7.7	Bachmann and Colombo (1984)[49]
25	N.D	8.0	Briand et al., (1983)[16]
4	N.D	8.0	Monastiri et al., (1993)[82]
160	N.D	9.5	Briand et al., (1983)[16]
		mRNA ABUNDANCE	
58	N.D		Briand et al., (1983)[16]
67	N.D		Ohtake et al., (1987)[17]
74	81		Dubois et al., (1988)[18]
26	N.D		Mawal et al., (1996)[19]

Percent residual activity and mRNA expression of OTC were calculated by comparing with the corresponding control mice. N.D indicates not determined.

coma although chronic cases are now known. There is a wide spectrum of clinical manifestations in heterzygote females, from an aversion of protein foods to recurrent hyperammonemic episodes resulting in death. This disease is the most common hereditary urea cycle disorder in children.

Briand et al.,[22] compared the enzyme activity, kinetics and immunochemistry of mutant mouse OTC with liver samples from human males with OTC deficiency. They found that the spf and spf^{ash} mouse strains corresponded with two of the five groups of mutations seen in humans. OTC deficiency is also expressed in small intestine and colon of the spf mice[23]. A highly significant ($p<0.001$) correlation is seen with the enzyme activity from all segments of the intestine and that of the liver. The pH dependence and kinetics of mucosal OTC are similar to the liver enzyme. This similarity of OTC deficiency provides a basis for the use of mucosal biopsies to confirm the human disease.

Blood and Urine Chemistry

Similar to human patients of OTC deficiency, the spf/Y males given normal protein diets show plasma ammonia levels 2 to 3 times higher than normal (Table 2), whereas no differences were seen with a low protein diet[24]. There is an absolute increase in liver pyrimidine synthesis, which causes the down-regulation of the activity of the orotate-metabolizing enzyme complex[25]. There is an increased synthesis of pyrimidine nucleotides in spf mouse livers[26], similar to that of human patients of congenital hyperammonemia[27]. Our laboratory has tested the values of urinary orotate as a clinical parameter to distinguish the female carriers of OTC deficiency[28]. In a pure bred population of spf/+ heterozygotes (crosses of +/Y x spf/spf), a wide variability was seen in liver OTC activity and orotate excretion, which overlapped the normal distribution curves of +/+ and spf/Y groups. These correlation studies indicated that urinary orotate as an index of hepatic enzyme deficiency is valuable only for heterozygotes having an OTC activity less than 50% of normal. This is similar to the situation in human female heterozygotes of OTC deficiency, who have to be given an allopurinol loading test to verify the orotate and orotidine excretion as the current test for confirming heterozygosity.

Serum Amino Acids

Besides studying the levels of serum glutamine, various authors have measured the levels of other amino acids in the serum samples obtained from congenitally hyperammonemic spf mice (Table 3). In adult spf mice, except for serum tryptophan and glutamine levels of all the other amino acids are significantly reduced. In Table 4, these results are being correlated with the levels seen in the brains of spf mice and shall be discussed in detail in the section on neurochemical pathology. As predictable, there is also a significant reduction in the urea cycle amino acids in the serum e.g. arginine, ornithine and citrulline.

Secondary Carnitine Deficiency

Our clinical studies at the Sainte-Justine hospital, had indicated that various patients of congenital hyperammonemia have a tendency to develop a secondary carnitine deficiency of plasma and urinary free carnitine and an excess of esterified carnitines, particularly when being given a sodium benzoate therapy[29]. We have found similar results in spf mice. Our detailed studies of muscle and liver free carnitine and various acyl-carnitine groups have indicated that spf/Y mice develop a secondary carnitine deficiency of total, free and short & medium chain acyl-carnitines ranging from a 30 to 60% depletion[30,31]. Since more than 90% of the body carnitine reserves reside in the muscle and liver, this finding is quite significant. As such the spf mouse may also be considered as a model of secondary carnitine deficiency, caused by chronic hyperammonemia.

NEUROCHEMICAL PATHOLOGY IN THE spf MOUSE

Metabolic Abnormalities

Cerebral ammonia and glutamine (Table 2). The neurochemical abnormalities in congenitally hyperammonemic spf mice may primarily be due to the elevated levels of cerebral ammonia and glutamine. As a result of OTC deficiency at the hepatic level, the synthesis of urea and thus the detoxification of blood ammonia is compromised in spf mice. Since the blood and brain ammonia levels are in dynamic equilibrium, elevated blood ammonia rapidly diffuses into the brain. Inoue et al.,[32] reported high ammonia levels in the brains of spf mice, in which hyperammonemia was prominent immediately after weaning (30–40 days) and the levels of brain ammonia decreased at 60–80 days of age. Based on this observation, they called the former age to be the hyperammonemic stage (HA) and the later age as an adaptive stage (Ad). They also observed that the levels of ammonia during the adaptive stage almost reached the control values. In our laboratory, however, all the neurochemical studies performed in spf mice during the adaptive stage[33,36] showed that the cerebral ammonia levels, although lower than the HA stage, remained significantly higher as compared to the control CD–1 mice. One possibility for this discrepancy could be the various methods of brain isolation and the biochemical estimation of cerebral ammonia, employed in these studies.

Hyperglutaminemia is a consistent phenomenon in spf mice[32,34]. Our studies reported a two fold increase in the brain glutamine levels during the adaptive stage of the spf mice and this was consistent with the earlier reports of Inoue et al.,[32] and Batshaw et al.,[37]. In brain, glutamine synthesis is the major pathway for the removal of ammonia, due to a compromised urea cycle. Under hyperammonemic conditions, higher brain ammonia levels would be followed by an enhanced synthesis of brain glutamine as a reaction to the excess ammonia. The enhanced glutamine synthesis in spf mice is akin to the human congenital OTC deficiency, wherein a 2 to 3 fold increase in brain glutamine was reported by proton MR spectroscopy[38]. The ammonia–induced glutamine accumulation in astrocytes of the congenitally hyperammonemic patients was suggested to be responsible for the cerebral edema and astrocytic modifications called 'Alzheimer type II astrocytosis'[39].

Table 2. Plasma and brain ammonia and glutamine levels in the congenitally hyperammonemic spf–mouse

AMMONIA		GLUTAMINE		
PLASMA	BRAIN	PLASMA	BRAIN	REFERENCES
(% OVER CONTROL)				
+70	N.D	+43	N.D	Qureshi et al., (1981)[1]
+167	N.D	N.D	N.D	Spector et al., (1983)[24]
+190	N.D	N.D	N.D	Gushiken et al., (1985)[79]
+94	N.D	N.D	N.D	Chaouloff et al., (1985)[50]
+197	N.D	+75	N.D	Batshaw et al., (1987)[2]
+131	+127	+33	+169	Inoue et al., (1987)[32]
+159	N.D	+40	+54	Batshaw et al., (1988)[37]
+59	+55	+451	+110	Ratnakumari et al., (1992)[33]
+225	+70	N.D	+56	Seiler et al., (1994)[81]

Percentage changes are calculated comparing the corresponding control mice. N.D indicates not determined.

Cerebral neutral amino acids (Table 3). In addition to the enhanced accumulation of cerebral glutamine, various reports have also indicated an increase of large neutral amino acids such as tyrosine, phenylalanine and tryptophan in the brains of spf mice[32]. These reports also suggested that the increased accumulation of cerebral glutamine could be responsible for the influx of large neutral amino acids into the brain, since the efflux of cerebral glutamine is mediated by the large neutral amino acid carrier, and this condition could cause disturbances in the neurotransmitter synthesis.

Our studies on the cerebral amino acid profiles in spf mice have also indicated significantly increased levels of brain alanine and aspartate[35]. Increased brain alanine in spf mice could possibly be due to an ammonia-induced inhibition of pyruvate oxidation and subsequent shunting of the pyruvate carbons through the transaminase pathway. Increased cerebral aspartate levels in spf mice were in contrast to those observed in acquired hyperammonemic models of chronic liver disease[40], where the cerebral aspartate levels are reduced. However, ammonia-induced inhibition of the malate-aspartate shuttle could possibly result in the suppression of aspartate aminotransferase which could cause accumulation of cerebral aspartate. Thus, increased aspartate levels in spf mice may be responsible for seizure activity often encountered in OTC deficiency.

Urea cycle amino acids and cerebral creatine. Our studies have shown decreased levels of cerebral arginine, ornithine and citrulline which may be a reflection of the depletion of the serum levels of these amino acids in spf mice (Table 3). Our previous report[41] in spf mice, had indicated depleted serum levels of arginine, ornithine and citrulline, as a consequence of OTC deficiency in the intestinal mucosa which exports the citrulline required for the synthesis of arginine. Our studies also indicated a depletion of cerebral levels of guanidinoacetic acid and creatine in spf mice for which arginine is a precursor[36]. This arises due to the fact that, in brain, creatine synthesis depends absolutely on the availability of arginine which is derived from intestinal citrulline. Since OTC mutation is also expressed in the intestine, the availability of the circulating citrulline is compromised, leading to a metabolic arginine deficiency in spf mice. This condition could further compromise not only the cerebral creatine levels but also the synthesis of cerebral nitric oxide (NO). The synthesis of NO is mediated by the enzyme nitric oxide synthase (NO synthase), whose activity was also found to be decreased in spf mice[36]. Depleted cerebral creatine due to arginine deficiency in conjunction with increased alanine concentration, due to the inhibition of pyruvate oxidation would certainly exert a deleterious effects on the cerebral mitochondrial energy metabolism.

Mitochondrial Energy Metabolism

Studies on the peripheral type benzodiazepine receptor densities as a parameter of mitochondrial membrane functions. As a part of the series of experimental studies performed in spf mice to identify the neurochemical abnormalities, our studies on the peripheral type benzodiazepine receptors (PTBR)[42], which are markers on the mitochondrial membrane, indicated significantly higher densities (number of binding sites) in brain and in peripheral organs such as liver, kidney and testis. In brain, PTBRs are preferentially associated with the astrocytic mitochondria[43]. Since the OTC deficiency is characterized by astrocytic proliferation leading to Alzheimer's type II astrocytosis, we suggested that the ammonia-induced alterations in the PTBR densities in spf mice could be an index of the disturbances in the mitochondrial membrane function. This could subsequently lead to alterations in the cerebral mitochondrial energy metabolism.

Alterations in the cerebral energy metabolites. The primary neurochemical abnormality as a consequence of high ammonia levels may be its interference with the brain energy metabolism[44]. Our studies on the congenitally hyperammonemic spf-mouse model[33] indicated significantly higher levels of cerebral glucose, lactate and a-KG, while levels of pyruvate, glutamate and ultimately the levels of ATP were decreased. These alterations in the cerebral energy metabolites severely affected the ratios of the reducing equivalents in which the cytosolic

Table 3. Amino acid levels in serum and brain of congenitally hyperammonemic spf–mouse

AMINO ACIDS	SERUM	BRAIN	REFERENCE
	% OVER CONTROL		
Neutral amino acids			
Tyrosine	–35	+117	Inoue et al., (1987)[36]
Phenylalanine	–25	+123	"
Methionine	—	+66	"
Valine	–32	—	"
Leucine	–21	—	"
Isoleucine	–27	—	"
Threonine	–58	—	"
Serine	–43	—	"
Alanine	—	+42–80	Ratnakumari et al (1994)[35]
Tryptophan	—	+74	Bachamann & Colombo (1984)[49]
	+35	+28	Chaouloff et al., (1985)
	+ 36	+44	Batshaw et al., (1988)[37]
	N.D	+100	Inoue et al., (1989)[51]
Basic amino acids			
Histidine	—	+140	Inoue et al., (1987)[32]
Urea cycle amino acids			
Arginine	–56	–65	Inoue et al., (1987)[32]
	–64	—	Batshaw et al., (1988)[37]
	–55	–65	Seiler et al., (1994)[81]
	N.D	–40	Ratnakumari et al., (1996)[36]
Ornithine	–45	–19	Batshaw et al., (1988)[37]
	–18	+ 50	Seiler et al., (1994)[81]
	N.D	–41	Ratnakumari et al., (1996)[36]
Citrulline	–80	B.D	Inoue et al., (1987)[32]
	–82	B.D	Batshaw et al., (1988)[37]
	–80	–22	Seiler et al., (1994)[81]
	N.D	–33	Ratnakumari et al., (1996)[36]
Neurotransmitter amino acids			
Glutamate	N.D	—	Inoue et al., (1987)[32]
	N.D	–33	Ratnakumari et al., (1994)[35]
GABA	N.D	+20–40	Ratnakumari et al., (1994)[35]
Aspartate	N.D	+55–66	Ratnakumari et al., (1994)[35]

Percentages are calculated comparing with the corresponding control mice. __ denotes no change. + denotes % increase in the concentration while – denotes % decrease in the concentration. N.D indicates not determined, while B.D indicates a value below detectable range.

NADH/NAD$^+$ ratio was elevated, subsequently depleting their ratio in the mitochondria. Cerebral levels of CoA–SH and acetyl–CoA were also decreased in spf mice[45].

The abnormalities in cerebral energy metabolites could be implicated in a direct effect of hyperammonemia on the glycolytic and citric acid cycle pathways. The increase observed in the cerebral glucose levels could be due to its decreased consumption in the brain. The increased cerebral lactate levels could be explained on the basis of an ammonia–induced inhibition of the pyruvate dehydrogenase complex, while the increased a–KG levels in the brains of spf–mice could be due to a decreased utilization in the transamination reaction and by the glutamate dehydrogenase. The reduced mitochondrial energy metabolism in spf mice is similar to that of acute hyperammonemic animal models[46,47], which further confirms that ammonia *per se* could be responsible for the compromised energy metabolism. The decreased levels of pyruvate could probably be the result of increased conversion to lactate and/or its reduced production by alanine aminotransferase. Our results on the increased cerebral alanine levels in spf mice, as discussed in the previous paragraphs, would support this concept.

Defective respiratory chain enzymes. Our studies on the increased cytosolic NADH/NAD$^+$ ratios and subsequent depletion of the same in mitochondria prompted us to further study the status of the electron transport chain, including the activities of respiratory chain complexes in spf mice[45]. These results indicated a progressive decline in the cytochrome C oxidase (COX; complex IV) activity in different cerebral regions of spf mice. The degree of reduction was non–significant at pre–weaning (3 weeks) stage, while it became significant in 6 weeks old mice with a 26 ± 3% reduction as compared to the normal CD–1 controls. At 40 weeks the spf mice showed a further decline (36–48%) in the activity of cerebral COX. In order to elucidate the cause of the decreased COX activity, we have studied the quantitative expression of the whole brain mRNA corresponding to sub–unit I of COX in mutant spf mice and the normal CD–1 controls. The relative abundance of COX I sub–unit mRNA showed a tendency to decrease in spf mice, subsequent to a decline in the cerebral ratios of mitochondrial NADH/NAD$^+$.

The observed decline in the COX activity in our present studies could be due to multiple synergistic effects of hyperammonemia, leading to a cascade of dysfunctions at the level of cerebral mitochondrial energy metabolism. In brain, the reducing equivalents generated in the cytosol, are preferentially transported into mitochondria by the malate–aspartate shuttle, which plays an important role in the transfer of reducing equivalents[48]. Several lines of evidence have indicated that excess ammonia directly interferes with malate–aspartate shuttle, via the inhibition of cytosolic malate dehydrogenase and aspartate aminotransferase, which would result in the accumulation of reducing equivalents in the cytosol and the depletion of the same in the mitochondria[47]. This metabolic block in the transfer of reducing equivalents could further compromise the mitochondrial ATP production, possibly through substrate–depleted inhibition of the respiratory chain enzymes and subsequent feedback effect on the transcription e.g. cytochrome C oxidase.

The ammonia–induced metabolic abnormalities in spf mice, epecially the alterations in the cerebral amino acid profiles and the levels of energy metabolites, would directly or indirectly lead to disturbances in the synthesis, maintenance and functioning of various neurotransmitters in the brain, which could result in a cascade of neuronal dysfunctions at the synaptic level.

Neurotransmitter Abnormalities

Alterations in the cerebral transport of tryptophan. A precursor for serotonin. Published results have repeatedly indicated that the cerebral levels of tryptophan, and its metabolite 5–hydroxy indoleacetic acid (5–HIAA), which are the precursors for the neurotransmitter serotonin, are elevated in brains of spf mice. Bachmann and Colombo[49] reported enhanced levels of tryptophan and 5–HIAA in forebrain, brain stem and in the striatum of 28 days old spf mice. They also reported a flux through increase of serotonin synthesis using probenecid, an inhibitor of 5–HIAA efflux from the brain, which suggested that the increased transport of tryptophan and 5–HIAA could directly be responsible for the excess synthesis of cerebral serotonin. This is because of the fact that, tryptophan hydroxylase is never saturated *in vivo* at the ambient tryptophan concentrations. Chaouloff et al.,[50] reported a similar increased transport of tryptophan into brain in spf mice, while Inoue et al.,[51] reported enhanced levels of both catecholamines, such as norepinephrine, dopamine and dihydroxyphenyl-acetic acid (DOPAC), and tryptophan, 5-HIAA and serotonin in different cerebral regions of spf mice. It was commonly implicated that the ammonia-induced excessive synthesis of cerebral glutamine in congenitally hyperammonemic spf mice, could be responsible for increased transport of tryptophan and the subsequent enhanced synthesis of cerebral serotonin. Our further studies[52] on the activities of monoamine oxidases (MAO_A and MAO_B), which are the enzymes of serotonin catabolism, indicated a decrease in the MAO_A activity in cerebellum and brain stem of spf mice, with a concomitant increase in the MAO_B activity. In brain, MAO_A utilizes serotonin and norepinephrine as substrates and is predominantly present in neurons, while the MAO_B utilizes ß-phenylamine and is localized in astrocytes. Our report[52] further suggested that the increased levels of 5-HIAA, previously observed in spf mice, could be of astrocytic origin rather than of neuronal serotonin oxidation. Our results also suggested that a prolonged inhibition of neuronal MAO_A activity in spf mice brain, could have an impact on the excessive stimulation of serotonin receptors and a further down regulation of the same in spf mice.

Alterations in serotonin receptors. Our collaborative studies with Robinson et al.,[53], indicated significant alterations in the agonistic binding sites of both $serotonin_2$ and $serotonin_{1A}$ receptors in the spf mice. Using [^{3}H]ketanserin (for $serotonin_2$) and 8-[^{3}H]-hydroxy (di-n-propylamino)tetralin (8-OH-DPAT) (for $serotonin_{1A}$), it was reported that the number of binding sites (Bmax) for the $serotonin_2$ receptors were decreased, with a concomitant increase of the $serotonin_{1A}$ binding sites in brains of spf mice. No significant differences were observed in the affinities for both receptor subtypes. Studies were also conducted on the behavioral responses mediated by these receptors, in which spf mice when injected with quipazine, an agonist for the $serotonin_2$ receptors, showed a significantly reduced head twitch-response, a phenomenon mediated by the $serotonin_2$ receptors. Similarly, hypothermia elicited by the administration of 8-OH-DPAT studied as a response mediated by the $serotonin_{1A}$ receptors, increased significantly in spf mice. These data further provided support for the link between congenital hyperammonemia and alterations in the serotoninergic system in spf mice, which is akin to the patients of congenital urea cycle disorders. The symptoms associated with anorexia and sleep disturbances, often shown by the children with urea cycle disorders, are believed to be due to alterations in the serotoninergic neurotransmission[54].

Excitotoxicity of Quinolinate. A metabolite of tryptophan. Quinolinic acid, a tryptophan metabolite is also increased in the brains of spf mice [55] and in the CSF of children suffering from congenital urea cycle disorders[56]. Quinolinate is a known excitotoxin that acts at the N-methyl-D-aspartate (NMDA) sub-type of glutamate receptors to cause a persistent stimulation. Studies in the spf mouse brain, indicated significantly elevated levels of quinolinate following an increase in the cerebral tryptophan and glutamine[55]. A severe loss of medium-spiny neurons was also reported in the striatum of spf mice. This is similar to the pathological conditions identified by Batshaw et al.[57], in patients of urea cycle disorders. It is well known that a persistent stimulation of NMDA receptors opens up a cascade of excitotoxic mechanisms, leading to a calcium-mediated neuronal degeneration in brain. Batshaw et al.,[56] suggested that enhanced quinolinic acid levels in congenitally hyperammonemic children could be responsible for the severe neuronal loss and alterations in the astrocytic morphology.

Developmental deficiency of the cholinergic system. The patients of ornithine transcarbamylase (OTC) deficiency are characterized clinically by occasional seizures and impairment of cognitive functions, accompanied by a progressive cerebral atrophy and alterations in the normal morphological structure of astrocytes, leading to Alzheimer's type II astrocytosis[58]. The survivors of neonatal hyperammonemic coma, progressively develop mental retardation and cognitive dysfunctions. It is well known that, in brain, cholinergic mechanisms play a crucial role in the cognitive processes[59]. Based on this hypothesis, we undertook a series of neurochemical studies of the cholinergic system in the spf mouse model. These studies were conducted at various developmental stages to elucidate the ammonia–induced pathological changes in the cholinergic neurotransmission. The results of our study[60], indicated no significant changes in the choline acetyltransferase (ChAT) activity in spf mice upto 21 days of age. However, beyond 21 days, a generalized delay in the development of the ChAT was observed in spf mice with a reduction of upto 63% in the cortex, 53% in the thalamus, 36% in the striatum, 25% in brain stem and 26% in hippocampus, as compared to the age–matched CD–1 controls. The high affinity choline uptake, which is supposed to be involved in the synthesis of acetylcholine, also showed a developmental decrease in spf mice as compared to the control mice. No significant developmental changes were observed in the acetylcholinesterase activities in spf mice. The possible explanation for the delayed development of cholinergic system in spf mice could be due to an ammonia–induced inhibition and/or a loss of trophic factors to mediate the differentiation and maintain the normal number of cholinergic neurons. It has already been reported that nerve growth factors (NGFs) play an important role in the differentiation and survival of forebrain cholinergic neurons[61]. In order to clear this concept, we attempted to determine the levels of ß–NGF in different cerebral regions of spf mice. These data indicated significantly reduced levels of ß–NGF in most of the brain regions of spf mice, parallel to the decreased ChAT activity, confirming that ammonia–induced depletion of the nerve growth factors could be responsible for the delayed development of ChAT activity. Batshaw et al.,[7] have recently reported behavioral abnormalities in spf mice. These results also correlate well with the behavioral abnormalities and mental retardation exibited by the children suffering from urea cycle disorders. Using passive avoidance learning tests, they reported that the spf mice had less ability to perform this task with respect to the normal controls. These results also strongly pointed out the possibility of an impaired synthesis of neurotransmitter acetylcholine in spf mice and a subsequent effect on the cholinergic receptors.

Cholinergic receptor alterations. Our studies on the delayed development of cholinergic parameters prompted us to further probe into the fate of the cholinergic receptors in the spf mouse model. We performed *in vivo* quantitative receptor autoradiographic studies[62] on the central muscarinic cholinergic M_1 and M_2 receptors using selective ligands, [^{3}H]pirenzepine (M_1 receptor ligand) and [^{3}H]–AFDX 384 (M_2 receptor ligand), in different cerebral regions of spf mice. These data indicated a selective increase in M_1 receptors with a concomitant decrease in the M_2 receptor densities in brains of spf mice as compared to the CD–1 controls. The degree of increase in M_1 sub–type of receptors was between 24–54%, while the degree of reduction in M_2 receptors was up to 60%. In brain, M_2 sub–type of cholinergic receptors are supposed to be present in the pre–synaptic neurons, while the localization of M_1 sub–type is predominantly on the post–synaptic neurons. This pattern of decreased pre–synaptic M_2 receptors and our earlier studies of reduced ChAT activity in the brains of spf mice are well correlated. The concomitant increase in the M_1 post–synaptic binding sites in our spf mouse model could be due to the up–regulation in response to the loss of pre–synaptic M_2 binding sites. However, these results together, pointed towards the assumption that there could be an ammonia–induced selective loss of presynaptic cholinergic neurons in the spf mice.

Evidence of cholinergic neuronal loss. Our parallel studies to establish if there was any selective cholinergic neuronal loss in the spf mice, revealed a loss of choline acetyltranferase (ChAT) positive neurons throughout the cerebral cortex, septal area and diagonal band of spf mice[63]. These studies were performed by immunohistochemical technique using a monoclonal antibody for ChAT in the selective areas mentioned above. The results clearly showed a decreased ChAT–positive neuronal cell count in spf mice brains as compared to CD–1 controls. Our studies on spf mouse model were similar to the neuropathological studies done in human OTC deficiency, which consistently revealed a significant neuronal loss in cerebral cortex, basal ganglia and thalamus while relatively sparing the cerebellum and brain stem regions[64,65]. However, the pathophysiological mechanisms responsible for a selective neuronal loss in congenital hyperammonemias have not been definitely established. The correlation between the degree of brain damage and duration of hyperammonemia, rather than the peak ammonia levels in both spf mice and in patients of OTC deficiency[60,66], strongly supports the hypothesis that a metabolite of ammonia rather than ammonia *per se*, could be responsible for the excitotoxic neuronal damage in both these cases. The other alternative in this regard could be quinolinic acid, a known excitotoxin, which was reported to be elevated both in spf mice[55] and in patients of urea cycle disorders[56]. It has been reported that intrastriatal injections of quinolinic acid lead to a decreased ChAT activity in a dose–dependent manner[67]. Whatever the mechanism, our observations conclusively indicated a cholinergic neurotransmitter dysfunction in spf mouse model which was similar to that of the patients of OTC deficiency..

Alterations in the tissue glutamic acid levels. Our studies on the regional amino acid changes in spf mice[35] indicated a reduced glutamate level, only in the cerebral cortex, but not in any other regions. During the process of ammonia detoxification, brain utilizes tissue glutamate and cellular ATP for the synthesis of glutamine, which could lead to a depletion of tissue glutamate pools. However, lack of significant depletion of brain glutamate, except in cerebral cortex, could be explained on the basis of glutamate metabolism which is highly compartmentalized in brain, with a relatively small portion of tissue glutamate being available for glutamine synthesis. The selective depletion of glutamate levels in cerebral cortex, could possibly be as a result of a loss of glutamatergic neurons as a consequence of ammonia–induced, energy depletion–mediated excitotoxicity in spf mice. Cortical neuronal loss is characteristic in patients of OTC deficiency[64,65]. Moreover, we have also reported a cholinergic neuronal loss in the forebrains of spf mice[63]. Our current studies are, therefore, focussed on studying the mechanisms of a possible excitotoxic neuronal loss in spf mice .

Alterations in the N–methyl–D–aspartate (NMDA) receptor functions. NMDA sub–type of glutamate receptors are known to play a major role in brain physiology and pathology. These receptors under physiological conditions, mediate the long term potentiation of neurons, a phenomenon involved in learning and memory process. However, under certain pathological conditions, possibly including hyperammonemias of different etiologies, excess stimulation of these receptors opens up a cascade of calcium–mediated neuronal dysfunctions and is the cause of devastating consequences to the neurons, leading to their death. In order to address the causal relationship of neuronal loss and NMDA receptors, we have extended our studies in the spf mouse model to evaluate NMDA receptor densities by *in vivo* quantitative receptor autoradiography, using the selective antagonist MK–801[68]. These data indicated significantly decreased densities of MK–801 binding sites in 16 out of 17 brain regions of spf mice as compared with the CD–1 controls.

One possible explanation for the reduction in MK–801 displaceable NMDA binding sites, could be the loss of glutamatergic neurons in the brains of congenitally hyperammonemic spf mice. In one way, this is supported by our results on the loss of cortical and hippocampal neurons of upto 20% in spf mice[63]. The second and most likely explanation could be the down–regulation of these receptors in response to excessive exposure to the endogenous ligands. The endogenous ligands for NMDA receptors could be glutamate and/or quinolinate. Reports in the literature have already indicated elevated levels of cerebral quinolinic acid in spf mice[55] and in patients of OTC deficiency[56]. Although elevated quinolinic acid could probably be a likely explanation for the down regulation of NMDA receptors, the direct excitotoxic effects of the glutamate neurotransmitter in congenital hyperammonemias cannot be ruled out. This argument may arise due to the fact that in hyperammonemic animal models of either the aquired (portacaval anastomosis)[69] or induced (injection of ammonium salts)[70] type, increased extracellular concentration of glutamate is a characteristic in the brain with a concomitant loss of NMDA binding sites. However, in our spf mouse model, the phenomenon of increased extracellular glutamate, whether responsible for the down regulation of NMDA receptors or not, awaits further experimentation.

Alterations in Na^+–K^+–ATPase activity. Our earlier observations[33,34] have demonstrated a cerebral depletion of ATP in spf mice. The possible explanation for such a decrease in ATP availability could be due to: (a) direct toxic effects of ammonia at the sites of ATP production via the inhibition of various enzymes of the citric acid cycle and oxidative phosphorylation, including the cytochrome C oxidase and/or (b) enhanced utilization of the cerebral ATP in the detoxification of ammonia e.g. glutamine synthesis and/or increased consumption in response to ammonia-induced hyperexcitability of the neuronal membranes. It has already been reported by *in vitro* and *in vivo* studies that ammonium ions can cause membrane hyperpolarization and alter the ionic shifts[44]. Na^+–K^+–ATPase (EC 3.6.1.3), a plasma membrane bound enzyme involved in the maintenance of membrane potentials in brain, accounts for upto 50% of the total brain oxidative metabolism[71] and is coupled to various neurotransmitter functions. In view of the consistent ATP depletion and neurotransmitter–related changes, particularly the glutamatergic function in spf mouse model, we assessed the Na^+–K^+–ATPase activity in both congenital (spf mouse) and acquired (portacaval anastomosis) hyperammonemic conditions. Our results indicated a significantly elevated Na^+–K^+–ATPase activity in different cerebral regions of both spf mice and portacaval shunted rats[72].

The mechanism by which ammonia may cause the activation of Na^+–K^+–ATPase is not clear. One possible explanation, that has been recently proposed[73], involves the calcium–induced protein kinase C mediated decrease in the phosphorylation of Na^+–K^+–ATPase. This enzyme, when less phosphorylated, is more active[74]. These findings suggest that, in the brains of both spf mice and portacaval shunted rats, Na^+–K^+–ATPase is less phosphorylated and is therefore more active. This has been further supported by the in vitro experiments conducted by Neary et al.,[75] who reported a decreased protein phosphorylation in cultured astrocytes exposed to millimolar concentrations of ammonia. The increased Na^+–K^+–ATPase activities in spf mice model could partially, if not completely, be responsible for the depleted ATP levels and other pathophysiological mechanism(s) in this animal model.

Current work on the glutamatergic excitotoxicity and energy depletion. As mentioned, the exact mechanism for the neuronal loss and the down regulation of the NMDA sub–type of glutamate receptors in spf mice is not completely known. However, the possible factors involved in these abnormalities e.g. elevation of cerebral quinolinate, have already been discussed. Alternatively, the possible involvement of enhanced extracellular glutamate at the nerve terminals is also indicated. Our current research studies on the parameters of excitotoxicity, therefore, include: (a) the effects of hyperammonemia on the ontogeny of the NMDA receptors in spf mice, (b) further evaluation of the parameters of excitotoxicity e.g. changes in the extra–cellular concentrations of transmitter glutamate, intracellular accumulation of calcium and the changes in the energy–mediated reuptake of transmitter glutamate. In addition, studies are also continuing to evaluate the energy availability at various points in the mitochondrial energy metabolism e.g. electron transport chain complexes other than complex IV, ATP transfer enzyme such as ATP–ADP translocase in spf mice, as a consequence of congenital hyperammonemia in spf mice. To neutralize these pathogenetic mechanisms, the effect of acetyl–L–carnitine therapy is being studied in detail.

CONCLUSIONS

Extensive studies on the spf mouse model from our laboratory, in conjunction with our collaborators and from those of independent research groups, provide valuable information on the neurochemical pathology of the congenital hyperammonemias. Most of the metabolic abnormalities present in the spf mouse model are found to be similar to the patients of congenital hyperammonemias, especially of urea cycle enzymopathies. These studies suggest that the elevated brain ammonia and glutamine are the chief culprits causing various neuropathological abnormalities, including the brain amino acid imbalances, alterations in the mitochondrial membrane properties and various energy metabolites that could alter the respiratory chain enzyme complexes and ultimately the ATP depletion. These dysfunctions could further lead to the neurotransmitter abnormalities including the serotoninergic functions, cholinergic dysfunctions and ultimately the glutamatergic excitotoxicity.

It is interesting to note that, from a neuropathological standpoint, many of these neurochemical abnormalities, observed in congenital hyperammonemias and in the spf mouse model, are similar to the neurodegenerative disorders e.g. Alzheimer's type dementia. Seiler[76] and Hoyer[77], have speculated that ammonia and/or its chief metabolites could also be causative factors in Alzheimer's type disorders. In addition, Beal[78] has stated that defective cerebral mitochondrial function(s), leading to a decreased energy production, might result in the triggering of the excitotoxic mechanisms ultimately leading to neurodegeneration as seen in the Alzheimer's type disorders.

Based on our studies, in conjunction with other reports on the neuropathological abnormalities in neurodegenerative disorders, we hypothesize that the congenital hyperammonemias might also be neurodegenerative disorders, induced by an ammonia-mediated energy depletion and amplified by excitoxicity leading to a progressive neuronal loss.

Acknowledgements

The authors wish to acknowledge the Medical Research Council (MRC), Canada and Sigma-Tau company, Italy for financial support, Ms. Diane leblanc and Ms. Elaine Larouche for the technical assistance and Ms. Micheline Patenaude for secretarial work. The authors would also like to thank various collaborators, particularly, Drs. Mark Batshaw, Roger Butterworth, Mike Robinson, Bart Marescau and Peter de Deyn, who participated in some of the studies on spf mice, conducted in our laboratory.

References

1. I.A. Qureshi, J. Letarte, and S.R. Qureshi, Congenital hyperammonemia (Model No. 235), in: Handbook of Animal Models of Human Disease, C. C. Capen, D. B Hackle, T. C Jones, G. Migaki ed., Fasc 11. Washington, D.C: Registry of Comparative Pathology, pp 2–4 (1981).
2. M.L. Batshaw, S.L. Hyman, C. Bachmann, I.A. Qureshi and J.T. Coyle, Animal Models of congenital hyperammonemia, in: Animal Models of Dementia, J.T.Coyle, ed., Alan. R. Liss, Inc, New York, pp 163–198 (1987).
3. I.A. Qureshi, Congenital hyperammonemia (Model No. 235) Supplemetal Update, in: Handbook of Animal Models of Human Disease, C. C. Capen, D. B Hackle, T. C Jones, G. Migaki, ed., Fasc 11. Washington, D.C: Registry of Comparative Pathology, pp 1–2 (1989).
4. I.A. Qureshi, Animal models of hereditary hyperammonemias, in: Neuromethods, Animal Models of Neurological Disease, II, A. Boulton., G. Baker and R. Butterworth, ed., The Humana Press Inc, New York pp 329–356 (1992).
5. R. Demars, S.L. LeVan, B.L. Trend and L.B. Russel, Abnormal ornithine carbamoyl-transferase in mice having the sparse-fur mutation. Proc. Natl. Acad. Sci, U.S.A. 73:1693–1698 (1976).
6. I.A. Qureshi, J. Letarte and R. Ouellet, Spontaneous animal models of ornithine transcarbamylase deficiency: Studies on serum and urinary nitrogen metabolites, in: Urea Cycle Diseases, A. Lowenthal, A. Mori and B. Marecau, ed., Plenum Press, New York, pp 173–183 (1983).
7. M.L. Batshaw, M. Yudkoff, B.A. McLaughlin, E. Gorry, N.J. Anegawa, I.A.S. Smith and M.B. Robinson, The sparse-fur mouse as a model of gene therapy in ornithine carbamoyltransferase deficiency, Gene Therapy. 2:743–749 (1995).
8. J.C. Pages, M. Andreoletti, M. Bennoun, C. Vons, J. Elcheroth, P. Lehn, D. Houssin, J. Chapman, P. Briand, R. Benarous, D. Franco and A. Weber, Efficient retroviral-mediated gene transfer into primary cultures of murine and human hepatocytes: Expression of LDL receptor, Human Gene Therapy 6:21–30 (1995).
9. S.E. Raper, Hepatocyte transplantation and gene therapy, Clin Transplantation. 9:249–254 (1995).

10. M.A. Morsy and C.T. Caskey, Ornithine transcarbamylase deficiency: A model for gene therapy, in: Hepatic Encephalopathy, Hyperammonemia, and Ammonia Toxicity, V. Felipo and S. Grisolia, ed., Plenum Press, New York, pp 145–154 (1994).
11. M.A. Morsy, J.Z. Zhao, T.T. Ngo, A.W. Warman, W.E. O'Brien and F.L. Graham, Patient selection may affect gene therapy success, J. Clin. Invest. 97:826–831 (1996).
12. X. Ye, M.B. Robinson, M.L. Batshaw, E.E. Furth, I. Smith and J.M. Wilson, Prolonged metabolic correction in adult ornithine transcarbamylase-deficient mice with adenoviral vectors, J. Biol. Chem. 271:3639–3646 (1996).
13. I.A. Qureshi, J. Letarte and R. Ouellet, Ornithine transcarbamylase deficiency in mutant mice I. Studies on the characterization of enzyme defect and suitability as animal model of human disease, Pediat. Res. 13:807–811 (1979).
14. G. Veres, R.A. Gibbs, S.E. Scherer and C.T. Caskey, The molecular basis of sparse-fur mouse mutation, Science. 237:415–417 (1987).
15. N.S. Cohen, C.W. Cheung and L. Raijman, Altered enzyme activities and citrulline synthesis in liver mitochondria from ornithine carbamoyltransferase-deficient sparse-fur^{ash} mice, Biochem. J. 257:251–257 (1989).
16. P. Briand, S. Mirira, M. Mori, L. Cathelineau, P. Kamoun and M. Talibana, Cell-free synthesis and transport of precursors of mutant ornithine carbamoyltransferases into mitochondria, Biochem. Biophys. Acta, 760:389–397 (1983).
17. A. Ohtake, M. Takayanagi, S. Yamamoto, H. Nakajima and M. Mori, Ornithine transcarbamylase deficiency in spf and spf-^{ash} mice: Genes, mRNA and mRNA precursors, Biochem. Biophys. Res. Commun. 146:1064–1070 (1987).
18. N. Dubois, C. Cavard, J.F. Chasse, P. Kamoun and P. Briand, Compared expression of ornithine transcarbamylase and carbamyl phosphate synthetase in liver and small intestine of normal and mutant mice, Biochim. Biophys. Acta. 950:321–328 (1988).
19. Y.R. Mawal, K.V. RamaRao and I.A. Qureshi, Enhanced expression of hepatic mitochondrial urea cycle enzymes and cytochrome C oxidase with chronic acetyl-L-carnitine treatment in spf mice with ornithine transcarbamylase deficiency, J. Biol. Chem. (submitted) (1996).
20. A. Russel, B. Levin, V.G. Oberholzer and L. Sinclair, Hyperammonemia. A new instance of an inborn enzymatic defect of the biosynthesis of urea, Lancet. 2:699–700 (1962).
21. E.M. Short, HO. Conn, P.J. Snodgrass, A.G.M. Campbell and L.E. Rosenberg, Evidence for X-linked dominant inheritance of ornithine transcarbamylase deficiency, N. Engl. J. Med. 288:7–12 (1973).
22. P. Briand, B. Francois, D. Rabier and L. Cathelineau, Ornithine transcarbamylase deficiencies in human males: Kinetic and immunochemical classification, Biochem. Biophys. Acta. 704:100–106 (1982).
23. I.A. Qureshi, J. Letarte and R. Ouellet, Expression of ornithine transcarbamylase deficiency in the small intestine and colon of sparse-fur mutant mice, J. Pediatr. Gastroenterol. Nutr. 4:118–124 (1985).
24. E.B. Spector and R.A. Mazzochi, The sparse-fur mouse: An animal model for a human inborn error of metabolism of the urea cycle, in: Orphan Drugs and Orphan Diseases: Clinical Realities and Public Policy, Alan R. Liss, Inc, New York, pp 86–96 (1983).
25. I.A. Qureshi, J. Letarte and R. Ouellet, Activity of orotate metabolizing enzyme complex and various urea cycle enzymes in mutant mice with ornithine trans-carbamylase deficiency, Experientia. 38:308–309 (1982).
26. S. Vasudevan, I.A. Qureshi, L. Mores, P.M. Rao, S. Rajalakshmi and D.S.R. Sarma, Abnormal hepatic nucleotide pools in sparse-fur (spf) mutant mice deficient in ornithine transcarbamylase, Biochem Med. Metabol. Biol. 47:274–278 (1992).
27. L. Vasudevan, I.A. Qureshi, M. Lambert, P. Rao, S. Rajalakshmi and D.S.R. Sarma, Nucleotide pool imbalances in the livers of patients with urea cycle disorders associated with increased levels of orotic acid, Biochem. Mol. Biol. Int. 35:685–690 (1995).
28. I.A. Qureshi, J. Letarte, S. Lebel and R. Ouellet, Variablite de l'active enzymatique et de l'acidurie orotique chez les souris spf/+ heterozygotes deficientes en ornithine transcarbamylase, Diabete. Metabolisme. 12:250–255 (1986).
29. J.C. Feoli-Fonseca, M. Lambert, G. Mitchell, S.B. Melançon, L. Dallaire, D.S. Millington and I.A. Qureshi, Chronic sodium benzoate therapy in children with inborn errors of urea synthesis: Effect on carnitine metabolism and ammonia nitrogen removal, Biochem. Mol. Med. 57:31–36 (1996).
30. A. Michalak and I.A. Qureshi, Carnitine musculaire chez les souris hyperammoniémiques: effect du traitement au benzoate de sodium, Can. J. Physiol. Pharmacol. 71:439–446 (1990).
31. A. Michalak and I.A. Qureshi, Profil des acylcarnitines hepatiques et musculares chez les souris chroniquement hyperammonemiques apres un traitment aigu avec le benzoate de sodium: etudes dose-response, Ann Biol Clin. 50:879–885 (1993).
32. I. Inoue, T. Gushiken, K. Kobayashi and T. Saheki, Accumulation of large neutral amino acids in the brains of sparse-fur mice at hyperammonemic state, Biochem Med. Metabol. Biol. 38:378–386 (1987).

33. L. Ratnakumari, I.A. Qureshi and R.F. Butterworth, Effects of congenital hyperammonemia on the cerebral and hepatic levels of the intermediates of energy metabolism in spf mice, Biochem. Biophys. Res. Commn. 184:746–751 (1992).
34. L. Ratnakumari, I.A. Qureshi and R.F. Butterworth, Effect of sodium benzoate on cerebral and hepatic energy metabolites in spf mice with congenital hyperammonemia, Biochem. Pharmacol. 45:137–146 (1993).
35. L. Ratnakumari, I.A. Qureshi and R.F. Butterworth, Regional amino acid neuro–transmitter changes in brains of spf/Y mice with congenital ornithine transcarbamylase deficiency, Metabol Brain Dis. 9:43–51 (1994).
36. L. Ratnakumari, I.A. Qureshi, R.F. Butterworth, B. Marescau and P.P. De Deyn, Arginine-related guanidino compounds and nitric oxide synthase in brain of ornithine transcarbamylase deficient spf mutant mouse: Effect of metabolic arginine deficiency, Neurosci. Lett. 215:153–156 (1996).
37. M.L. Batshaw, S.L. Human, J.T. Coyle, M.B. Robinson, I.A. Qureshi, E.D. Mellits and S. Quaskey, Effect of sodium benzoate and sodium phenylacetate on brain serotonin turnover in the ornithine transcarbamylase-deficient sparse–fur mouse, Pediatr. Res. 23:368–374 (1988).
38. A. Conelly, J.H. Cross, D.G. Gadien, J.V Hunter, F.J. Kirkham and J.V. Leonard, Magnetic resonance spectrocopy shows increased brain glutamine in ornithine trans–carbamylase deficiency, Pediatr. Res. 33:77–81 (1993).
39. S.W. Brusilow and A.L. Horwich, Urea cycle enzymes, in: Metabolic and Molecular Bases of Inherited Disease, C.R. Scriver, A.L. Beaudet, W.S. Sly and D. Valle ed., McGraw Hill, New York, pp 1187–1232, (1995).
40. J.F. Giguere and R.F. Butterworth, Amino acid changes in regions of CNS in relation to function in experimental portal–systemic encephalopathy, Neurochem. Res. 9:1309–1321 (1984).
41. I.A. Qureshi, B. Marescau, M. Levy, P.P. DeDeyn, J. Letarte and A. Lowenthal, Serum and urinary guanidino compounds in sparse–fur mutant mice with ornithine transcarbamylase deficiency, in: Guanidines 2, A. Mori, B.D. Cohen and H. Koide, ed., Plenum Press, New York, pp 45–51 (1989).
42. V.L.R. Rao, I.A. Qureshi and R.F. Butterworth, Increased densities of binding sites for peripheral–type benzodiazepine receptor ligand [^{3}H]PK 11195 in congenital ornithine transcarbamylase–deficient sparse–fur mouse, Pediatr. Res. 6:777–780 (1993).
43. R.R.H. Anholt, Mitochondrial benzodiazepine receptors as potential modulators of intermediary metabolism, Trend. Pharmacol Sci. 7:506–511 (1986).
44. A.J.L. Cooper and F. Plum, Biochemistry and physiology of brain ammonia, Physiol Rev. 67:440–519 (1987).
45. K.V. Rama Rao, Y.R. Mawal and I.A. Qureshi, Progressive decrease of cerebral cytochrome C oxidase activity in spf mice: Effect of acetyl–L–carnitine in restoring the ammonia–induced cerebral energy depletion, Neurosci. Lett (accepted with revision) 1996.
46. L. Ratnakumari, G.Y.C.V. Subbalaxmi and Ch.R.K. Murthy, Acute effects of ammonia on the enzymes of citric acid cycle in rat brain, Neurochem. Int. 8:115–120 (1986).
47. L. Ratnakumari and Ch.R.K. Murthy, Activities of pyruvate dehydrogenase, enzymes of citric acid cycle and aminotransferases in the subcellular fractions of cerebral cortex in normal and hyperammonemic rats, Neurochem. Res. 14:221–228 (1989).
48. B. Hindfelt, F. Plum and T.E. Duffy, Effect of acute ammonia intoxication on cerebral energy metabolism in rats with porta–caval shunts, J. Clin. Invest. 59:386–396 (1977).
49. C. Bachmann and J.P. Colombo, Increased tryptophan and 5–hydroxyindoleacetic acid in the brain of ornithine carbamoyltransferase deficient sparse–fur mice, Pediatr. Res. 18:372–375 (1984).
50. F. Chaouloff, D. Laude, E. Mignot, P. Kamoun and J.L. Elghozi, Tryptophan and serotonin turnover rate in the brain of genetically hyperammonemic mice, Neurochem. Int. 7:143–153 (1985).
51. I. Inoue, T. Shimizu, T. Saheki, T. Noda and T. Fukuda, Serotonin–and catecholamine–related substances in the brain of ornithine transcarbamylase–deficient sparse–fur mice in the hyperammonemic state: Comparision of two procedures for obtaining brain extract, decapitation and microwave irradiation, Biochem Med. Metabol Biol, 42:232–239 (1989).
52. V.L.R. Rao, I.A. Qureshi and R.F. Butterworth, Activities of monoamine oxidase–A and–B are altered in the brains of congenitally hyperammonemic sparse–fur (spf) mice, Neurosci. Lett. 170:27–30 (1994).
53. M.B. Robinson, N.J. Anegawa, E. Gorry, I.A. Qureshi, J.T. Coyle, I. Lucki and M.L. Batshaw, Brain serotonin$_2$ and serotonin$_{1A}$ receptors are altered in the congenitally hyperammonemic sparse fur mouse, J. Neurochem. 58:1016–1022 (1992).
54. S.L. Hyman, J.C. Parke and C. Porter, Anorexia and altered serotonin metabolism in a patient with argininosuccinic aciduria, J. Pediatr. 108:705–709 (1986).
55. M.B. Robinson, K. Hopkins, M.L. Batshaw, B.A. McLaughlin, M.P. Heyes and M.L. Oster–granite, Evidence of excitotoxicity in the brain of the ornithine carbamoyltransferase deficient sparse fur mouse, Dev. Brain. Res. 90:35–44 (1995).
56. M.L. Batshaw, M.B. Robinson, K. Heyland, S. Djali and M.P. Heyes, Quinolinic acid in children with congenital hyperammonemia, Ann Neurol. 34:676–681 (1993).
57. M.L. Btashaw, Inborn errors of urea synthesis, Ann Neurol. 35:133–141 (1994).
58. S.W. Brusilow and A.L. Horwich, Urea cycle enzymes, in: Metabolic and Molecular Bases of Inherited Disease, C.R. Scriver, A. L. Beaudet, W.S. Sly and D. Valle, ed., McGraw Hill, New York, pp 1187–1232 (1995).

59. D.S. Olton, Dementia: Animal models of the cognitive impairments following damage to the basal forebrain cholinergic system, Brain Res. Bull. 25:499–502 (1990).
60. L. Ratnakumari, I.A. Qureshi, D. Maysinger and R.F. Butterworth, Developmental deficiency of the cholinergic system in congenitally hyperammonemic spf mice: Effect of acetyl–L–carnitine, J. Pharmacol. Exp. Ther. 274:437–443 (1995).
61. H.J. Martinez., C.F. Dreyfus., G.M. Jonakait and I.B. Black, Nerve growth factor promotes cholinergic development in brain striatal cultures, Proc. Natl. Acad. Sci. U.S.A. 82: 7777–7781 (1985).
62. L. Ratnakumari., I.A. Qureshi and R.F. Butterworth, Central muscarinic cholinergic M1 and M2 receptor changes in congenital ornithine transcarbamylase deficiency, Pediatr Res, 40: 25–28 (1996).
63. L. Ratnakumari., I.A. Qureshi and R.F. Butterworth, Evidence of cholinergic neuronal loss in brain in congenital ornithine transcarbamylase deficiency, Neurosci. Lett, 178: 63–65 (1994).
64. C.L. Dolman., R.A. Clasen and K. Dorovini–Zis, Severe cerebral damage in ornithine transcarbamylase deficiency, Clin. Neuropathol. 7: 10–15 (1988).
65. B.N. Harding., J.V. Leonard and M. Erdohazi, Ornithine transcarbamylase deficiency. A neuropathological study, Pediatrics. 141: 215–220 (1984).
66. M. Msall., P.S. Monahan., N. Chapanis and M.L. Batshaw, Cognitive development in children with inborn errors of urea synthesis. Acta. Pediatr (Jpn). 30: 435–441 (1988).
67. J. Alberch., E. Perez–Navarro., N.E. Calvo and J. Marsal, Trophic factors protect neostriatal cholinergic neurons against quinolinic acid lesion, Soc. Neurosci. Abstr. 19: 276.12 (1993).
68. L. Ratnakumari., I.A. Qureshi and R.F. Butterworth, Loss of [^{3}H]MK801 binding sites in brain in congenital ornithine transcarbamylase deficiency, Metabol Brain Dis. 10: 249–255 (1994).
69. F. Moroni, G. Lombardi, V. Carla, D. Pelligrini, G.L. Carassale and C. Cortesini, Content of quinolinic acid and other tryptophan metabolites increases in brains of rats used as experimental models of hepatic encephalopathy, J. Neurochem. 46:869–874 (1986).
70. V.L. Raghavendra Rao, A.K. Agrawal and Ch. R.K. Murthy, Ammonia–induced alteration in glutamate and muscimol binding to cerebellar synaptic membranes, Neurosci. Lett. 130:251–259 (1991).
71. J. Astrup, P. Sorensen and H. Sorensen, Oxygen and glucose consumption related to Na^{+}–K^{+}–transport in canine brain, Stroke. 12:726–730 (1981).
72. L. Ratnakumari, R. Audet, I.A. Qureshi and R.F. Butterworth, Na^{+},K^{+}–ATPase activities are increased in brain in both congenital and aquired hyperammonemic syndromes, Neurosci. Lett. 197:89–92 (1995).
73. E. Kosenko, Y. Kaminsky, E. Gran, M.D. Minara, M.G. Grisolia, S. Grisolia and V. Felipo, Brain ATP depletion induced by acute ammonia intoxication in rats is mediated by activation of the NMDA receptor and Na^{+},K^{+}–ATPase, J. Neurochem. 63:2172–2178 (1994).
74.. A.M. Bartello, A. Aperia, S.I. Walaas, A.C Nairn and P. Greengard, Phosphorylation of catalytic subunit of Na^{+}–K^{+}–ATPase inhibits the activity of the enzyme, Proc. Natl. Acad. Sci. USA. 88:11359–11362 (1991).
75. J.T. Neary, L–OB. Norenberg, M.P. Gutierrez and M.D. Norenberg, Hyperammonemia causes altered protein phosphorylation in astrocytes, Brain Res. 437:161–164 (1987).
76. N. Seiler, Is ammonia a pathogenetic factor in Alzheimers disease, Neurochem Res. 18:235–245 (1993).
77. S. Hoyer, Possible role of ammonia in the brain in dementia of Alzheimer type, in: Hepatic Encephalopathy and Hyperammonemia and Ammonia Toxicity, V. Felipo and S. Grisolia ed. Plenum Press, New York, pp 197–208 (1994).
78. F.M. Beal, Does impairment of energy metabolism result in excitotoxic neuronal death in neurodegenerative illnesses, Ann. Neurol. 31:119–130 (1992).
79. T. Gushiken, N. Yoshimura and T. Saheki, Transient hyperammonemia during aging in ornithine transcarbamylase–deficient, sparse–fur mice , Biochem. Int. 11:637–643 (1985).
80. C. Malo, I.A. Qureshi and J. Letarte, Postnatal maturation of enterocytes in sparse–fur mutant mice, Am. J. Physiol. 250:G177–184 (1986).
81. N. Seiler, C. Grauffel, G. Daune–Anglard, S. Sarhan and B. Knodgen, Decreased hyperammonemia and orotic aciduria due to inactivation of ornithine aminotransferase in mice with a hereditary abnormal ornithine carbamoyltransferase, J. Inher. Metab. Dis. 17:691–703 (1994).
82. K. Monastiri, D. Rabier and P. Kamoun, Prenatal diagnosis of ornithine transcarbamylase deficiency: Results in spf^{ash} mice, Prenatal Diagnosis. 13:441–447 (1993).

ABNORMAL GENE EXPRESSION CAUSING HYPERAMMONEMIA IN CARNITINE-DEFICIENT JUVENILE VISCERAL STEATOSIS (JVS) MICE

Takeyori Saheki, Mineko Tomomura, Masahisa Horiuchi, Yasushi Imamura, Akito Tomomura, Dewan Md. Abdullah Abu Musa, and Keiko Kobayashi

Department of Biochemistry, Faculty of Medicine, Kagoshima University
8-35-1 Sakuragaoka, Kagoshima 890, Japan

1. Introduction

Autosomal recessive juvenile visceral steatosis (JVS) was discovered in C3H.OH mice in 1985 by Hayakawa et al. (1, 2). The mutant mice showed symptoms very similar to those of Reye's syndrome, such as fatty liver, hyperammonemia, hypoglycemia and growth retardation. About 70% of the mice died at about 30 days of age. From the symptoms, carnitine deficiency was postulated and verified by analysis of serum and organs. Concentrations of both free and acylcarnitine were found to be very low (10 to 20% of the controls) in every organ examined (3). No abnormal carnitine derivatives were detected in the urine. These results together with the therapeutic effect of carnitine (4) indicate that the mice are a novel animal model of primary systemic carnitine deficiency. Thereafter, careful observation of JVS mice revealed cardiac hypertrophy (5), the most typical symptom in the human disease (6). Further studies showed that the primary defect is most probably in the renal carnitine transport system (7) and that the gene, *jvs*, is located on chromosome 11 (8). We analyzed the urea cycle enzymes to investigate hyperammonemia in JVS mice and found its pathogenesis novel and interesting (9). On the other hand, hyperammonemia is one of the symptoms in several inherited diseases of fatty acid metabolism (6, 10-12) and its pathogenesis in relation to urea cycle is not known. JVS mice can provide a means to solve the problem.

2. The Urea Cycle in JVS Mice in Infancy

We became interested in JVS mice when we found the activities of all urea cycle enzymes in the liver of JVS mice reduced to low levels during development (Fig. 1): 57% of control at 15-17 days to 11% at 25 days in carbamoylphosphate synthetase (CPS), 86% to 30% in ornithine carbamoyltransferase (OCT), 56% to 23% in argininosuccinate synthetase (ASS), and about 70% to 40% in argininosuccinate lyase (ASL) and arginase (9). On the other hand, at 25 days, the concentration of N-acetylglutamate was much higher in the liver of JVS mice than control (134 ± 35 nmol/g liver vs. 60 ± 20 nmol/g liver, respectively; n = 4). Thus, the hyperammonemia in JVS mice is associated with the reduction of all urea cycle enzyme activities. The reduction of the activities was parallel to the reduction of the enzyme amounts (9). The enzyme activities of glycolysis such as aldolase and lactate dehydrogenase and the rate of β-oxidation from palmitic acid in the homogenate supplemented with carnitine were higher in the liver of JVS mice than in the

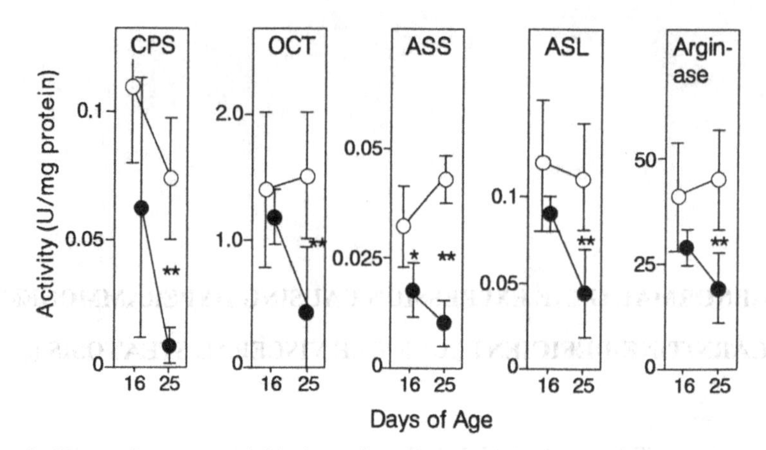

Figure 1. Urea cycle enzyme activities in the liver of control (O) and JVS (●) mice at 16 (15-17) days and 25 days of age. Values are the means ± SD (n = 9-11). From (9).

controls (9), indicating that the reduction of the urea cycle enzymes is not due to liver damage.

We analyzed mRNA coding for urea cycle enzymes along with several other mRNAs expressed in the liver by Northern blot analysis (13). The mRNAs of four urea cycle enzymes (CPS, OCT, ASS and ASL) tested at 25 days of age were remarkably reduced in the liver of JVS mice, as shown in Fig. 2 (13). Other liver-selective mRNAs such as albumin, serine dehydratase (SDH) and tyrosine aminotransferase (TAT) were low in JVS mice but glyceraldehyde 3-phosphate dehydrogenase (GAPDH) (13) and aldolase A (14) were high. Time-course experiments on the mRNA levels in the liver showed that CPS and ASS mRNAs increased during infancy in control mice but not in JVS mice (13, 15). The differences were significant at 15 days (see Fig. 5).

Run-on assay showed that the transcription of the urea cycle enzyme genes is suppressed (13). The suppressed transcription can account for the reduced mRNA levels of CPS, ASS and ASL, although some other factors seem to be necessary for the reduced OCT mRNA level.

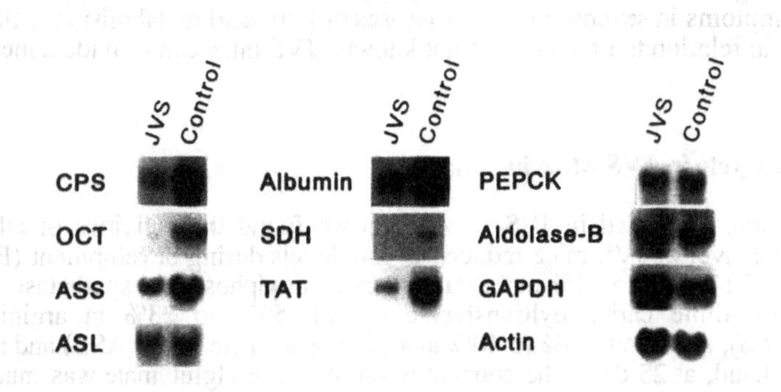

Figure 2. Northern blot analysis of total RNA from the liver of JVS and control mice. Total RNA (20 μg) isolated from mouse liver at 25 days of age was analyzed by Northern blot hybridization with probes; CPS, OCT, ASS, ASL, albumin, SDH, TAT, PEPCK, aldolase B, GAPDH and β-actin. From (13).

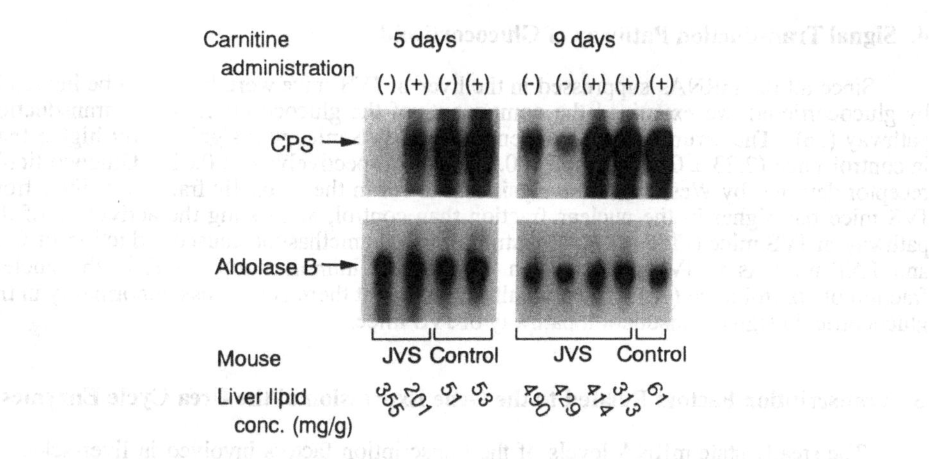

Figure 3. Effect of carnitine administration on CPS and aldolase B mRNAs revealed by Northern blot analysis and on lipid concentration in the liver. Total RNA (20 μg) isolated from mice treated with carnitine (+) or saline (-) for 5 or 9 days from 10 days after birth was applied to each lane. From (4).

3. The Effect of Carnitine Administration

Administration of carnitine at a dose of 1 mg per day from 10 days of age for 9 days caused complete normalization of CPS mRNA level (Fig. 3), although the lipid content in the liver was not normalized (4). This was probably due to the difference in the dose of carnitine necessary for normalization of gene expression and fatty liver. Since none of the carnitine-administered mice died, this was found to be a good way of breeding JVS mice.

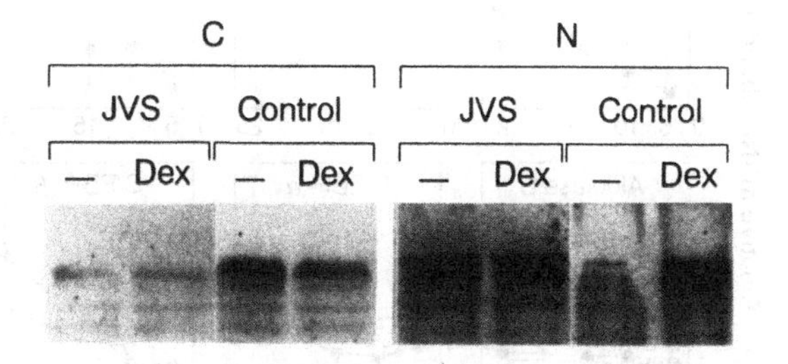

Figure 4. Relative amounts of glucocorticoid receptor protein and its intracellular localization in the liver of JVS and control mice at 25 days. Glucocorticoid receptor protein in cytosolic (C) and nuclear (N) fractions was determined after treatment with dexamethasone (Dex) or saline (-) for 30 min in control and JVS mice. In each experiment, 30 μg of protein of each fraction was electrophoresed on 7% SDS-polyacrylamide gel and immunoblotting with anti-GR antibody. From (16).

4. Signal Transduction Pathway of Glucocorticoid

Since all the mRNAs suppressed in the liver of JVS mice were known to be inducible by glucocorticoid, we examined the components of the glucocorticoid signal transduction pathway (16). The serum cortisol concentration in JVS mice was significantly higher than in control mice (2.23 ± 0.05 vs. 1.03 ± 0.04 ng/dl, respectively; $P < 0.01$). Glucocorticoid receptor detected by Western blot analysis was lower in the cytosolic fraction of liver from JVS mice but higher in the nuclear fraction than control, suggesting the activation of the pathway in JVS mice (Fig. 4). Administration of dexamethasone caused induction of CPS and TAT mRNAs in JVS mice and an elevation of immunoreactive GR in the nuclear fraction of control mice (16). These results suggest that there is no gross abnormality in the glucocorticoid signal transduction pathway of JVS mice.

5. Transcription Factors Related to the Gene Expression of the Urea Cycle Enzymes

The steady-state mRNA levels of the transcription factors involved in liver-selective gene expression were compared in control and JVS mice by Northern blot analysis at 25 days, when CPS mRNA was very low in JVS mice (15). The mRNA contents of HNF-4 in the liver of JVS mice were lower than control, and C/EBP-α was approximately half of the control level, but C/EBP-β and HNF-3α were slightly higher. There was no difference in HNF-1 between the two groups of mice. Figure 5 shows the developmental changes of the transcription factor mRNAs by slot blot analysis. CPS and the transcription factor mRNAs tested increased in the control liver during development but aldolase B mRNA did not. HNF-4 and C/EBP-α mRNA increased more slowly in JVS mice and were significantly lower in JVS mice than control at 25 days, while CPS mRNA in JVS mice was already significantly lower at 15 days. C/EBP-β mRNA content in the liver of JVS mice was higher than the control (but not significant), and there was no difference in developmental changes in HNF-1 and aldolase B mRNAs between the two groups. These results suggest that reduced amounts of C/EBP-α and HNF-4 may play a role in the decreased expression of the genes for urea cycle enzymes in infancy.

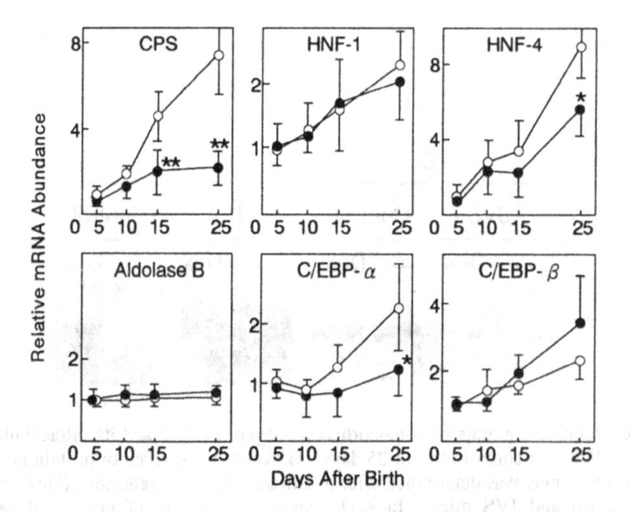

Figure 5. Developmental changes in the contents of CPS, aldolase B and liver-selective transcription factor mRNAs. Total RNA was isolated from livers of JVS (●) and control (O) mice at the ages indicated. The mRNA content was quantitated by slot blot hybridization analysis. Values are presented as means ± SD (n=6) in relative abundance units taking the control at 5 days as 1. *$P < 0.05$, **$P < 0.01$. From (15).

6. Enhanced Expression of Proto-oncogenes, c-jun and c-fos, and Activation of AP-1 DNA Binding Activity in the Liver of JVS Mice

During the experiments, we noticed that the disordered gene expression (suppression of liver-selective genes and activation of glycolytic enzyme genes) in the liver of JVS mice is similar to that in cancer or cancer-bearing liver. We observed that mRNA levels of proto-oncogenes, c-jun and c-fos, were high in JVS mice (14). α-Fetoprotein and aldolase A mRNA levels were also high (14). As shown in Fig. 6A, DNA binding activity of AP-1, the product of c-jun and c-fos genes, were markedly higher in JVS mice than in control at 7 days of age and increased till at least 25 days during development of JVS mice (16). Treatment of JVS mice with one mg of L-carnitine twice a day for 2 days caused a significant decrease in AP-1 activity, and treatment for 5 days caused a dramatic decrease to the same level as in control mice (Fig. 6B). These results together with the the results shown in Fig. 3 indicate that AP-1 activation and the expression of urea cycle enzymes are inversely proportional and that the change of AP-1 activity precedes the change of urea cycle enzyme expression.

7. Urea Cycle in Adulthood of JVS Mice and Effect of Starvation

JVS mice show growth retardation recognizable from 2 weeks and remarkable at 4 weeks, with concurrent reduction of urea cycle enzymes. As described previously, about 70% of JVS mice die by 5 weeks, but the rest survive the crisis. They begin to gain body weight rapidly and reach the control level at 46 days of age (15). They show urea cycle enzyme activities comparable to those of the controls, indicating that the reduction of the urea cycle enzymes is reversible and also suggesting that the symptoms such as hyperammonemia and growth retardation are limited to infancy.

To test whether JVS mice suffer from any disorder in the urea cycle in adulthood, we forced 8-week-old JVS mice to starve for 48 h and compared several parameters between fed and starved conditions (15). The liver of fed JVS mice looked less fatty at 8 weeks than at 4 weeks and was a little heavier than the control. On the other hand, 48 h starvation caused about 50% loss of liver weight in control mice and almost no change in JVS mice.

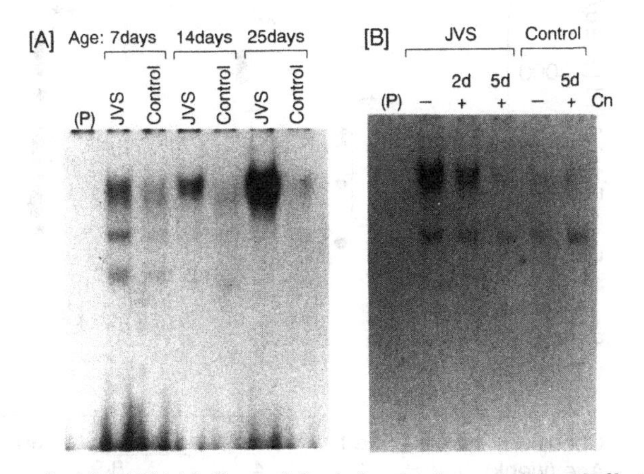

Figure 6. Changes in AP-1 DNA binding activity during development (A) and effect of carnitine administration on AP-1 DNA binding activity (B) determined by gel mobility-shift assay. Liver nuclear extracts from JVS and control mice at 7, 14 and 25 day (A), and from JVS mice at 15 days of age treated with carnitine (+) for 2 days or 5 days or saline (-) for 5 days before sacrifice (B) were incubated with ^{32}P-labeled oligonucleotide containing AP-1 binding site. (P), probe only. From (16).

Table 1. Effects of starvation for 48 h on hepatic lipid content and blood hormone levels in control and JVS mice at 8 weeks

	Control		JVS	
	Fed	Starved	Fed	Starved
Hepatic lipid (mg/g)	46.1 ± 5.2	42.1 ± 2.9	107.9 ± 35.3[a]	309.6 ± 71.7[b, c]
Insulin (ng/ml)	1.38 ± 0.37	< 0.38[a]	1.05 ± 0.65	< 0.38
Glucagon (pg/ml)	81.5 ± 22.8	92.3 ± 29.7	93.3 ± 29.1	159.5 ± 71.4
Cortisol (μg/dl)	1.24 ± 0.32	1.49 ± 0.14	1.34 ± 0.24	1.95 ± 0.48[d]

Data are expressed as the mean ± SD. [a] $P < 0.05$ compared with fed control mice; [b] $P < 0.01$ compared with fed JVS mice; [c] $P < 0.01$ compared with starved control mice; [d] $P < 0.05$ compared with starved control mice. From (15).

The color of the liver of JVS mice changed from reddish in fed mice to whitish in starved mice. The hepatic lipid concentration of control mice was not altered by the starvation (Table 1). On the other hand, the lipid concentration of JVS mice was twice that of the control mice under fed conditions, and was remarkably increased by the starvation. The level under starvation was comparable to that at 15 days (4). There were no significant differences in the concentrations of serum insulin, plasma glucagon and serum cortisol under fed conditions between control and JVS mice. The starvation caused a large decrease in the insulin concentration and no significant change in the glucagon concentration in both groups of mice. The cortisol concentration was significantly increased in JVS mice but did not change in control mice (Table 1).

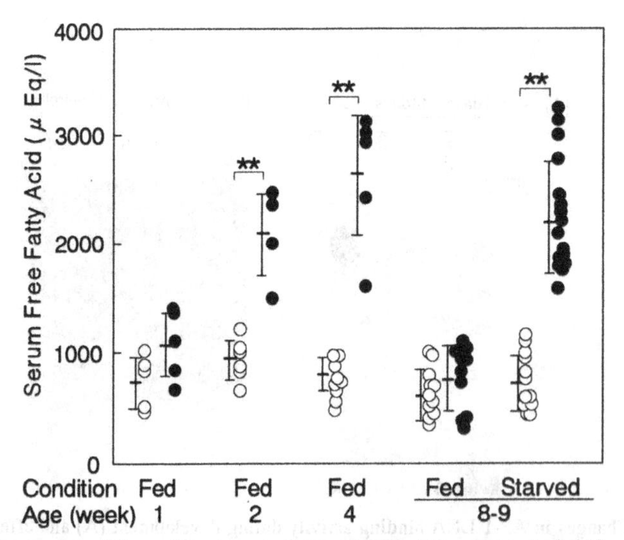

Figure 7. Serum free fatty acid concentrations of JVS (●) and control (O) mice during development and effect of starvation. Serum was taken from JVS and control mice at various ages under fed or 48 h starved conditions. $**P < 0.01$. From (15).

As shown in Fig. 7, serum free fatty acid concentration in JVS mice increased during development and reached three times the control level at 4 weeks. At 8 weeks, however, the fatty acid fell to the control level under fed conditions. Starvation for 48 h caused a great elevation of the free fatty acid concentration in JVS mice, almost to the level at 4 weeks, but no change in control mice (15).

CPS, ASS and GAPDH mRNA levels in the liver of fed JVS mice were comparable to those of the control mice at 8 weeks (Fig. 8). Starvation for 48 h doubled the CPS and ASS mRNA concentrations in the liver of control mice, but the effect was not significant in the liver of JVS mice. On the other hand, GAPDH mRNA increased under 48 h starvation in both groups, but more markedly in JVS mice. Thus, JVS mice show expression of urea cycle enzyme genes comparable to that in control mice in fed states, but the expression is insensitive to starvation stress.

The HNF-4 mRNA content under fed conditions was the same in control and JVS mice, and increased about four-fold in control mice and two-fold in JVS mice after the 48 h starvation (Fig. 8). The HNF-4 mRNA of starved JVS mice was significantly lower than that of control. Very similar results were observed for the C/EBP-β mRNA of control and JVS mice. On the other hand, there was no significant difference in C/EBP-α mRNA content between control and JVS mice and no significant change after the starvation. These results indicate that HNF-4 and C/EBP-β as well as urea cycle enzymes are less sensitive to starvation in JVS mice and suggest that the low response of these two transcription factors may be in part responsible for the low or zero response of urea cycle enzyme genes during starvation.

As described previously, AP-1 DNA binding activity increased in the liver of JVS mice during development (16), accompanied by increased c-jun and c-fos mRNA concentration (14). Figure 9 shows that AP-1 binding activity was low in the nuclear extracts from the liver both of control and JVS mice under fed conditions. The starvation stimulated AP-1 binding activity remarkably in JVS mice and slightly in control mice. There were no differences and no changes in Sp-1 DNA binding activity under fed and starved conditions of control and JVS mice. Northern blot analysis showed no difference in the mRNA level of c-jun, a component of AP-1, between control and JVS mice under fed conditions (data not shown). The starvation doubled the levels in both groups, but there was no difference between the groups. Again, activated AP-1 DNA binding activity were inversely related to the low response of the urea cycle enzyme genes.

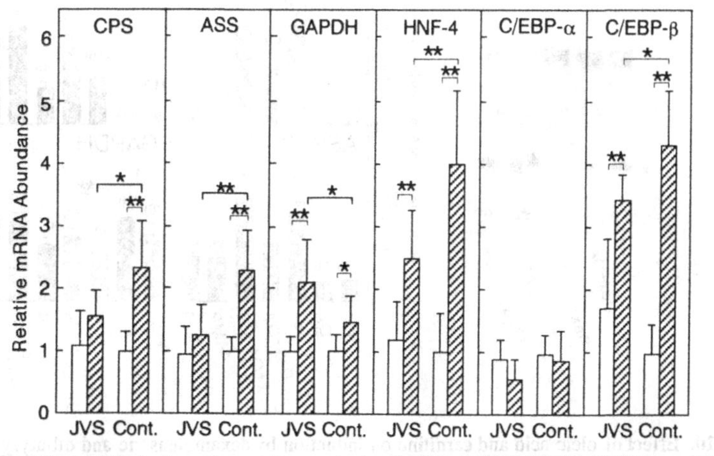

Figure 8. Effect of 48 h starvation on the contents of CPS, ASS, GAPDH, HNF-4, and C/EBP-α and -β mRNAs in the liver of JVS and control mice at 8 weeks. The mRNA contents in fed (open boxes) and starved (hatched boxes) mice were quantitated by slot blot hybridization analysis. Values are expressed as means ± SD (n = 8 or 9) in relative absorbance units taking the control under fed conditions as 1. From (15).

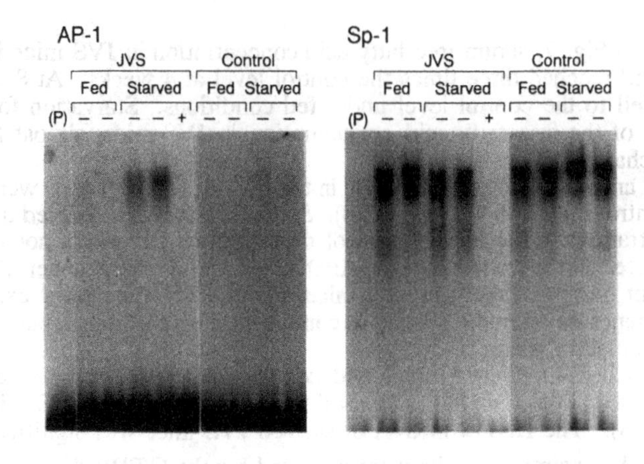

Figure 9. Effect of 48 h starvation on AP-1 and Sp-1 DNA binding activities in the nuclear extract from livers of JVS and control mice. DNA binding activities were assayed as described in Fig. 6. (P), probe only.

8. Long-Chain Fatty Acids as a Candidate for the Suppressor of Glucocorticoid Induction of Urea Cycle Enzyme Genes

All these results suggest that long-chain fatty acids, which cannot be metabolized properly in carnitine-deficient JVS mice and which accumulate in the sera of infant and starved adult JVS mice, may be a suppressor of glucocorticoid induction of urea cycle enzyme genes. We tested this possibility by using rat primary cultured hepatocytes (17).

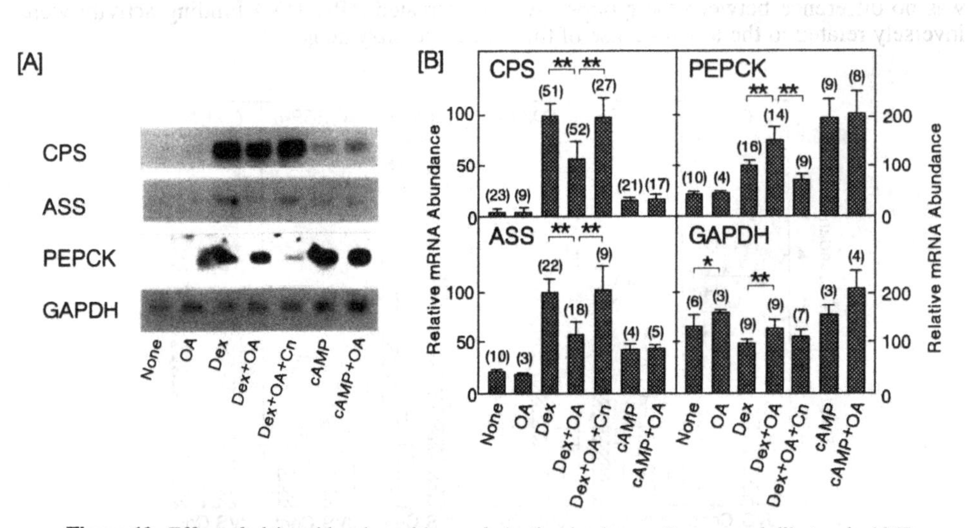

Figure 10. Effect of oleic acid and carnitine on induction by dexamethasone and dibutyryl cAMP of CPS, ASS, PEPCK and GAPDH mRNAs in the primary cultured rat hepatocytes. The mRNA contents were quantitated by slot blot hybridization analysis and values are presented as means ± SD in relative abundance with dexamethasone (Dex) as 100. Concentrations of reagents used are 0.5 mM oleic acid (OA), 10 nM Dex, 1 mM carnitine (Cn), and 10 μM dibutyryl cAMP (cAMP). Numbers in figure denote numbers of experiments. Statistically significant differences between the groups with and without oleic acid or carnitine are shown in figure; $^{*}P < 0.05$ and $^{**}P < 0.01$. From (17).

We examined the effect of oleic acid on CPS, ASS, phosphoenolpyruvate carboxykinase (PEPCK) and GAPDH mRNAs in the primary cultured hepatocytes with and without dexamethasone and dibutyryl cAMP (Fig. 10). Addition of 0.5 mM oleic acid (OA) to the medium caused almost no changes in mRNA amounts. Addition of 10 nM dexamethasone (Dex) caused approximately 30-fold, 5-fold and 2-fold increases in CPS, ASS and PEPCK mRNAs, respectively. Further addition of oleic acid (Dex + OA) suppressed the induction by dexamethasone of CPS and ASS mRNAs, and enhanced that of PEPCK mRNA. Addition of 1 mM carnitine to the system (Dex + OA + Cn) relieved the suppression by oleic acid of CPS and ASS induction and relieved the enhancement of PEPCK induction. Oleic acid showed no effect on the induction of CPS, ASS and PEPCK by 10 μM dibutyryl cAMP. In the case of GAPDH, dexamethasone caused a slight decrease in the mRNA content and dibutyryl cAMP caused a slight increase. Oleic acid caused a slight increase in the content irrespective of dexamethasone and dibutyryl cAMP. TAT mRNA increased like CPS and ASS mRNAs (data not shown). Thus, oleic acid specifically suppresses the induction by glucocorticoid of a group of genes. These changes in the mRNA of the enzymes caused by oleic acid seem to mimic those in the liver of JVS mice (13, 18).

We tested the specificity of fatty acids (Fig. 11). The induction of CPS mRNA by dexamethasone was not influenced by the addition of saturated medium-chain fatty acids (carbon-chain length less than 14). Saturated fatty acids having a carbon chain longer than 16 showed suppressive effects and the presence of double bonds enhanced the suppressive effect. With all fatty acids, addition of 1 mM carnitine reversed the effect almost completely. This suggests that the effect of fatty acids results partly from the shortage of carnitine in the primary cultured hepatocytes (19) causing the accumulation of fatty acids and that the addition of carnitine stimulates the metabolism by converting the fatty acids into fatty acylcarnitine. Addition of 0.5 mM lauric acid (12:0) or salicylic acid which were noneffective but may compete with an effective fatty acid for CoA to be further metabolized did not have any effect on the suppression (data not shown). All these results

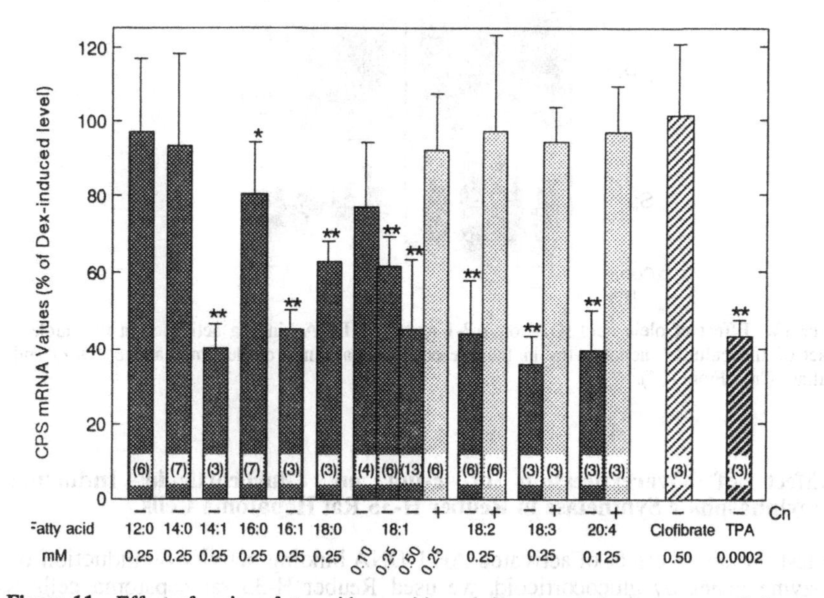

Figure 11. Effect of various fatty acids, carnitine, clofibrate and phorbor ester on induction by dexamethasone of CPS mRNA in the cultured hepatocytes. Fatty acids indicated with numbers of carbon and double bond or phorbor ester (TPA) were added to the medium with 10 nM dexamethasone (Dex) at the concentration indicated without (-) or with (+) 1 mM carnitine (Cn). Values are presented as means ± SD. Numbers in columns denote numbers of experiments. Statistically significant differences from the value of Dex only (100 ± 11.7; n=8) are shown in figure, *P < 0.05 and **P < 0.01. From (17).

suggest that free fatty acids, but not their metabolites, are the mediators. The spectrum of fatty acids affecting the induction seems to be similar to that for protein kinase C activation. Unsaturated long-chain fatty acids such as oleic acid and arachidonic acid have been reported to activate protein kinase C (20, 21). TPA (0.2 μM), a potent protein kinase C activator, suppressed glucocorticoid induction of CPS (Fig. 11). We do not have conclusive information on this mechanism, because protein kinase C inhibitors showed no consistent results (data not shown) and the suppression was caused by saturated long-chain fatty acids such as palmitic acid and stearic acid which have been reported not to activate protein kinase C (20, 21). Addition of clofibrate, a peroxisome proliferator, had no effect on the induction of CPS.

We assayed the AP-1 DNA binding activity by gel shift analysis of the nuclear fractions from the cultured hepatocytes under the conditions described in Fig. 12. AP-1 DNA binding activity observed under basal conditions was reduced by the addition of dexamethasone (Dex). Addition of oleic acid with dexamethasone (Dex + OA) enhanced the activity at 12 h but the effect was not clear at 24 h. Further addition of carnitine (Dex + OA + Cn) reduced the effect of oleic acid partially at 3 h (data not shown) and completely to the level of dexamethasone (Dex) at 12 h. Oleic acid only (OA) caused almost no change in the DNA binding activity. Sp-1 DNA binding activity was not affected by these treatments. These results suggest that the activated AP-1 DNA binding activity mediates suppression of urea cycle enzyme genes by fatty acids in cultured hepatocytes, although the AP-1 DNA binding activity was not so remarkably activated as in JVS mice *in vivo*.

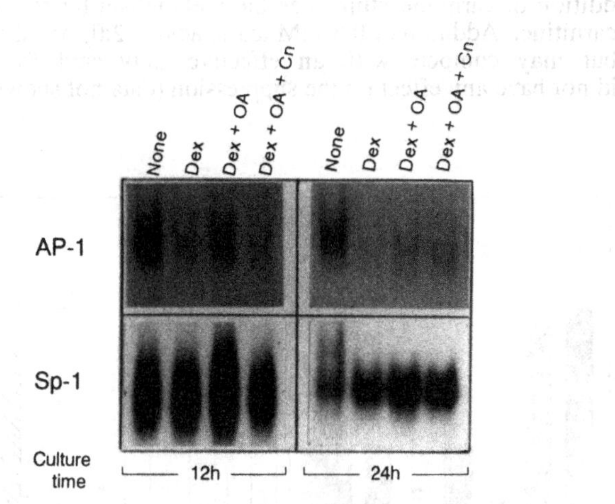

Figure 12. Effect of oleic acid (OA) on AP-1 and Sp-1 DNA binding activities in the nuclear extract of the cultured hepatocytes in the presence and absence of dexamethasone (Dex) and carnitine (Cn). From (17).

9. Effect of Overexpression of c-jun on Glucocorticoid Induction of Carbamoylphosphate Synthetase in Reuber H-35 Rat Hepatoma Cells

To test the direct effect of activated AP-1 DNA binding activity on induction of urea cycle enzyme genes by glucocorticoid, we used Reuber H-35 rat hepatoma cells which express CPS gene. The cells were transfected with a vector expressing rat c-jun cDNA (pCAGGS/c-jun) under cytomegalovirus enhancer and β-actin promoter elements (22). Fig. 13 shows the results of Northern blot analysis. Treatment with 1 nM dexamethasone for 15 h induced CPS mRNA in the cells transfected with a vector not carrying c-jun (pCAGGS) about 7-fold from the basal level. On the other hand, the induction levels of CPS mRNA by dexamethasone in the cells transfected with pCAGGS/c-jun were about 50% those of the cells transfected with pCAGGS. These results again strongly suggest that the product of proto-oncogene c-jun, AP-1, causes the suppression of glucocorticoid induction of urea cycle enzyme genes.

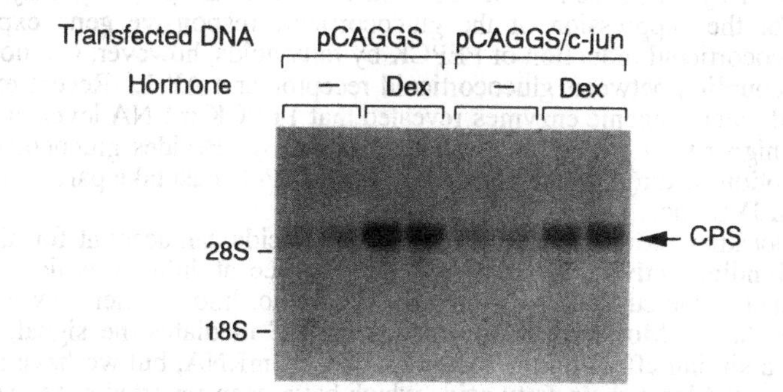

Figure 13. Effect of c-jun overexpression on dexamethasone induction of CPS in Reuber H-35 cells. Cells (10^6) were transfected by calcium-phosphate coprecipitation with 10 μg of expression vector carrying rat c-jun cDNA (pCAGGS/c-jun) or vector (pCAGGS) DNA only. After transfection, cells were washed and refed with serum-free medium containing 1 nM dexamethasone (Dex). After 15 h incubation, RNA was isolated and analyzed by Northern blot hybridization analysis.

10. Mechanisms of Suppression of Urea Cycle Enzyme Genes in JVS Mice

The expression of urea cycle enzyme genes is governed by a number of liver-selective transcription factors (23). Binding sites for the transcription factors have been sought to explain the liver-selective expression of the urea cycle enzymes: HNF-4 binding sites were found in OTC (24, 25) and CPS (26) genes; and C/EBP binding sites in OTC (24), CPS (27) and arginase (28, 29) genes. Nishiyori et al. (30) demonstrated that HNF-4 and C/EBP-β are important for the activation of the OTC gene. An imperfect CRE and half-sites of GRE have been found in the enhancer region of the CPS gene, and substitutional mutations in these sites strongly affected hormone-induced expression (26). The urea cycle enzymes, however, are induced by glucocorticoid with delayed onset which depends on *de novo* protein synthesis (31), suggesting that the glucocorticoid receptor does not act directly on the genes. Gotoh et al. (28) reported that C/EBP binding sites are present in the delayed glucocorticoid-responsive enhancer of the arginase gene. Matsuno et al. (32) showed that C/EBP-β is induced by glucocorticoid and glucagon, and suggested that the accumulated C/EBP-β protein is involved in secondary activation of target genes such as the urea cycle enzyme genes in response to the hormones in the liver.

Low mRNA levels of the liver-selective transcription factors, HNF-4 and C/EBP-α, at infancy, and low response of HNF-4 and C/EBP-β mRNAs to starvation in adulthood are probably involved in the suppressed expression of the urea cycle enzyme genes. But the CPS and ASS mRNA levels changed earlier and more remarkably than the transcription factors, and AP-1 DNA binding activity decreased earlier than the CPS mRNA increase after carnitine administration. These results suggest that AP-1 is involved more directly in the regulation of the urea cycle enzyme gene expression.

The results presented in this paper suggest that the mechanisms of suppression of urea cycle enzyme genes in JVS mice are as follows: JVS mice cannot utilize long-chain fatty acids but accumulate them in serum because the mice are carnitine-deficient owing to defective renal carnitine reabsorption. Fatty acid accumulation is remarkable in infancy and during starvation in adulthood when fatty acids are the major energy source. Long-chain fatty acids mediate a signal to activate AP-1, which causes suppression of glucocorticoid induction of urea cycle enzyme genes together with other liver-selective genes such as albumin and TAT. The cross coupling between glucocorticoid receptor and AP-1, suggested by Yang-Yen et al. (33) and Schüle et al. (34, 35), may be a possible mechanism for the suppression of the glucocorticoid-responsive gene expression. The enhanced glucocorticoid induction of PEPCK by fatty acids, however, can not be explained by the cross coupling between glucocorticoid receptor and AP-1. Recent experiments on glycolytic and gluconeogenic enzymes revealed that PEPCK mRNA levels in JVS mice are significantly higher than control at 2 weeks of age (18). Besides glucocorticoid receptor, some transcription factor(s) which also interact with AP-1 must take part in the altered gene expressions in JVS mice.

We do not know now whether long-chain fatty acids can account for all the activated AP-1 DNA binding activity in the liver of JVS mice at infancy which is much more remarkable than in the cultured hepatocytes. We do not know either how long-chain fatty acids activate AP-1. Most probably protein kinase C mediates the signal, since phorbor ester showed a similar effect on the induction of CPS mRNA, but we have no explanation as to why saturated long-chain fatty acids which have been reported not to activate protein kinase C also suppressed glucocorticoid induction of CPS in cultured hepatocytes and why we did not get consistent results with protein kinase C inhibitors.

Further analyses are under way to elucidate the mechanism of the fatty acid effect on gene expression and to examine its connection with the pathophysiology of JVS mice *in vivo.*

As described in the Introduction, the pathogenesis of hyperammonemia in JVS mice is novel. We suggest that the pathogenesis of hyperammonemia seen in a number of disorders in fatty acid oxidation may be the same as in carnitine deficiency.

Acknowledgement

We thank Mr. M. Gore for critical reading of the manuscript and Ms. M. Tanaka for secretarial assistance. This work was supported by Grants-in-Aid for Scientific Research (08670182 and 08770106) from the Ministry of Education, Science and Culture of Japan.

References

1. Koizumi, T., Nikaido, H., Hayakawa, J., Nonomura, A., and Yoneda, T., 1988, Infantile disease with microvesicular fatty infiltration of viscera spontaneously occurring in the C3H-H-2^0 strain of mouse with similarities to Reye's syndrome. Lab. Anim. **22:** 83-87.
2. Hayakawa, J., Koizumi, T., and Nikaido, H., 1990, Inheritance of juvenile visceral steatosis (jvs) found in C3H-H-2^0 mice. Mouse Genome **86:** 261.
3. Kuwajima, M., Kono, N., Horiuchi, M., Imamura, Y., Ono, A., Inui, Y., Kawata, S., Koizumi, T., Hayakawa, J., Saheki, T., and Tarui, S., 1991, Animal model of systemic carnitine deficiency: analysis in C3H-H-2^0 strain mouse associated with juvenile visceral steatosis. Biochem. Biophys. Res. Commun. **174:** 1090-1094.
4. Horiuchi, M., Kobayashi, K., Tomomura, M., Kuwajima, Y., Imamura, Y., Koizumi, T., Nikaido, H., Hayakawa, J., and Saheki, T., 1992, Carnitine administration to juvenile visceral steatosis mice corrects the suppressed expression of urea cycle enzymes by normalizing their transcription. J. Biol. Chem. **267:** 5032-5035.

5. Horiuchi, M., Yoshida, H., Kobayashi, K., Kuriwaki, K., Yoshimine, K., Tomomura, M., Koizumi, T., Nikaido, H., Hayakawa, J., Kuwajima, M., and Saheki, T., 1993, Cardiac hypertrophy in juvenile visceral steatosis (JVS) mice with systemic carnitine deficiency. FEBS Lett. **326:** 267-271.
6. Roe, C. R., and Coates, P. M., 1995, Mitochondrial fatty acid oxidation in: *The Metabolic and Molecular Bases of Inherited Disease* (Scriver, C. R., Beaudet, A. L., Sly, W. S., and Valle, D., eds) pp. 1501-1533, McGraw-Hill Inc., New York.
7. Horiuchi, M., Kobayashi, K., Yamaguchi, S., Shimizu, N., Koizumi, T., Nikaido, H., Hayakawa, J., Kuwajima, M., and Saheki, T., 1994, Primary defect of juvenile visceral steatosis (*jvs*) mouse with systemic carnitine deficiency is probably in renal carnitine transport system. Biochim. Biophys. Acta **1226:** 25-30.
8. Nikaido, H., Horiuchi, M., Hashimoto, N., Saheki, T., and Hayakawa, J., 1995, Mapping of *jvs* (juvenile visceral steatosis) gene, which causes systemic carnitine deficiency in mice, on Chromosome 11. Mammalian Genome **6:** 367-370.
9. Imamura, Y., Saheki, T., Arakawa, H., Noda. T., Koizumi, T., Nikaido, H., and Hayakawa, J., 1990, Urea cycle disorder in C3H-H-2° mice with juvenile steatosis of viscera. FEBS Lett. **260:** 119-121.
10. Pande, S. V., and Murphy, M. S. R., 1994, Carnitine-acylcarnitine translocase deficiency: implications in human pathology. Biochim. Biophys. Acta **1226:** 269-276.
11. Vianey-Saban, C., Stremler, N., Paut, O., Buttin, T., Divry, P., Zabot, M. T., Camboulives, J., Mathieu, M., and Mousson, B., 1995, Infantile form of carnitine palmitoyltransfease II deficiency in a girl with rapid fatal onset. J. Inherit. Metab. Dis. **18:** 362-363.
12. Rufini, S., Bragetti, P., Brunelli, B., Campolo, G., and Lato, M., 1993, Non-ketotic hypoglycemia caused by carnitine palmitoyltransferase I deficiency. Pediatr. Med. Chir. **15:** 63-66.
13. Tomomura, M., Imamura, Y., Horiuchi, M., Koizumi, T., Nikaido, H., Hayakawa, J., and Saheki, T., 1992, Abnormal expression of urea cycle enzyme genes in juvenile visceral steatosis (jvs) mice. Biochim. Biophys. Acta **1138:** 167-171.
14. Tomomura, M., Nakagawa, K., and Saheki, T., 1992, Proto-oncogene c-jun and c-fos messenger RNA increase in the liver of carnitine-deficient juvenile visceral steatosis (jvs) mice. FEBS Lett. **311:** 63-66.
15. Tomomura, M., Tomomura, A., Dewan, M. A. A. M., Horiuchi, H., Takiguchi, M., Mori, M., and Saheki, T., 1997, Suppressed expression of the urea cycle enzyme genes in the liver of carnitine-deficient juvenile visceral steatosis (JVS) mice in infancy and during starvation in adulthood. J. Biochem. in press.
16. Tomomura, M., Imamura, Y., Tomomura, A., Horiuchi, M., and Saheki, T., 1994, Abnormal gene expression and regulation in the liver of jvs mice with systemic carnitine deficiency. Biochem. Biophys. Acta **1226:** 307-314.
17. Tomomura, M., Tomomura, A., Dewan, M. A. A. M., and Saheki, T., 1997, Long-chain fatty acids suppress the induction of urea cycle enzyme genes by glucocorticoid action. FEBS Lett. in press.
18. Hotta, K., Kuwajima, M., Ono, A., Nakajima, H., Horikawa, Y., Miyagawa, J., Namba, M., Hanafusa, T., Horiuchi, M., Nikaido, H., Hayakawa, J., Saheki, T., Kono, N., Noguchi, T., and Matsuzawa, Y., 1996, Disordered expression of glycolytic and gluconeogenic liver enzymes of juvenile visceral steatosis mice with systemic carnitine deficiency. Diabetes Res. Clin. Practice **32:** 117-123.
19. Christiansen, R. Z., and Bremer, J., 1976, Active transport of butyrobetaine and carnitine into isolated liver cells. Biochim. Biophys. Acta **448:** 562-577.
20. McPhail, L. C., Clayton, C. C., and Snyderman, R., 1984, A potential second messenger role for arachidonic acid: activation of Ca^{2+}-dependent protein kinase. Science **224:** 622-625.
21. Murakami, K., Chan, S. Y., and Routtenberg, A., 1986, Protein kinase C activation by cis-fatty acid in the absence of Ca^{2+} and phospholipids. J. Biol. Chem. **261:** 15424-15429.
22. Niwa, H., Yamamura, K., and Miyazaki, J., 1991, Efficient selection for high-expression transfectants with a novel eukaryotic vector. Gene **15:** 193-199.

23. Takiguchi, M., and Mori, M., 1995, Transcriptional regulation of genes for ornithine cycle enzymes. Biochem. J. **312:** 649-659.
24. Murakami, T., Nishiyori, A., Takiguchi, M., and Mori, M., 1990, Promoter and 11-kilobase upstream enhancer elements responsible for hepatoma cell-specific expression of the rat ornithine transcarbamylase gene. Mol. Cell. Biol. **10:** 1180-1191.
25. Kimura, A., Nishiyori, A., Murakami, T., Tsukamoto, T., Hata, S., Osumi, T., Okamura, R., Mori, M., and Takiguchi, M., 1993, Chicken ovalbumin upstream promoter-transcription factor (COUP-TF) represses transcription from the promoter of the gene for ornithine transcarbamylase in a manner antagonistic to hepatocyte nuclear factor-4 (HNF-4). J. Biol. Chem. **268:** 11125-11133.
26. Christoffels, V. M., van den Hoff, M. J. B., Moorman, A. F. M., and Lamers, W. H., 1995, The far-upstream enhancer of the carbamoyl-phosphate synthetase I gene is responsible for the tissue specificity and hormone inducibility of its expression. J. Biol. Chem. **270:** 24932-24940.
27. Howell, B. W., Lagace, M., and Shore, G. C., 1989, Activity of the carbamylphosphate synthetase I promoter in liver nuclear extracts is dependent on a cis-acting C/EBP recognition element. Mol. Cell. Biol. **9:** 2928-2933.
28. Gotoh, T., Haraguchi, Y., Takiguchi, M., and Mori, M., 1994, The delayed glucocorticoid-responsive and hepatoma cell-selective enhancer of the rat arginase gene is located around intron 7. J. Biochem. **115:** 778-788.
29. Takiguchi, M., and Mori, M., 1991, In vitro analysis of the rat liver-type arginase promoter. J. Biol. Chem. **266:** 9186-9193.
30. Nishiyori, A., Tashiro, H., Kimura, A., Akagi, K., Yamamura, K., Mori, M., and Takiguchi, M., 1994, Determination of tissue specificity of the enhancer by combinatorial operation of tissue-enriched transcription factors. Both HNF-4 and C/EBP-β are required for liver-specific activity of the ornithine transcarbamylase enhancer. J. Biol. Chem. **269:** 1323-1331.
31. Nebes, V. L., and Morris, S. M. Jr., 1988, Regulation of messenger ribonucleic acid levels for five urea cycle enzymes in cultured rat hepatocytes: Requirements for cyclic adenosine monophosphate, glucocorticoids, and ongoing protein synthesis. Mol. Endocrinol. **2:** 444-451.
32. Matsuno, F., Chowdhury, S., Gotoh, T., Iwase, K., Matsuzaki, H., Takatsuki, K., Mori, M., and Takiguchi, M., 1996, Induction of the C/EBP-β gene by dexamethasone and glucagon in primary-cultured rat hepatocytes. J. Biochem. **119:** 524-532.
33. Yang-Yen, H. -F., Chambard, J. -C., Sun, Y. -L., Smeal, T., Schmidt, T. J., Drouin, J., and Karin, M., 1990, Transcriptional interference between c-jun and the glucocorticoid receptor: Mutual inhibition of DNA binding due to direct protein-protein interaction. Cell **62:** 1205-1215.
34. Schüle, R., Rangarajan, P., Kliewer, S., Ransone, L. J., Bolado, J., Yang, N., Verma, I. M., and Evans, R.M., 1990, Functional antagonism between oncoprotein c-jun and the glucocorticoid receptor. Cell **62:** 1217-1226.
35. Schüle, R., and Evans, R, M., 1991, Cross-coupling of signal transduction pathways: Zinc finger meets leucine zipper. Trends in Genet. **7:** 377-381.

HYPERAMMONAEMIA WITHOUT PORTAL SYSTEMIC SHUNTING DOES NOT RESEMBLE HEPATIC ENCEPHALOPATHY

Robert A.F.M. Chamuleau and Birgit A.P.M. Vogels

Laboratory of Experimental Internal Medicine
Academic Medical Center
University of Amsterdam, The Netherlands

INTRODUCTION

During our experimental studies on the role of ammonia in the pathogenesis of hepatic encephalopathy[1] we did the interesting observation: a 20 times increased blood ammonia concentration caused no symptoms of encephalopathy in SHAM-operated rats, but it did definitely in portacaval shunted (PCS) rats.

Increased ammonia levels were obtained by ammonium-acetate bolus infusion (0.5 mmol per kg bw) followed by a maintenance infusion (2.8 mmol per kg bw/hr) during 6 hours. SHAM-operated rats with ammonium-acetate infusion (AI- NORM rats) needed a higher dose of ammonium-acetate infusion (6.5 mmol/kg/bw/h) than PCS rats (AI-PCS) to maintain the same high blood ammonia concentration (Fig 1).

Diagnosis and grading of encephalopathy were based on clinical grading (Table I and Fig 2) and a more objective measure like quantitative changes in the EEG power density spectrum: the so called left index (Figure 3) and the mean dominant frequency (MDF, Fig 4).[2]

The striking difference in encephalopathy symptomatology between the two experimental models (AI-NORM versus AI- PCS) prompted us to further analysis of their blood, cerebral cortex and cerebral spinal fluid (CSF) concentrations of ammonia and amino acids.
Ammonia was measured by use of the blood ammonia checker 2 (Kyoto Daiichi Kagaku Co Ltd.)[3]. Amino acid concentrations were measured in plasma by HPLC analysis as described by van Eik et al.[4]

By means of a cisterna magna canula[5,6] CSF was obtained and intracranial pressure (ICP) measured. Finally brain water content was calculated by subtracting dry from wet brain weight after sacrificing the animals.

Statistical analysis was performed by means of repeated measurement analysis of variant (ANOVA) for blood ammonia concentrations, clinical grading and EEG activity, and Student's t-test for blood ammonia concentration at the start of the infusion, brain and CSF ammonia concentrations, amino acid concentrations, ICP and brain water content. P values < 0.05 were considered to be significant.

Advances in Cirrhosis, Hyperammonemia, and Hepatic Encephalopathy
Edited by Felipo and Grisolía, Plenum Press, New York, 1997

Table 1. Stages in experimental hepatic encephalopathy

clinical grade 0	normal behaviour
clinical grade 1	mild lethargy
clinical grade 2	decreased motor activity, poor gesture control, diminished response to pain stimuli
clinical grade 3	severe ataxia: no spontaneous righting reflex
clinical grade 4	no righting reflex to pain stimuli
clinical grade 5	no reaction to pain stimuli

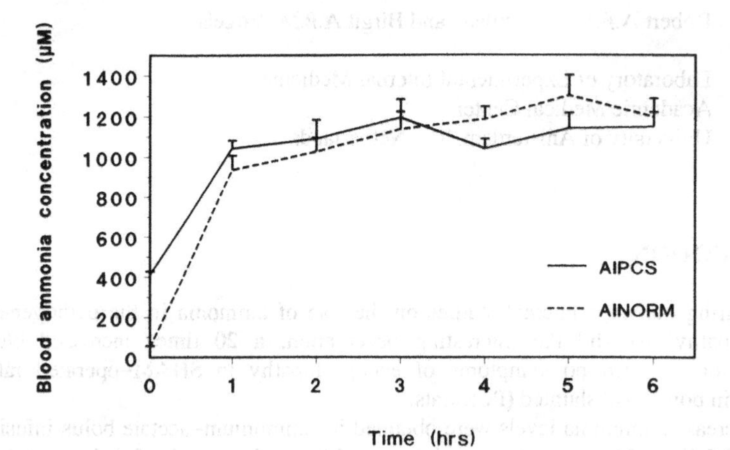

Figure 1. Blood ammonia concentration in AI–PCS rats and AI–NORM rats (mean ± sem).

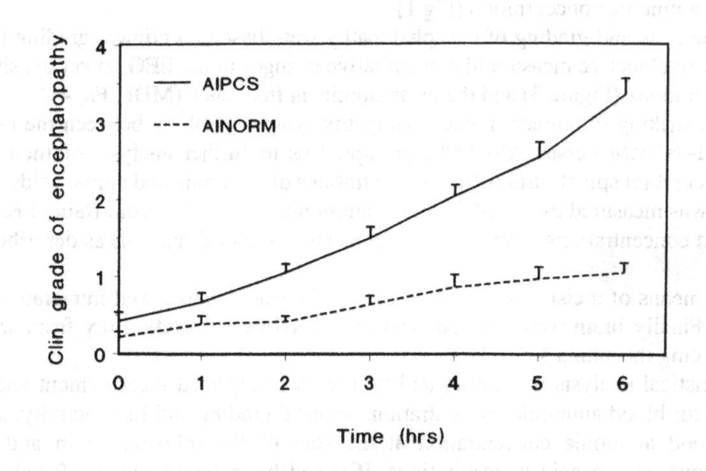

Figure 2. Clinical grade of encephalopathy in AI–PCS rats and AI–NORM rats (mean ± sem).

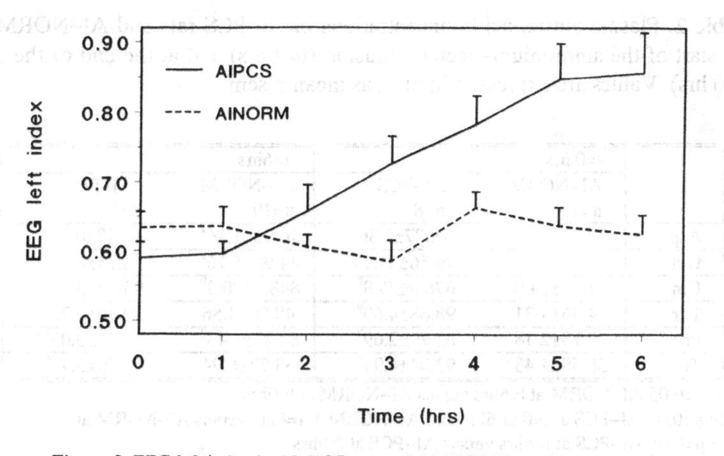

Figure 3. EEG left index in AI–PCS rats and AI–NORM rats (mean ± sem).

RESULTS AND DISCUSSION

At the end of the experiments, when the difference in ecephalopathy was greatest the following interesting results were obtained, when comparing AI–PCS and AI–NORM rats at T=6 hrs.

1. A significant increase in plasma tyrosine concentration of AI–PCS rats (Table 2).

2. Significantly higher cerebral cortex concentrations in AI–PCS rats of Gln , Tyr, Phe and Trp (Table 3).

3. Significantly higher increases of CSF concentrations of Asp, Glu, Gln, Tyr, Phe, and Trp in AI–PCS rats (Table 4).

4. Significantly higher increases in brain water content and ICP in AI–PCS rats (Table 5).

From these data it is obvious that hyperammonaemia is not the sole factor causing encephalopathy and that PCS has an important and probably essential contribution to its

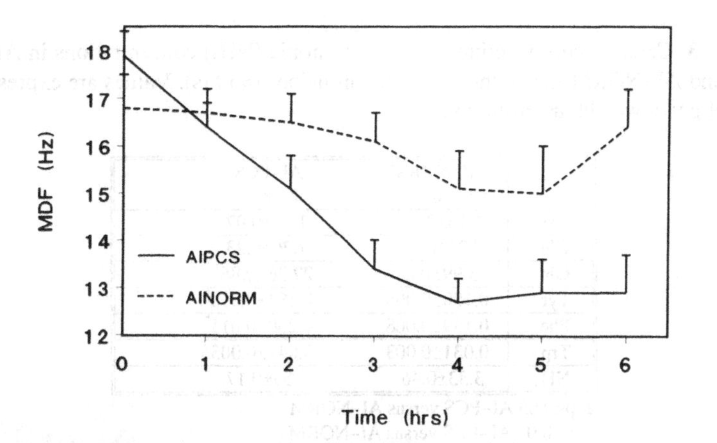

Figure 4. Mean dominant frequency (MDF) in AI–PCS rats and in AI–NORM rats (mean ± sem).

Table 2. Plasma amino acid concentrations in AI–PCS rats and AI–NORM rats at the start of the ammonium–acetate infusion (t=0 hrs) and at the end of the infusion (t=6 hrs). Values are expressed in mM, as mean ± sem

	t=0 hrs		t=6hrs	
	AI–NORM n=10	AI–PCS n=8	AI–NORM n=10	AI–PCS n=8
Asp	17.32±1.78	18.77±1.36	10.91±1.16^{a}	13.48±0.80^{c}
Glu	62.94±6.36	76.56±11.10	44.95±5.16^{a}	58.15±6.39
Gln	512.1±24.0	678.6±25.8^{b}	848.4±80.3^{b}	954.2±39.7^{bd}
Tyr	54.36±1.31	98.88±4.60^{b}	48.90±4.56	70.90±3.25^{bde}
Phe	49.75±2.18	82.79±2.69^{b}	89.23±4.43^{b}	99.42±3.03^{bd}
Trp	58.58±1.43	93.04±4.94^{b}	63.77±6.94	61.59±3.41^{d}

a: $p<0.05$ AI–NORM at t=6hrs versus AI–NORM at t=0hrs
b: $p<0.01$ AI–PCS at t=0 or 6hrs and AI–NORM at t=6hrs versus AI–NORM at t=0hrs
c: $p<0.05$ AI–PCS at t=6hrs versus AI–PCS at t=0hrs
d: $p<0.01$ AI–PCS at t=6hrs versus AI–PCS at t=0hrs
e: $p<0.05$ AI–PCS at t=6hrs versus AI–NORM at t=6hrs

pathogenesis. However, the question remains: what is the mechanism of encephalopathy in AI–PCS rats and how does PCS contribute to this mechanism?

For the time being our hypothesis is given in Fig 5.

In agreement with others[7] we have attributed an important role to increased brain glutamine concentrations.

Based on our experimental data we propose the following sequence of events.The significantly higher increase of cerebral cortex and CSF glutamine concentrations in AI– PCS rats results in higher concentrations of both cerebral cortex aromatic amino acids Phe, Tyr, Trp (taken together as AAA) and CSF concentrations of AAA, Glu and Asp. Increased cerebral cortex AAA concentrations can contribute to changes in neurotransmission as has been postulated by the false neurotransmitter hypothesis.[8,9]

Furthermore the extra large increase of intracellular cerebral cortex glutamine concentration will promote osmotic cell swelling by exhaustion of compensatory mechanisms of cell volume regulation[10,11] and will induce increased concentrations of extracellular Glu and Asp which in turn

Table 3. Cerebral cortex amino acid and ammonia (NH_3) concentrations in AI–PCS rats and AI–NORM rats at the end of the infusion (t=6 hrs). Values are expressed in mmol/g wet weight, as mean ± sem

	AI–NORM N=10	AI–PCS N=8
Asp	1.16±0.08	1.30±0.07
Glu	7.91±0.17	7.76±0.23
Gln	23.99±0.68	27.26±0.86^{a}
Tyr	0.100±0.005	0.184±0.010^{b}
Phe	0.159±0.008	0.260±0.011^{b}
Trp	0.031±0.003	0.047±0.003^{b}
NH_3	3.33±0.46	3.53±0.17

a: $p<0.05$ AI–PCS versus AI–NORM
b: $p<0.01$ AI–PCS versus AI–NORM

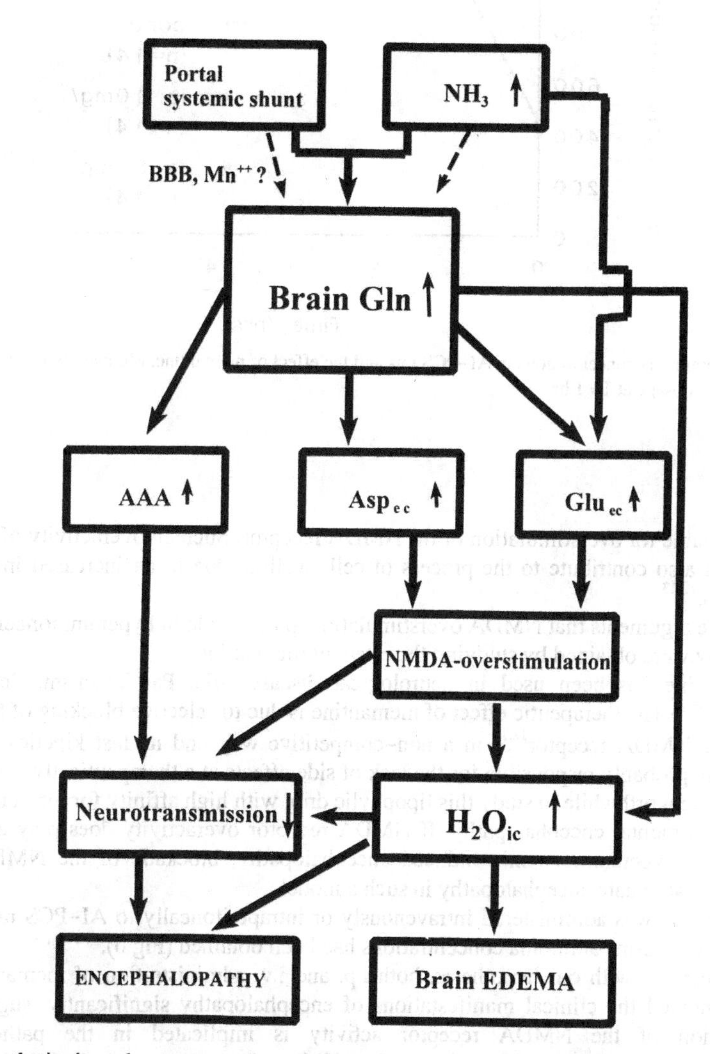

Figure 5. Hypothesis about the sequence of events during hyperammonemia induced encephalopathy in PCS rats. Abbreviations: BBB=blood brain barrier; Gln=glutamine; AAA= aromatic amini acids; Asp=aspartate; Glu=glutamate; ec=extracellular; ic=intracellular; NMDA= N–methyl–D–aspartate.

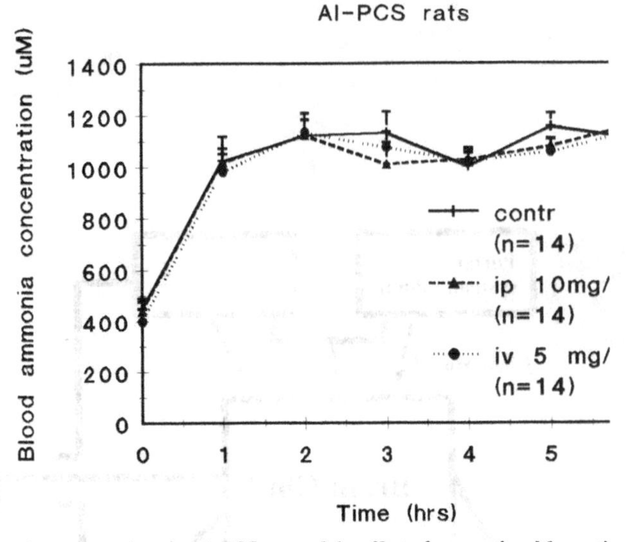

'igure 6. Blood ammonia concentrations in AI–PCS rats and the effect of memantine. Memantine is given either i.p. or v. in the indicated dosage at T= 1 hr.

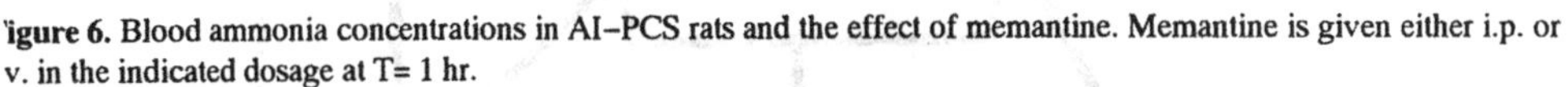

nay be responsible for overstimulation of the NMDA receptor. Such an overactivity of the NMDA eceptor might also contribute to the process of cell swelling due to an increased influx of ions Na^{+},Ca^{2+}, Cl^{-}).[12,13]

Positive arguments that NMDA overstimulation plays a role in hyperammonaemia induced ncephalopathy were obtained by studying the effect of memantine.

Memantine has been used in neurological diseases like Parkinsonism, dementia and erebral coma.[14,17] The therapeutic effect of memantine is due to selective blocking of the open ion hannel of the NMDA receptor[12,13] in a non–competitive way and its fast kinetics and voltage lependency are probably responsible for the lack of side effects at a therapeutically used dosage. It eemed therefore worthwhile to study this lipophylic drug with high affinity for the central nervous ystem in experimental encephalopathy. If NMDA receptor overactivity does play a role in the athogenesis of hyperammonaemia induced encephalopathy, blockade of the NMDA receptor ould be able to attenuate encephalopathy in such a model.

Memantine was administered intravenously or intraperitoneally to AI–PCS rats at t=1 hr, vhen stable high plasma ammonia concentrations had been obtained (Fig 6).

In agreement with our hypothesis, both i.p. and i.v. administration of memantine in AI–PCS rats attenuated the clinical manifestations of encephalopathy significantly, suggesting that ver–stimulation of the NMDA receptor activity is implicated in the pathogenesis of yperammonaemia– induced encephalopathy. In addition, the improvement in EEG after NMDA eceptor blockade suggests that NMDA receptor activation is associated with changes in EEG ctivity. Indications of excitatory amino acids induced alterations in EEG activity have been eported by Kuchiwaki et al.[18]

There was a significant effect on clinical grade, EEG left index, and MDF in comparison to AI– PCS rats receiving saline (Fig 7). This was associated with a significant decrease of CSF Glu Fig 8) and prevention of the increase in ICP and brain water content (Table 5).

Despite high blood ammonia concentrations, brain water content and ICP were ignificantly decreased in AI– PCS rats after memantine administration. This suggests that the mprovement and clinical manifestations of encephalopathy in AI–PCS rats may be at least artially due to a reduction in cell swelling.

Table 4. CSF amino acid and ammonia (NH_3) concentrations in AI–PCS rats and AI–NORM rats at the start of the ammonium–acetate infusion (t=0 hrs) and at the end of the infusion (t=6 hrs). Values are expressed in mM, as mean ± sem

	t=0 hrs		t=6 hrs	
	AI–NORM N=5	AI–PCS N=5	AI–NORM N=5	AI–PCS N=5
Asp	2.86±0.53	4.82 ± 0.65^{a}	9.93 ± 0.45^{b}	18.42 ± 2.66^{ace}
Glu	7.05±1.47	28.98 ± 0.65^{a}	36.99 ± 4.13^{b}	120.9 ± 17.62^{ace}
Gln	469.2±30.1	2543 ± 494.0^{a}	2651 ± 643.0^{b}	9164 ± 914.8^{ace}
Tyr	5.57±0.41	25.90 ± 4.46^{a}	13.23 ± 0.92^{b}	31.19 ± 2.46^{bf}
Phe	4.24±0.46	18.32 ± 2.70^{a}	20.63 ± 0.90^{b}	32.96 ± 3.33^{ace}
Trp	1.02±0.21	4.40 ± 0.41^{b}	3.85 ± 0.50^{b}	8.04 ± 0.41^{bdf}
NH_3	24.6±3.28	172 ± 13.7^{b}	535 ± 75^{b}	552 ± 37^{bd}

a: $p<0.05$ AI–PCS at t=0 or 6hrs versus AI–NORM at t=0hrs
b: $p<0.01$ AI–PCS at t=0 or 6hrs and AI–NORM at t=6hrs versus AI–NORM at t=0hrs
c: $p<0.05$ AI–PCS at t=6 hrs versus AI–PCS at t=0 hrs
d: $p<0.01$ AI–PCS at t=6 hrs versus AI–PCS at t=0 hrs
e: $p<0.05$ AI–PCS at t=6 hrs versus AI–NORM at t=6 hrs
f: $p<0.01$ AI–PCS at t=6 hrs versus AI–NORM at t=6 hrs

Furthermore, memantine treatment resulted in a smaller or even no increase in CSF Glu concentrations. This can be explained by the fact that stimulation of NMDA receptor activity also promotes glutamate release, which is in agreement with the data of Bustos et al.[19] They showed that addition of NMDA to the dialysate induced a release of Glu and Asp to the extracellular compartment, measured by in vivo brain dialysis in rats. After administration of MK 801, another non–competitive NMDA receptor antagonist, the increase of Glu and Asp in brain dialysate was inhibited, indicating that NMDA receptor activity enhances the release of Glu and Asp.

The stimulation of Glu release by NMDA receptor activity might be mediated b may be y nitric oxide (NO), which is increased after NMDA receptor activity by stimulation of NO synthase. Montague et al.[20] have shown that NMDA receptor mediated NO production and its diffusion into the extracellular compartment induces a release of Glu. Blockade of NO synthase resulted in an inhibition of Glu release.

In summary, the present data indicate that overstimulation of NMDA receptor activity by increased extracellular concentrations of the excitatory amino acids Glu and Asp, contributes to the pathogenesis of hyperammonaemia–induced encephalopathy. Furthermore, the results suggest that non–competitive NMDA receptor antagonists like memantine are of potential therapeutic value for portosystemic encephalopathy in man.

Table 5. Brain water content (in %) and ICP (mmHg) in normal rats (NORM), AI– NORM rats and AI–PCS rats. Memantine was administered to AI–PCS rats at T=1hr either i.p. 10 mg/kg bw or i.v. 5 mg/kg bw

	NORM N=6	AI–NORM N=10	AI–PCS contr N=7	AI–PCS mem ip N=7	AI–PCS mem iv N=7
CP	2.0±0.4	2.4±0.6	$8.5\pm2.0^{b,c}$	2.3±1.3	4.4±2.8
% water	80.90±0.07	81.39 ± 0.15^{a}	$81.96\pm0.14^{b,c}$	81.31 ± 0.10^{d}	81.24 ± 0.14^{d}

ANOVA (one way procedure) was used for differences between the experimental groups
a: $p<0.05$ AI–NORM versus NORM
b: $p<0.001$ AI–PCS versus NORM
c: $p<0.001$ AI–PCS versus AI–NORM
d: $p<0.05$ versus control AI–PCS Table 5

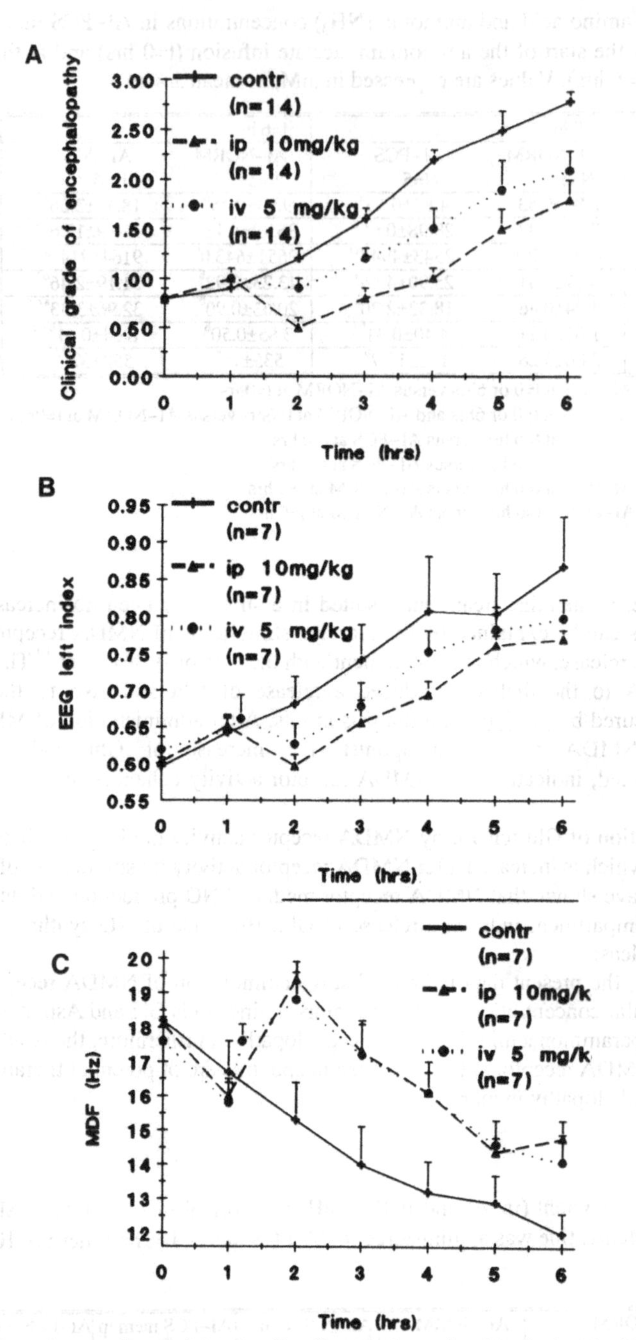

Figure 7. The effect of memantine administration (i.p. 10 mg/kg bw or i.v. 5 mg/kg bw) in AI–PCS rats on a. clinical grade of encephalopathy,b. EEG left index, and c. mean dominant frequency (MDF).(Values are expressed as mean ± sem. Statistical analysis was performed by means of repeated measurement ANOVA. Clinical grade and EEG left index were significantly lower in memantine treated rats compared to controls: $p<0.05$. MDF was significantly higher in memantine treated rats compared to controls: $p<0.0001$).

Finally there is still an open question: why are cerebral cortex and CSF Gln concentrations significantly higher increased in AI–PCS rats compared to AI–NORM rats? It is well known that an increase in brain Gln and AAA concentrations is already present after one day PCS in rats [9,21,22] and that the increase is even more pronounced in subacute liver failure with brain glutamine concentrations of 20 – 25 mM.[23,26]

The following explanations are available for the rise in brain glutamine concentration after PCS:

1. Increased brain glutamine synthesis by glutamine synthase (GS).
2. Inhibition of brain glutaminase activity.
3. Decreased glutamine efflux from brain to blood.

The last explanation seems unlikely, since it has been suggested[7] and shown[27] that glutamine efflux is increased after portal systemic shunting.

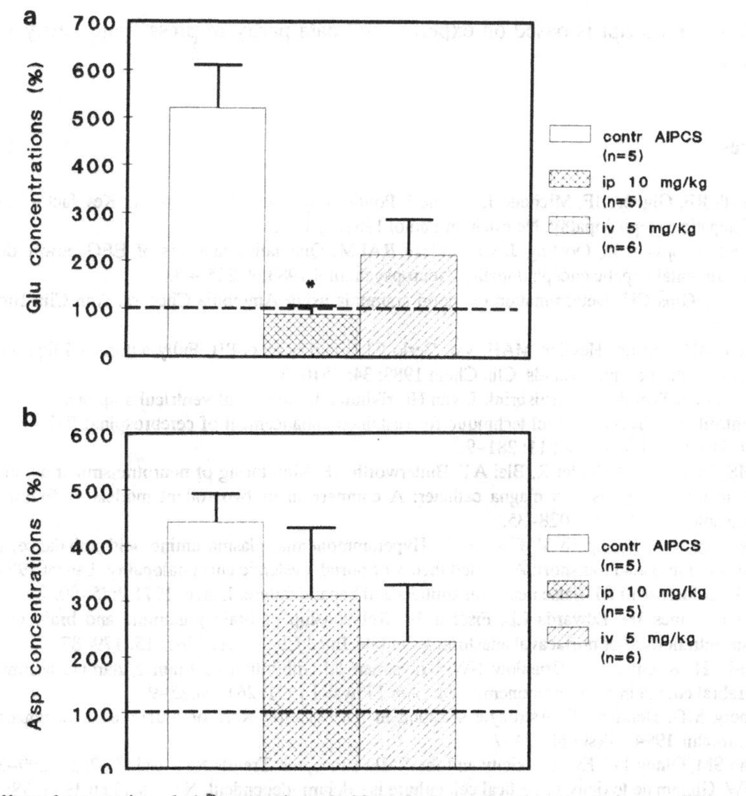

Figure 8. The effect of memantine administration (i.p. 10–20 mg/kg bw or i.v. 5 mg/kg bw) on a. CSF concentrations of glutamate and aspartate in AI–PCS rats at the end of the experiment (expressed as percentage of initial value in each rat, mean ± sem. Statistical analysis was performed by Student's T-test. CSF glutamate concentrations were significantly lower in memantine treated rats compared to controls: $p<0.01$. CSF aspartate concentrations were not significantly different in memantine treated rats compared to controls).

The other two explanations are both possible, because increased brain ammonia concentrations can inhibit glutaminase activity ($K_i = 0.6$mM)[28] and can stimulate GS (K_m value of ammonia is 180 mM).[29] But is has been suggested that GS activity is already maximal at normal brain ammonia levels (0.2–0.3 mmol/kg ww) and several studies have found no change or even less GS activity in brain tissues of PCS rats.[30,31] However, GS activity is usually measured in vitro under optimal conditions with enzyme saturating concentrations. ^{15}N–MRS studies of Kanamori et al.[32,34] showed that the in vivo activity of brain GS in rats (3,5 mmol/hr/g) was only 1–2% of the in vitro activity (275–350 mmol/hr/g) which suggests that substrates and/or co–factors other than ammonia kinetically limit GS activity in vivo.

A recent clinical study of Krieger et al.[35] has shown that blood and brain concentrations of manganese, one of the cofactors of GS, are increased in chronic HE. Therefore, it can be concluded that portal systemic shunting can induce increased cerebral glutamine concentrations by inhibition of glutaminase through increased ammonia concentrations and by stimulation of glutamine synthesis through increased ammonia and GS co–factor concentrations. Unfortunately we did not measure brain manganese in our experimental model. Such an analysis will be the subject of future research.

NOTE

This manuscript is based on experimental data partly in press[36] and partly submitted[37] for publication.

References

1. Butterworth RF, Giguère JF, Michaud J, Lavoie J, Pomier Layrargues G. Ammonia: Key factor in the pathogenesis of hepatic encephalopathy. Neurochem Pathol 1987; 6: 1–12.
2. Popken RJ, Kropveld D, Oosting J, Chamuleau RAFM. Qualitative analysis of EEG power density spectra in experimental hepatic encephalopathy. Neuropsychobiol 1983; 9: 235–43.
3. Huizenga JR, Gips CH. Determination of blood ammonia using Ammonia Checker. Ann Clin Biochem 1983; 20: 187–9.
4. Van Eijk HMH, van der Heyden MAH, van Berlo CLH and Soeters PB. Fully automated liquid chromatographic determination of amino acids. Clin Chem 1988; 34: 2510–3.
5. Boer GJ, van der Woude TP, Kruisbrink J, van Heerikhuize J. Successful ventricular application of the miniaturized controlled–delivery Accurel technique for sustained enhancement of cerebrospinal fluid peptide levels in the rat. J Neusoci Meth 1984; 11: 281–9.
6. Swain MS, Bergeron M, Audet R, Blei AT, Butterworth RF. Monitoring of neurotransmitter amino acids by means of an indwelling cisterna magna catheter: A comparison of two rodent models of fulminant liver failure. Hepatology 1992; 16: 1028–35.
7. James JH, Jeppsson B, Ziparo V, Fischer JE. Hyperammonemia, plasma amino acid imbalance, and blood–brain barrier amino acid transport: A unified theory of portal–systemic encephalopathy. Lancet 1979; 13: 772–5.
8. Fischer JE, Baldessarini RJ. False neurotransmitters and hepatic failure. Lancet 1971;2:75–80.
9. Jeppsson B, James JH, Edwards LL, Fischer JE. Relationship of brain glutamine and brain neutral amino acid concentrations after portacaval anastomosis in rats. Eur J Clin Invest 1985; 15: 179–87.
10. Takahashi H, Koehler RC, Brusilow SW, Traystman RJ. Inhibition of brain glutamine accumulation prevents cerebral edema in hyperammonemic rats. Am J Physiol 1991; 261: H825–9.
11. Norenberg MD, Bender AS. Astrocyte swelling in liver failure: Role of glutamine and benzodiazepines. Acta Neurochir 1994; 60(suppl): 24–7.
12. Rothman SM, Olney JW. Excitotoxicity and the NMDA receptor. Trends Neurosci 1987; 10: 299–302.
13. Choi DW. Glutamate toxicity in cortical cell culture is calcium–dependent. Neurosci Lett 1985; 58: 293–7.
14. Chen HV, Pelligrini JW, Aggarwal SK, Lei SZ, Warach S, Jensen FE Lipton SA. Open–channel block of N–methyl–D–aspartate (NMDA) responses by memantine: therapeutic advantage against NMDA receptor–mediated neurotoxicity. J Neurosci 1992;12:4427–4436.
15. Herrero JF, Headly PM, Parsons CG. Memantine selectively depresses NMDA receptor–mediated responses of rat spinal neurons in vivo. Neurosci Lett 1994;165:37–40.
16. Parsons CG, Quack G, Bresink I, Baran L, Przegalinski E, Kostowski W, Krzascik P, Hartmann S, Danysz W. Comparison of the potency, kinetics and voltage–dependency of a series of uncompetitive NMDA receptor antagonists in vitro with anticonvulsive and motor impairment activity in vivo. Neuropharmacology 1995; 34: 1239–1258.
17. Müller WE, Mutschler E, Riederer P. Noncompetitive NMDA receptor antagonists with fast open–channel blocking kinetics and strong voltage–dependency as potential therapeutic agents for Alzheimer's dementia. Pharmacopsychiatry 1995; 28: 113–124.

18. Kuchiwaka H, Inao S, Yamamato M, Yoshida K, Sugita K. An assessment of progression of brain edema with amino acid levels in cerebrospinal fluid and changes in electroencephalogram in an adult cat model of cold brain injury. Acta Neurochir 1994;60(s):62–64.
19. Bustos G, Abarca J, Forray MI, Gysling K, Bradberry CW, Roth RH. Regulation of excitatory amino acid release by N-methyl-D-aspartate receptors in rat striatum: in vivo microdialysis studies. BRES 1992; 585: 105–15.
20. Montague PR, Gancayo CD, Winn MJ et al. Role of NO production in NMDA receptor mediated neurotransmittor release in cerebral cortex. Science 1994;263:973–977.
21. Hawkins RA, Jessy J, Mans AM, De Joseph MR. Effect of reducing brain glutamine synthesis on metabolic symptoms of hepatic encephalopathy. J Neurochem 1993; 60: 1000–6.
22. Mans AM, de Joseph MR, Donald WD, Vina JR, Hawkins RA. Early establishment of cerebral dysfunction after portacaval shunting. Am J Physiol 1990; 259: E104–10.
23. Blei AT, Olafsson S, Therrien G, Butterworth RF. Ammonia-induced brain edema and intracranial hypertension in rats after portacaval anastomosis. Hepatology 1994; 19: 1437–44.
24. Bosman DK, Deutz NEP, De Graaff AA, vd Hulst RWN, van Eijk HMH, Boveé WMMJ, Maas MAW et al. Changes in brain metabolism during hyperammonemia and acute liver failure: results of a comparative 1H-NMR spectroscopy and biochemical investigation. Hepatology 1990; 12: 281–90.
25. Swain M, Butterworth RF, Blei AT. Ammonia and related amino acids in the pathogenesis of brain edema in acute ischemic liver failure in rats. Hepatology 1992; 15: 449–53.
26. Mans AM, De Joseph MR, Hawkins RA. Metabolic abnormalities and grade of encephalopathy in acute hepatic failure. J Neurochem 1994; 63: 1829–38.
27. De Jong CHC, Deutz NEP, Soeters PB. Cerebral cortex ammonia and glutamine metabolism in two rat models of chronic liver insufficiency-induced hyperammonemia: influence of pair-feeding. J Neurochem 1993; 60: 1047–57.
28. Benjamin AM. Control of glutaminase activity in rat brain cortex in vitro: influence of glutamate, phosphate, ammonium, calcium and hydrogen ions. Brain Res 1981; 208: 363–77.
29. Cooper AJL, Plum F. Biochemistry and physiology of brain ammonia. Physiol Rev 1987; 67: 440–519.
30. Butterworth RF, Girard G, Giguère JF. Regional differences in the capacity for ammonia removal by brain following portacaval anastomosis. J Neurochem 1988; 51: 486–90.
31. Girard G, Butterworth RF. Effect of portacaval anastomosis on glutamine synthetase activities in liver, brain, and skeletal muscle. Dig Dis Sci 1992; 7: 1121–6.
32. Kanamori K, Ross BD. ^{15}N NMR measurement of the in vivo rate of glutamine synthesis and utilization at steady state in the brain of the hyperammonemic rat. Biochem J 1993; 289: 461–8.
33. Kanamori K, Parivar F, Ross BD. A ^{15}N NMR study of in vivo cerebral glutamine synthesis in hyperammonemic rats. NMR in Biomed 1993; 6: 21–6.
34. Kanamori K, Ross BD, Kuo EL. Dependence of in vivo glutamine synthetase activity on ammonia concentration in rat brain studied by ^{1}H–^{15}N heteronuclear multiple quantum coherence-transfer NMR. Biochem J 1995; 311: 681–8.
35. Krieger D, Krieger S, Jansen O, Gass P, Theilmann L, Lichtnecker H. Manganese and chronic hepatic encephalopathy. Lancet 1995; 346: 270–4.
36. Vogels BAPM, van Steynen B, Maas MAW,Jorning GGA, Chamuleau RAFM. The effects of ammonia and portal-systemic shunting on brain metabolism, neurotransmission and intracranial hypertension in hyperammonemia-induced encephalopathy. J Hepatol 1996;24:in press
37. Vogels BAPM, Maas MAW, Daalhuisen J, Quack G, Chamuleau RAFM. Memantine, a non-competitive NMDA-receptor antagonist improves hyperammonemia-induced encephalopathy and acute hepatic encephalopathy in rats. Hepatology 1996;submitted.

MAGNETIC RESONANCE SPECTROSCOPY IN THE STUDY OF HYPERAMMONEMIA AND HEPATIC ENCEPHALOPATHY

Keiko Kanamori, Stefan Bluml and Brian Ross

Huntington Medical Research Institute and California Institute of Technology Pasadena and Schulte Medical Research Institute, Santa Barbara, California

INTRODUCTION

^{1}H MRS offers an interesting new noninvasive tool with which to monitor some limited aspects of brain chemistry in man [1]. The application of the method to the elucidation of HE has, in addition to the hoped for ability to demonstrate the central role of glutamine (Gln), provided two new insights into the disease. The first is the possible role of cerebral choline-containing compounds (Cho). This might have been anticipated from the role of liver in glycerophosphate and lipid biosynthesis. The second observation was without precedent and still awaits an explanation: This is the significant occurrence of cerebral myo-inositol (mI) depletion [2].

While the sensitive ^{1}H and ^{31}P MRS provides valuable information on changes in cerebral metabolite concentrations under normal and pathological conditions, including acute HE of Reye's syndrome [3,4], ^{13}C and ^{15}N, which have low natural abundance, are useful for measuring the flux of selected metabolites in intact brain using isotopically enriched precursors. ^{13}C MRS has provided interesting information on the rate of TCA-cycle and 2-oxoglutarate-glutamate exchange in animal and human brains in vivo [5]. ^{15}N MRS has proved useful for measuring the in vivo rates of glutamine synthetase (GS), phosphate-activated glutaminase (PAG) and glutamate dehydrogenase (GDH) in rat brain [6]. The second part of this Review describes findings of the isotope-chase method [7] and in vivo ^{15}N and ^{1}H-^{15}N HMQC MRS developed in our laboratory to explore mechanisms of acute HE, in rats.

HUMAN HEPATIC ENCEPHALOPATHY

Most of our clinical studies have been designed to look for a mechanism of mI depletion, an explanation for its role in HE and possible implications of this new cerebral pathology for treatment of HE. As we have reported previously, cerebral [Cho] falls in patients with liver disease, or HE, and recovers, with a considerable 'overshoot' after successful liver transplantation [8]. Because Cho determined with 1H MRS includes two phosphorylated choline metabolites,

PC (phosphorylcholine) and GPC (glycerophosphorylcholine) the true nature of this metabolic response has had to await the development of new methods of clinical MRS.

Method 1

Quantitative 31P MRS was performed on a standard GE Clinical MR scanner 1.5T, using an external reference, and the same correction for brain water, csf volume and brain 'dry-matter' as was developed for 1H MRS [9,10]. Absolute concentrations of phosphocreatine (PCr), ATP, inorganic phosphate (Pi) and intracellular pH of patients with HE (verified by reduced mI in 1H MRS) were compared with age-related normal controls.

Method 2

Quantitative proton decoupled 31P MRS (QPDC^{31}P) was performed with the addition of a second amplifier to the otherwise standard GE Signa 1.5T MR scanner, in the same subjects to a) separate the PC from phosphoethanolamine (PE), the other principal component of the unresolved phosphomonoester (PME), and GPC from glycerophosphoryl ethanolamine (GPE) in the unresolved phosphodiester (PDE); and b) to quantify each of these four metabolites [11].

Results

Proof that mI Depletion Is a Marker for Sub Clinical Hepatic Encephalopathy.

A blind study was undertaken to compare ^{1}H MRS vs. clinical diagnosis of HE [12]. For the purposes of this trial, the definition of SCHE (and of HE) was established using neuropsychiatric tests (NPsy) devised by previous workers in this field. mI depletion (>2 SD below mean in either parietal white matter or in occipital gray matter cortex) with or without the other two changes (namely reduced Cho; increased a- and / or b, g-glutamine plus glutamate (Glx)) was sufficient for a positive diagnosis of SCHE or HE in this trial. MRS appears to be sensitive to both HE and SCHE, and can be used with 94% sensitivity, twice that of 'clinical' (Parsons-Smith) diagnosis alone. It is not suggested that ^{1}H MRS alone can distinguish between SCHE and HE. Figure 1 shows an additional feature of ^{1}H MRS, which is that metabolite changes appear to grade the severity of HE.

Myoinositol as an osmolyte in HE? The evidence of mI as a cerebral osmolyte in man is fairly compelling, but circumstantial. Thus, in a single infant with severe hypernatremia, mI was twice the normal concentration at presentation, falling to near normal over 36 days, as serum sodium returned to normal [13]. Conversely, in a study of 10 hyponatremic adults, cerebral [mI] was significantly reduced, recovering slowly towards normal in the 5 individuals who were re-examined after effective treatment [14].

In a single case of severe hyponatremia followed by Haussinger et al. [15] the ratio of mI/Cr was reduced. However, as we saw above, [Cr] may be reduced by hyponatremia, so the ratio of the two metabolites must be treated with caution.

Origin of the changes in cerebral [Cho] in patients with chronic HE: Studies with Quantitative ^{1}H decoupled ^{31}P MRS.

Parallel changes in cerebral [Cho] were noted by [13]; and by [14] in the same studies, suggesting that Cho also functions as a cerebral osmolyte.

In the small number of patients with chronic HE so far examined, [PCr] was not different from normal. Absolute [PCr] obtained in Method 1 was used to quantify the remaining metabolites in Method 2. The precision of the PC and GPC assay was verified by comparing [Cho] obtained in ^{1}H MRS, with the sum of PC + GPC in both patients and controls. A preliminary finding is that

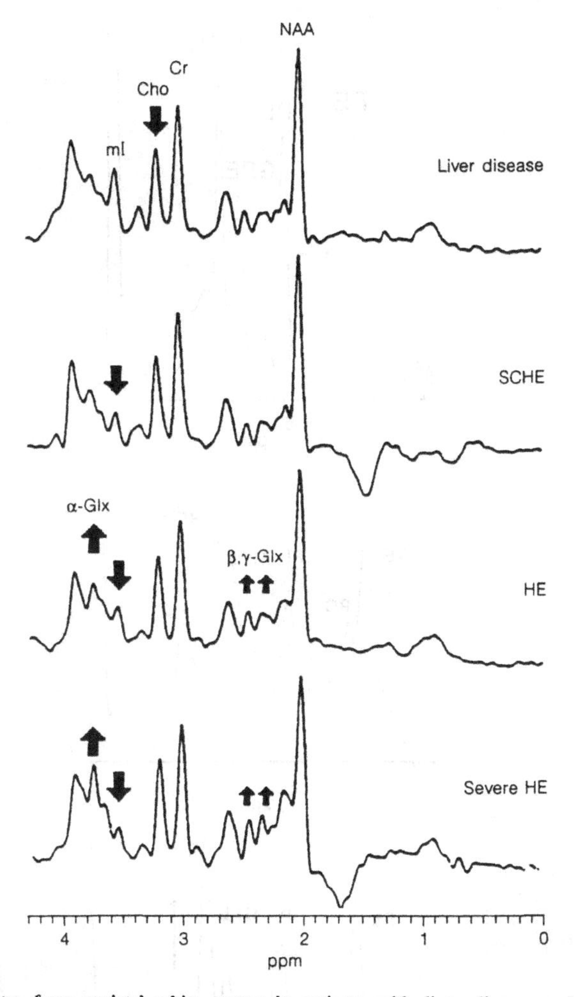

Figure 1. ^{1}H MR spectra from parietal white matter in patients with liver disease, only, subclinical hepatic encephalopathy (SCHE) and clinical hepatic encephalopathy (HE). Metabolites are identified from their chemical shift (scale in parts per million: ppm), while their concentrations are proportional to peak height and/or area; spectra are scaled to the Cr (phosphocreatine plus creatine) peak. Other abbreviations: NAA= N–acetyl aspartate; Glx= glutamine, with a contribution from glutamate; Cho= choline containing metabolites; mI= myo–inositol. Arrows indicate significant elevation or reduction of metabolite concentration.

in HE, that some but not all of the reduction in cerebral [Cho] is accounted for by a significant reduction in [GPC]; PC is well conserved (Fig 2). This finding is in accordance with a finding in brain in HE post–mortem in man and in brain extracts of portacaval shunt rats, analyzed by HPLC, of reduced GPC [16].

Conclusion

We suspect that, since GPC has been recognized previously as a renal and cerebral osmolyte, this new finding with QPDC^{31}P MRS is generally supportive of the foregoing discussion concerning mI, that chronic human HE is in part, a disturbance of cerebral osmo–regulation.

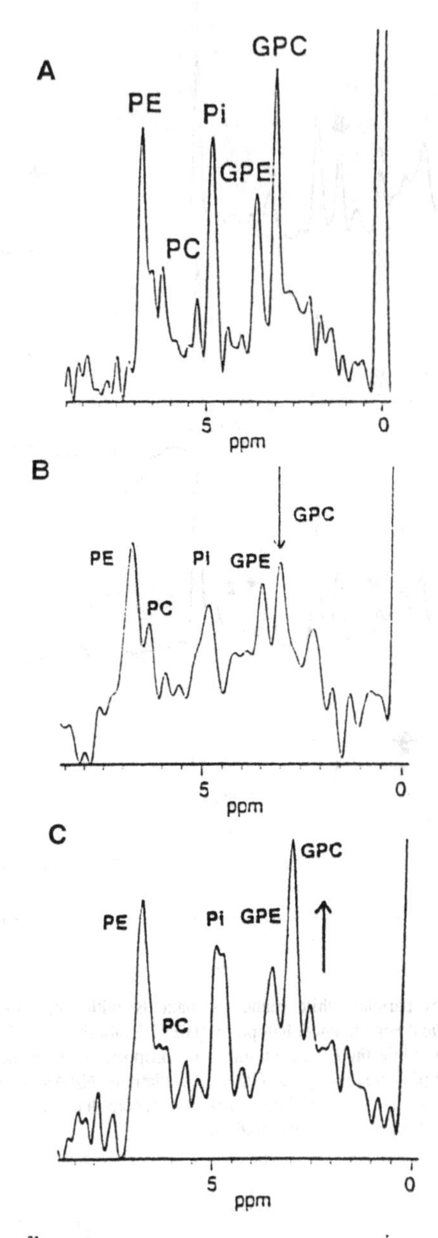

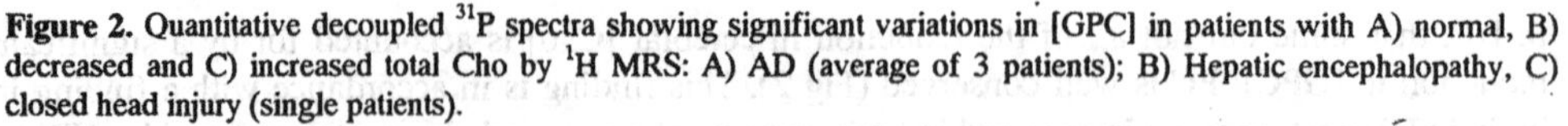

Figure 2. Quantitative decoupled ^{31}P spectra showing significant variations in [GPC] in patients with A) normal, B) decreased and C) increased total Cho by ^{1}H MRS: A) AD (average of 3 patients); B) Hepatic encephalopathy, C) closed head injury (single patients).

MRS FOR STUDY OF GLU AND GLN FLUX IN VIVO

The objective was to determine the rates of synthesis and turnover of neurotransmitters and their precursors implicated in the etiology of hepatic encephalopathy (HE). This was to be accomplished through measurement of in vivo activities of glutamine synthetase (GS), an astrocytic marker enzyme, and glutamate decarboxylase (GAD), a neuronal marker enzyme, in the brain of hyperammonemic rat. A novel feature was that the measurements are performed by ^{15}N and/or $^{1}H-^{15}N$ heteronuclear multiple quantum coherence (HMQC) transfer MRS. The results were expected to provide useful information on the in vivo rate of ammonia (NH_3) removal and glutamine (GLN) synthesis in astrocytes, on the rate of GABA turnover in nerve terminals and on the effect of hyperammonemia on the neuronal glutamate (GLU) pool. It was anticipated that the results would contribute to evaluation of the following proposed mechanisms for the etiology of HE, viz., that hyperammonemia causes HE through (a) neurotoxic effect of NH_3; (b) through accumulation of GLN; (c) through depletion of neurotransmitter GLU; or (d) through increased GABA turnover resulting in increased neural inhibition.

In vivo GS activity

We undertook a) measurement of in vivo GS activity by ^{15}N and ^{1}H–^{15}N HMQC NMR under various degrees of hyperammonemia; b) study of factors regulating GS activity in vivo; and c) correlation with neuro–behavioral symptoms to evaluate whether ammonia toxicity or glutamine accumulation is responsible for encephalopathy observed under hyperammonemia.

Because of the relatively low [5–^{15}N]glutamine concentrations achieved at near–physiological [NH_3], selective in vivo ^{1}H–^{15}N HMQC observation of brain metabolites was a necessary prerequisite.

Feasibility of in vivo ^{1}H–^{15}N HMQC [17]. The amide protons of [5–^{15}N]glutamine were selectively observed in vivo in the brains of anaesthetized, spontaneously–breathing rats after intravenous $^{15}NH_4^+$ infusion, by phase–cycled ^{1}H–^{15}N HMQC transfer NMR at 200 MHz for ^{1}H. The peak intensity of the nonlabile upfield amide proton was proportional to brain [5–^{15}N]glutamine concentration. The ^{15}N–decoupled amide proton signal was observed in vivo in 2 min of acquisition at brain [5–^{15}N]glutamine concentration of 7.7 ± 0.4 mmol/g and in 17–34 min at 2.0 ± 0.1 mmol/g. Phase–cycled HMQC was shown to be effective in selective observation of [5–^{15}N]glutamine amide protons in vivo with cancellation of all protons not coupled to ^{15}N (Fig. 3). Sensitivity of detection was substantially improved by ^{15}N–decoupling of the amide protons, as predicted in our previous application. The result suggested that the method will be useful for kinetic study of glutamine synthesis in rat brain at near–physiological concentrations of brain ammonia.

Ammonia dependence of in vivo GS activity [18]. Dependence of in vivo rate of glutamine synthesis on substrate ammonia concentration was studied in rat brain by ^{1}H–^{15}N

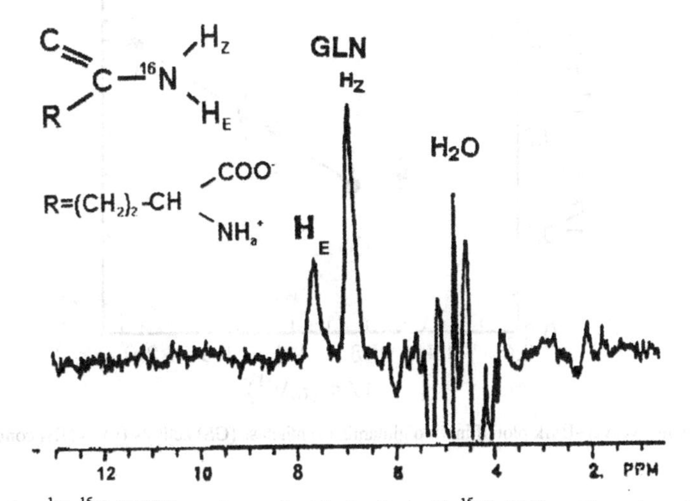

Figure 3. An in vivo ^{1}H–^{15}N HMQC spectrum of rat brain. Brain [5–^{15}N] GLN amide protons, H_Z and H_E, are selectively observed.

HMQC transfer NMR in combination with biochemical techniques. In vivo rates were measured at various steady–state blood and brain ammonia concentrations within the range of 0.4–0.55 mmol/g and 0.86–0.98 mmol/g respectively, after low-rate intravenous $^{15}NH_4^+$ infusion to ^{15}N-enrich brain glutamine, followed by $^{14}NH_4^+$ infusion (isotope chase). The in vivo rate (v) was 3.3– 4.5 mmol/h per g of brain at blood ammonia concentrations (s) of 0.4 – 0.55 mmol/g. Linear increase of 1/v with 1/s permitted estimation of in vivo glutamine synthetase (GS) activity at physiological blood ammonia level to be 0.4–2.1 mmol/h per g. The observed ammonia dependence strongly suggested that, under physiological condition, in vivo GS activity is kinetically limited by sub-optimal in situ concentration of ammonia as well as of glutamate and ATP.

Correlation of neurobehavioral symptoms of encephalopathy with brain ammonia and glutamine concentrations and the rate of ammonia removal by GS in vivo [6]. Correlation among in vivo glutamine synthetase (GS) activity, brain ammonia and glutamine concentrations and severity of encephalopathy was examined in hyperammonemic rats to obtain quantitative information on the capacity of GS to control these metabolites implicated in the etiology of HE. Awake rats were observed for neurobehavioral impairments, after ammonium acetate infusion to attain steady–state blood ammonia concentration of 0.9 mmol/g (group A) or 1.3 mmol/g (group B). As encephalopathy progressed from grade III to IV, brain ammonia increased from 1.9 to 3.3 mmol/g ($P<0.05$), then decreased to 1.3 mmol/g ($P<0.01$) on recovery to grade III. In contrast, brain glutamine concentration was 26, 23 and 21 mmol/g respectively. NH_4^+–infused rats pretreated with L–methionine DL–sulfoximine, an inhibitor of GS, reached grade IV when brain ammonia and glutamine were 3.0 and 5.5 mmol/g respectively. The results, summarized in [6], clearly show that severity of encephalopathy correlates with brain ammonia, but not glutamine.

In vivo GS activities, determined from the rate of increase of brain [5–^{15}N]glutamine observed by ^{1}H–^{15}N HMQC MRS were 6.8 ± 0.7 mmol/h/g and 6.2 ± 0.6 mmol/h/g at blood ammonia concentrations of 0.9 and 1.3 mmol/g respectively. Hence, the in vivo activity, shown previously to increase with blood ammonia over a range of 0.4 – 0.64 mmol/g, approaches saturation when blood ammonia reaches 0.9 – 1.3 mmol/g (Fig 4). This is likely to be the major cause of the observed accumulation of brain ammonia and the onset of grade IV encephalopathy.

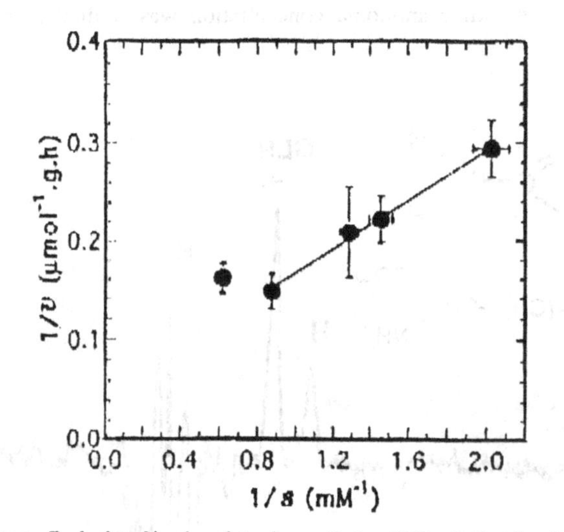

Figure 4. A lineweaver–Burk plot of in vivo glutamine synthetase (GS) activity (v) vs NH_3 concentration (s).

Significance of the results. In hepatic encephalopathy (HE), a metabolic disease of the brain caused by malfunction of the liver, decreased ammonia removal in the liver results in hyperammonemia and diffusion of excess ammonia into the brain. Multiple factors contribute to pathogenesis of HE, and mechanisms responsible for the pathogenesis are unresolved. There is substantial evidence that primary causes are disturbances of: a) cerebral ammonia metabolism and b) GABAergic neurotransmission. The study reported here resolves one of the controversial issues, viz. whether neurotoxicity of ammonia itself, or the concomitant accumulation of glutamine is the major factor in the pathogenesis of severe encephalopathy observed under acute hyperammonemia. Ammonia is metabolized to glutamine by glutamine synthetase (GS) in the brain. Our results show that severity of encephalopathy correlates with brain ammonia concentration and saturation of GS activity in vivo, but not with brain glutamine concentration. Hence, the results support the ammonia neurotoxicity theory. The study, using $^{1}H-^{15}N$ HMQC NMR to measure GS activity at metabolic steady–state in intact animals, provides, for the first time, quantitative evidence for the level of hyperammonemia at which GS activity levels off, resulting in accumulation of neurotoxic level of ammonia.

The effect of hyperammonemia on neuronal GLU pool – evaluation of glutamate depletion hypothesis

According to this hypothesis, hyperammonemia disturbs cerebral metabolism of the excitatory neurotransmitter glutamate, because ammonia removal by GS results in the loss of equimolar glutamate. Furthermore, ammonia–mediated inhibition of glutaminase may prevent replenishment of glutamate from glutamine in nerve terminals [19,20]. As a result, the neurotransmitter pool of glutamate is depleted and leads to symptoms of HE [19,21,22]. Modest but consistent decrease in whole–brain glutamate has been found in animal models of acute and chronic hyperammonemia as well as in autopsied brain tissues from patients dying in hepatic coma [23,24]. The key question is whether the decrease occurs predominantly in select compartments such as astrocytes or nerve terminals, and is extensive enough to affect the neurotransmitter pool of glutamate which is stored in vesicles and is replenished from the cytoplasmic pool. A quantitative evaluation of fluxes through various pathways of glutamate formation and depletion in brain compartments had not been possible because of lack of relevant information [25]. We hoped to contribute to a better understanding of glutamate flux through measurement of the rates of glutamate depletion and replenishment in an intact brain under normal and hyperammonemic conditions.

Glutamate depletion from astrocytes. The rate of glutamate depletion from astrocytes through the GS reaction under various degrees of hyperammonemia have now been measured. They are summarized in Table 1.

GLU synthesis by phosphate–activated glutaminase (PAG) [26]. PAG catalyzes the reaction:

$$\text{Glutamine} + H_2O \longrightarrow \text{Glutamate} + NH_4^+$$

PAG is predominantly a neuronal enzyme, particularly enriched in glutamatergic nerve terminals. This pathway is thought to play an important role in providing the neurotransmitter pools of GLU and possibly of GABA. However, in vivo activity of PAG in intact brain had not been measured previously.

We measured the in vivo activity of PAG in the brain of hyperammonemic rat by monitoring progressive decrease in brain [5–^{15}N]glutamine, PAG–catalyzed production of $^{15}NH_4^+$ and its subsequent assimilation into glutamate, using ^{15}N NMR. The in vivo PAG activity was 0.9 – 1.3 mmol/h/g, < 1% of the in vitro activity. The result suggested strong in situ inhibition of PAG by GLU and NH_3 .

Table 1. In vivo rates of GLU–producing and GLU–utilizing pathways

Tissue levels (mmol/g)		In vivo rate (mmol/g/h)		
Blood NH_3	Brain GLU	Glutamate production		Glutamate utilization
Blood $[NH^3]$	Brain [GLU]	PAG	GDH	GS
0.4 ± 0.02	9.2± 0.6	0.9–1.3	0.76–1.1	3.3 ± 0.3
0.55 ± 0.02	9.2± 0.7		1.1–1.2	4.5 ± 0.5
0.64 ± 0.06	9.3± 0.3			4.8 ± 0.3
0.89 ± 0.06	7.5–7.8			6.8 ± 0.7
1.37 ± 0.08	6.7–7.1			6.2 ± 0.6

GLU synthesis by glutamate dehydrogenase (GDH) [7]. GDH catalyzes the reversible reaction:

$$NH_3 + 2\text{–oxoglutarate} + NAD(P)H \longrightarrow \text{Glutamate} + NAD(P)^+$$

GDH is present in both astrocytes and neurons. GDH is believed to contribute to the synthesis of the metabolic and neurotransmitter pools of GLU, but its in vivo activity was not known. The in vivo GDH activity in the direction of reductive amination was measured in rat brain at steady–state concentrations of brain ammonia and GLU after intravenous infusion of the substrate $^{15}NH_4^+$. The in vivo GDH activity was 0.76 – 1.17 mmol/h/g at a brain ammonia concentration of 0.87±0.055 mmol/g, and 1.1–1.2 mmol/h/g at 1.0±0.1 mmol/g. Comparison of the observed in vivo GDH activity with the in vivo GS and PAG activities suggested that, under mild hyperammonemia, GDH–catalyzed de novo synthesis can provide a minimum of 19% of the GLU pool that is recycled from neurons to astrocytes through the glutamate–glutamine cycle.

Rates of glutamate synthesis and depletion in vivo---summary of results to date; Table 1 summarizes the rates of glutamate synthesis by PAG and GDH and of glutamate depletion by GS under various levels of hyperammonemia. At steady–state blood ammonia concentration of 0.4 ± 0.02 mmol/g, the rate of glutamate synthesis was 0.9–1.3 mmol/h/g by the PAG pathway and 0.76 – 1.1 mmol/g/h by the GDH pathway. Hence, the combined rate of glutamate synthesis through the two pathways is 1.7 to 2.4 mmol/h/g. The rate of glutamate depletion through the GS pathway was 3.3 mmol/h/g. Thus, if PAG and GDH were the only pathways of glutamate synthesis, glutamate depletion at the rate of 0.9 – 1.6 mmol/h/g is expected even under mild hyperammonemia. Whole brain glutamate after 3–4 h of sustained hyperammonemia at this level was 9.2 mmol/g, only 10% lower than that in normal brain (10.2 mmol/g). Hence it is likely that the third pathway of glutamate synthesis, transamination from other amino acids contributes to the replenishment of glutamate. Measurement of the transamination rate in intact brain is now in progress.

Significance of the results -- in vivo regulation of GS, PAG & GDH: ^{15}N and ^{1}H–^{15}N HMQC NMR studies of rat brain have provided important novel information regarding the in vivo rates of glutamine synthetase (GS), phosphate–activated glutaminase (PAG) and glutamate dehydrogenase (GDH). The in vivo rates were shown to be nearly 2 orders of magnitude lower than the in vitro rates measured in brain homogenates under enzyme–saturating concentrations of the substrates. The difference could most reasonably be attributed to subsaturating in situ concentrations of substrates and cofactors (GS and GDH) and strong in situ inhibition of enzyme activity (PAG). The results highlight the importance of measuring metabolite flux in intact brain.

The wealth of new data in human and experimental hepatic encephalopathy arising from in vivo MRS techniques poses a new question. What is the relationship between events identified in chronic human HE, most conveniently viewed as adaptations of astrocyte metabolism and volume regulation, and the profound changes in glutamate, glutamine and ammonia metabolism, which result from saturation of glutamine synthetase in vivo? The residual biochemical changes in treated patients may be the result of ammonia toxicity or the cause of heightened susceptibility to the toxic effects of ammonia. It seems highly likely that an examination using all of described MRS techniques, of the relevant enzyme rates in patients and animals with chronic HE may throw light on this still tantalizing question.

Key Words: Hepatic coma, Magnetic Resonance Spectroscopy, Glutamine; Myoinositol; Cholines, Hyperamonemia; Nitrogen-15, HMQC

References

1. Ross, B.D., R. Kreis, and T. Ernst, Clinical tools for the 90's: magnetic resonance spectroscopy and metabolite imaging. Eur. J. Radiol, 1992. 14: p. 128-140.
2. Kreis, R., N.A. Farrow, and B.D. Ross, Diagnosis of hepatic encephalopathy by proton magnetic resonance spectroscopy. Lancet, 1990. 336: p. 635-6.
3. Ernst, T., B.D. Ross, and R. Flores, Cerebral MRS in infant with suspected Reye's syndrome (Lett). Lancet, 1992. 340: p. 486.
4. Ross, B.D. and T. Michaelis, MR spectroscopy of the brain: Neurospectroscopy, in Clinical Magnetic Resonance Imaging, R.R. Edelman, J.R. Hesselink, andM.I. Zlatkin, Editor. 1996, W. B. Saunders Company: Philadelphia. p. 928-981.
5. Shulman, R.G., et al., Nuclear magnetic resonance imaging and spectroscopy of human brain function. Proc. Natl. Acad. Sci. USA, 1993. 90: p. 3127-3133.
6. Kanamori, K., et al., Severity of hyperammonemic encephalopathy correlates with brain ammonia level and saturation of glutamine synthetase in vivo. J. Neurochem, 1996. 67: p. 1584 - 1594.
7. Kanamori, K. and B.D. Ross, Steady-state in vivo glutamate dehydrogenase activity in rat brain measured by ^{15}N NMR. J. Biol. Chem, 1995. 270(42): p. 24805-809.
8. Ross, B.D., E.R. Danielsen, and S. Bluml, Proton MRS: The new gold standard for diagnosis of clinical and sub-clinical hepatic encephalopathy? Digestive Diseases, 1996. 14(1): p. 30-39.
9. Kreis, R., T. Ernst, and B.D. Ross, Absolute quantitation of water and metabolites in the human brain. Part II: Metabolite concentrations. J. Magn. Reson, 1993. 102(1): p. 9-19.
10. Bluml, S., et al. Creatine kinase and free-energy of ATP hydrolysis in normal and diseased human brain. in Proceedings, 4th Society of Magnetic Resonance. 1996. New York:
11. Bluml, S. and B. Ross, Clinical Application of Quantitative Proton Decoupled 31P MRS in Normal and Diseased Human Brain. International Society for Magnetic Resonance in Medicine Fifth Scientific Meeting, 1997. (In Press).
12. Ross, B.D., et al., Subclinical hepatic encephalopathy: Proton MR spectroscopic abnormalities. Radiology, 1994. 193: p. 457-463.
13. Lee, J.H., E. Arcinue, and B.D. Ross, Organic osmolytes in the brain of an infant with hypernatremia. N. Eng. J. Med, 1994. 331(7): p. 439-442.
14. Videen, J.S., et al., Human cerebral osmolytes during chronic hyponatremia: A proton magnetic resonance spectroscopy study. J. Clin. Invest, 1995. 95: p. 788-793.
15. Haussinger, D., et al., Proton magnetic resonance spectroscopy studies on human brain myo-inositol in hypo-osmolarity and hepatic encephalopathy. Gastroenterology, 1994. 107: p. 1475-1480.
16. Moats, R.A., et al., Decrease in cerebral inositols in rats and humans. Biochem. J, 1993. 295(1): p. 15-18.
17. Kanamori, K., B.D. Ross, and J. Tropp, Selective, in vivo observation of [5-^{15}N]glutamine amide protons in rat brain by ^{1}H-^{15}N heteronuclear multiple-quantum-coherence transfer NMR. J. Magn. Reson, 1995. B, 107(2): p. 107-115.
18. Kanamori, K., B.D. Ross, and E.L. Kuo, Dependence of in vivo glutamine synthetase activity on ammonia concentration in rat brain studied by ^{1}H-^{15}N heteronuclear multiple-quantum coherence-transfer NMR. Biochem. J, 1995. 311: p. 681-688.
19. Bradford, H.F. and H.K. Ward, Glutamine as a metabolic substrate for isolated nerve-endings: Inhibition by ammonium ions. Biochem. Soc. Trans, 1975. : p. 1223-1227.
20. Kvamme, E. and K. Lenda, Regulation of glutaminase by exogenous glutamate, ammonia and 2-oxoglutarate in synaptosomal enriched preparation from rat brain. Neurochem Res, 1982. 7(6): p. 667-678.
21. Hamberger, A., B. Hedquist, and B. Nystrom, Ammonium ion inhibition of evoked release of endogenous glutamate from hippocampal slices. J. Neurochem, 1979. 33: p. 1295-1302.

22. Theoret, Y., et al., Effects of ammonium chloride on synaptic transmission in the rat hippocampal slice. Neurosci, 1985. 14: p. 798–806.

23. Hindfelt, B., F. Plum, and T.E. Duffy, Effect of acute ammonia intoxication on cerebral metabolism in rats with portacaval shunts. J. Clin. Invest, 1977. 59(March): p. 386–396.

24. Lavoie, J., et al., Amino acid changes in autopsied brain tissue from cirrhotic patients with hepatic encephalopathy. J Neurochem, 1987. 49: p. 692–697.

25. Erecinska, M. and I.A. Silver, Metabolism and role of glutamate in mammalian brain. Prog. Neurobiol, 1990. 35: p. 245–296.

26. Kanamori, K. and B.D. Ross, In vivo activity of glutaminase in the brain of hyperammonaemic rats measured by ^{15}N nuclear magnetic resonance. Biochem. J, 1995. 305: p. 329–336.

OSMOSIGNALLING AND OSMOLYTES IN LIVER AND ASTROCYTES

Dieter Häussinger, Ulrich Warskulat and Freimut Schliess

Medizinische Universitätsklinik Düsseldorf
Heinrich-Heine-Universität Düsseldorf
Moorenstrase 5
D-40225 Düsseldorf/Germany

INTRODUCTION

In recent years it became clear that the regulation of cell function involves another important controlling parameter, i.e. the cellular hydration state. Cell hydration can change within minutes under the influence of hormones, nutrient supply and oxidative stress and such a short-term modulation of cell volume within a narrow range acts per se as a potent signal which modifies cellular metabolism and gene expression (for reviews see [1-3]). Indeed, several effects of amino acids and hormones are apparently mediated by alterations of cell hydration. The intracellular signalling mechanisms which link the osmotic water shift across the plasma membrane to cell function are understood only in part, however, osmosignalling pathways have been identified, whose interruption by suitable inhibitors leads to an uncoupling of cell swelling from the metabolic response of the cell. Organic osmolytes interfere with cell hydration and can modify the function of liver parenchymal and non-parenchymal cells. This article briefly reviews our recent work on osmosignalling in hepatocytes and astrocytes and the role of organic osmolytes.

OSMOSIGNALLING IN HEPATOCYTES AND H4IIE HEPATOMA CELLS

The hepatocellular hydration state is now recognized as an important physiologic determinant of cell function. Hormones and nutrients exert in part their effects on metabolism and gene expression in liver by a modification of cell volume [1-3]. This creates an elegant control mechanism which helps to adapt cellular metabolism to alterations of the environment (substrate, tonicity, hormones, oxidative stress). In view of the multiple and potent effects of cell hydration on cell function, the question arises as to how cell volume changes are sensed and how the signal is transduced to the level of cell function. Little is known about the structures that sense the changes in cell hydration. Because cell volume/hydration is a physical property of the cell, sensing could occur physically and/or mechanically. One hypothesis is that hydration changes will affect the concentrations of one or more intracellular constituents, which may act to regulate volume-regulatory transport systems and/or intracellular signalling pathways. One intruiging model postulates that the extent of macromolecular crowding, i.e. the cytosolic protein concentration will determine the tendency of intracellular macromolecules to associate with the plasma membrane and thereby affect their enzymatic activity [4,5]. Other candidates for mechanical cell volume sensing include the cytoskeleton, recently identified ion conductance regulator proteins in non-hepatic tissues [6] and stretch-activated cation and anion channels (for review see [7]). Recently, histidine kinases have been identified in yeast, which are putative integral membrane proteins and may act as osmosensors [8]. The signal is transduced by autophosphorylation and subsequent phosphate transfer to an aspartate residue in the receiver domain of a cognate response regulator molecule that regulates a MAP-kinase-like protein kinase cascade. As yet, a counterpart in liver has not been identified.

Little more is known about the intracellular signalling events which couple changes in liver cell hydration to cell function, although the picture is still incomplete. Current interest focusses on the osmotic regulation of mitogen-activated protein (MAP-) kinases and related protein kinases, such as Jun-kinases (Jnk). MAP-kinases are serine/threonine kinases, which are activated by dual phosphorylation at threonine and tyrosine residues (for reviews see [9-11]). In rat hepatoma cells [12] and rat hepatocytes [13] Erk-1 and Erk-2, two members of the MAP-kinase family are activated in response to hypoosmotic and amino acid-induced cell swelling (fig. 1). A signal transduction sequence, which is initiated by the osmotic water shift across the plasma membrane and ultimately leads to changes in cell function, has been identified in rat liver cells [12,13]. Here, hypoosmotic cell swelling results within one minute in a pertussis-toxin, cholera toxin- and genistein-sensitive, but protein kinase C- and Ca^{2+} independent phosphorylation of the MAP-kinases Erk-1 and Erk-2. This suggests that liver cell swelling leads to a G-protein-mediated activation of a yet unidentified tyrosine kinase, which acts to activate a pathway towards MAP-kinases.

MAP-kinases have multiple protein substrates [9,10], such as the microtubule-associated proteins MAP-2 and Tau, other protein kinases, such as S6 kinase and trans-

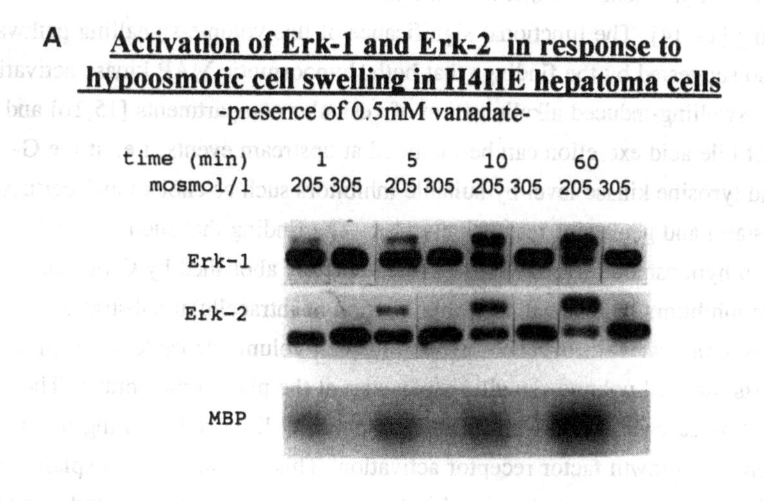

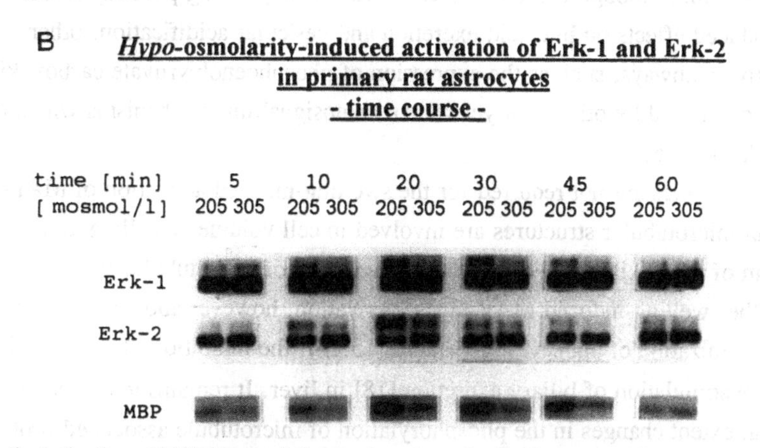

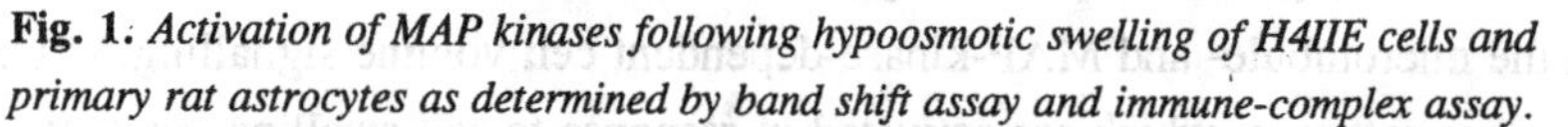

Fig. 1. *Activation of MAP kinases following hypoosmotic swelling of H4IIE cells and primary rat astrocytes as determined by band shift assay and immune-complex assay.*
Cells were incubated in normoosmotic (305 msomol/l) or hypoosmotic (205 mosmol/l) media for the time periods indicated. Erk-1 and Erk-2 are activated within minutes of hypoosmotic swelling as revealed by the appearence of a second, phosphorylated protein band. In these band shift assays, total protein extracts were analysed in western blots using specific antibodies against Erk-1 and Erk-2, respectively. MAP-kinase activation is also shown directly by immune complex assays using the myelin basic protein (MBP) as phosphorylation substrate and the antibody against Erk-2 as described in [12,19].

cription factors such as c-Jun. In fact, the swelling-induced activation of MAP kinases is followed by an increased phosphorylation of c-Jun, which may explain -due to autoregulation of the c-jun gene- the increase in c-jun mRNA levels 30min after the onset of cell swelling [12,14]. The functional significance of this volume-signalling pathway in liver is also suggested by the findings that both, hypoosmotic MAP kinase activation as well as the swelling-induced alkalinization of vesicular compartments [15,16] and stimulation of bile acid excretion can be inhibited at upstream events, i.e. at the G-protein and tyrosine kinase level by suitable inhibitors such as cholera and pertussis toxin, erbstatin and genistein, respectively [13]. The finding that such metabolic responses to hypoosmotic liver swelling are completely abolished by G-protein and tyrosine kinase inhibitors indicates that simple dilution of intracellular substrates following the osmotic water shifts cannot explain the cell volume-dependence of metabolism and suggests that cell volume signalling may start at the plasma membrane. The intracellular signalling cascade which is initiated in response to liver cell swelling resembles that triggered by growth factor receptor activation. This similarity may explain why cell swelling acts like an anabolic signal in liver with respect to protein and carbohydrate metabolism. Although the above-mentioned osmosignalling pathway mediates the swelling-induced effects on bile acid excretion and vesicular acidification, other osmosensitive pathways, such as the expression of phosphoenolpyruvate carboxykinase are apparently controlled by other, not yet known osmosignalling mechanisms which do not involve MAP-kinases.

Intact microtubules are not required for the swelling-induced activation of MAP-kinases, but microtubular structures are involved in cell volume signalling at a step downstream of MAP-kinases. For example, disruption of microtubules by colchicine does not inhbit the swelling-induced MAP-kinase activation, however abolishes the swelling-induced alkalinization of endocytotic vesicles [15,16], the inhibition of proteolysis [17] and the stimulation of biliary excretion [18] in liver. It remains to be established to what extent changes in the phosphorylation of microtubule associated proteins are involved in the microtubule- and MAP-kinase-dependent cell volume signalling. On the other hand, other pathways which are activated in response to cell swelling, such as stimulation of glycine oxidation or of the pentose phosphate shunt are not affected following microtubule disruption.

In H4IIE cells, hyperosmotic cell shrinkage leads to an activation of Jun-kinases and an induction of CL100 (also known as MAP kinase phosphatase-1, MPK-1). CL100 is a dual-specificity protein phosphatase which inactivates a delayed hyperosmolarity-induced MAP-kinase signal (Schliess, Heinrich and Häussinger, manuscript submitted). However, the functional relevance of the hyperosmolarity-induced signal transduction pathway remains to be established.

OSMOSIGNALLING IN ASTEROSYTES AND C6 GLIOMA CELLS

Like in primary hepatocytes and H4IIE hepatoma cells, also hypoosmotic exposure of primary astrocytes and C6 glioma cells induces MAP kinase activation [19,20] (fig. 1). However, the upstream signalling events, which lead to MAP kinase activation are different. Hypoosmotic swelling of primary astrocytes leads to a biphasic Ca^{++} signal, which is characterized by an initial, transient peak being followed by a sustained elevation of the intracellular Ca^{++} concentration ("plateau") [21,22]. The initial peak is largely derived from an intracellular IP_3-, but not ryanodine-sensitive pool, whereas the plateau phase of Ca^{++} elevation is due to Ca^{++} entry from the extracellular space via capacitative entry and influx through nimodipine-sensitive Ca^{++} channels [19,23]. The sustained plateau-like elevation of intracellular Ca^{++}, but not the initial peak, is mandatory for the hypoosmolarity-induced MAP kinase activation in primary astrocytes [19]. On the other hand, hypoosmotic activation of MAP-kinases is not affected by inhibitors of tyrosine kinases, protein kinase C or of G-proteins, but is abolished in presence of PI_3-kinase inhibitors such as wortmannin or following activation of protein kinase A [19]. All these inhibitors were without effect on the swelling-induced Ca^{++} signal in astrocytes. The findings suggest that hypoosmotic astrocyte swelling activates MAP-kinases in a Ras/Raf-dependent and PI_3-kinase-dependent way which is initiated by a swelling-induced Ca^{++} signal. Protein kinase C, phospholipase C, tyrosine kinases and G-proteins do apparently not play a role in cell volume signalling towards MAP kinases in astrocytes [19].

Also hypoosmotic exposure of C6 glioma cells activates MAP-kinases and leads to an increase of the cytosolic free Ca^{++} concentration due to Ca^{++} influx from the extracellular space. However, in contrast to astrocytes there is no initial spike-like Ca^{++} transient [20]. Omission of extracellular Ca^{++} abolishes the hypoosmolarity-induced elevation of intracellular Ca^{++}, however, the MAP-kinases signal is preserved. Thus, in C6 glioma cells the hypoosmolarity-induced increase in intracellular Ca^{++} is not required for osmosignalling towards MAP-kinases as it is observed in astrocytes. Like in astrocytes, MAP kinase activation in C6 glioma cells is abolished following protein kinase A activation, indicating the involvement of the Ras/Raf pathway [20]. Neither wortmannin nor inhibitors of protein kinase C, phospholipase C, tyrosine kinases or G-proteins abolished osmosignalling towards MAP kinases. These data show that hepatocytes, astrocytes, hepatoma and glioma cells respond with an activation of the MAP-kinases Erk-1 and Erk-2 following hypoosmotic cell swelling, however, marked differences exist with respect to the upstream signalling events when these cell types are compared. The data also show that extrapolation of findings obtained in glioma cells to the situation in astrocytes may be misleading. Fig. 2 summarizes our current knowledge on osmosignalling towards MAP kinases in hepatocytes and astrocytes.

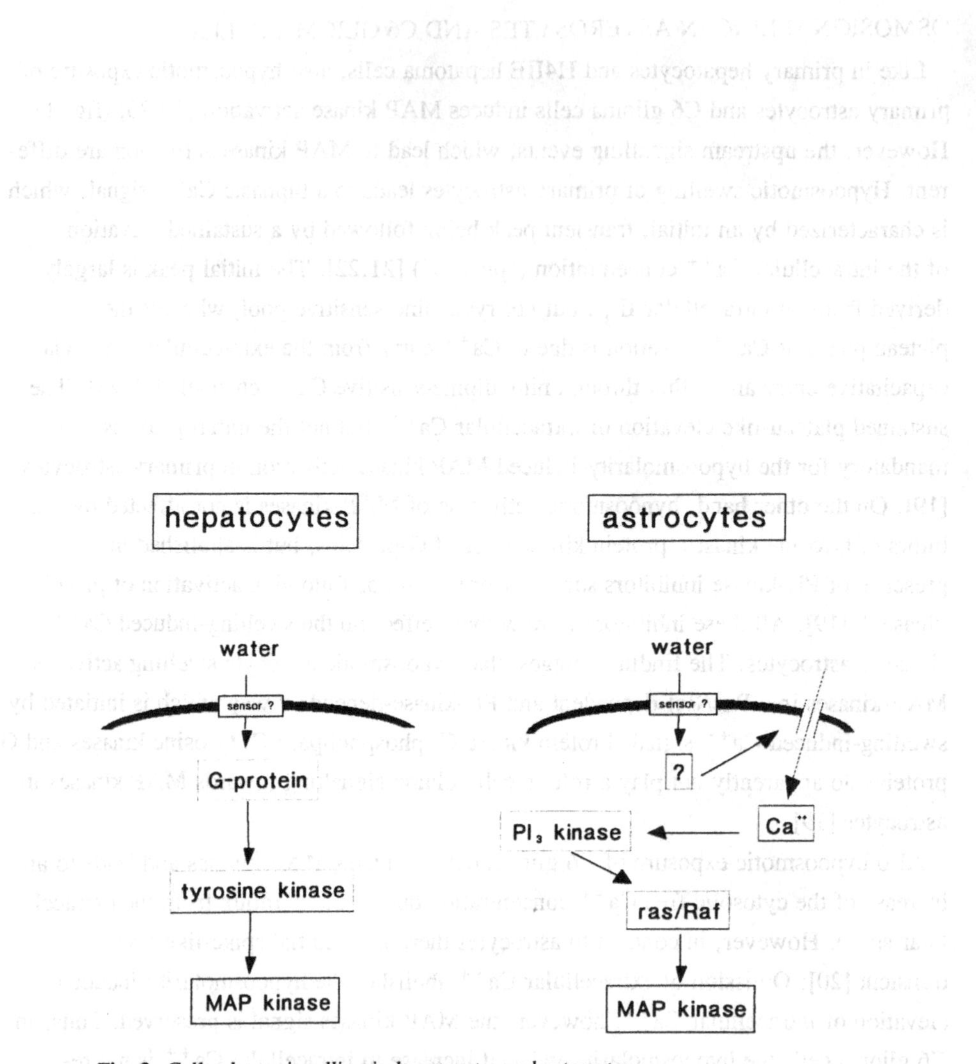

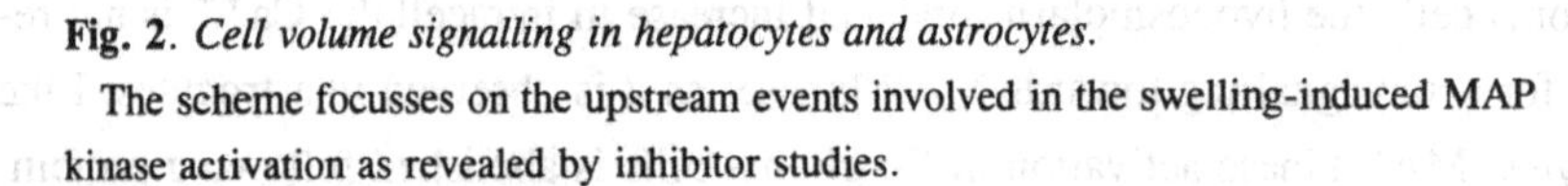

Fig. 2. *Cell volume signalling in hepatocytes and astrocytes.*
The scheme focusses on the upstream events involved in the swelling-induced MAP kinase activation as revealed by inhibitor studies.

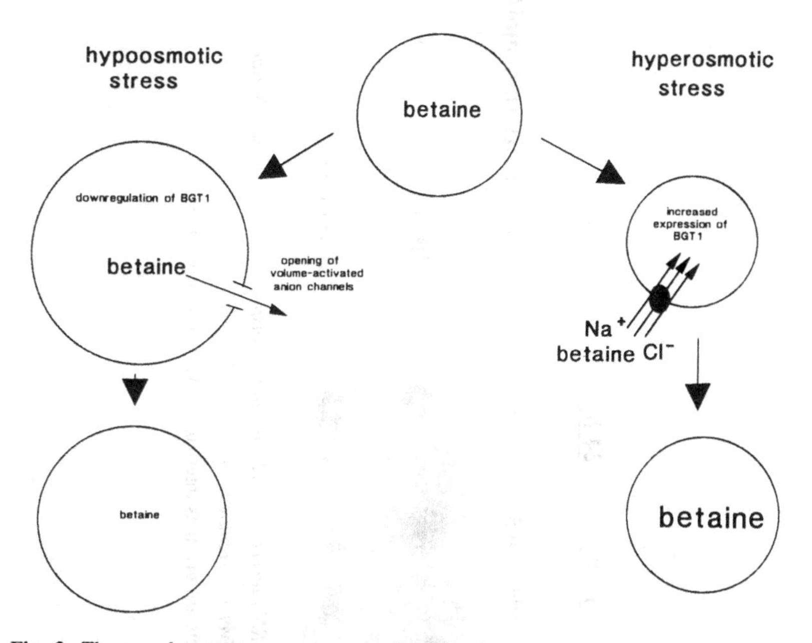

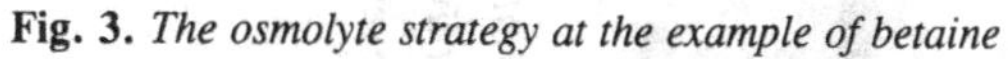

Fig. 3. *The osmolyte strategy at the example of betaine*

Hyperosmotic exposure leads to the induction of the betaine transporter BGT1 and cumulative uptake of betaine into the cell in order to increase cell volume. Hypoosmotic exposure leads to a rapid efflux of betaine from the cells via volume activated organic anion channels and a downregulation of BGT1.

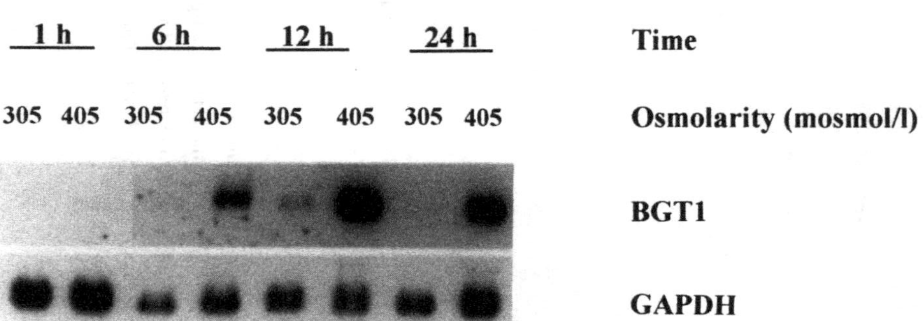

Fig. 4. *Induction of mRNA levels for BGT1 (betaine transporter) in lipopolysaccharide-(LPS)-stimulated rat liver macrophages (Kupffer cells)*
GAPDH mRNA levels are given as internal standard. From ref. [33].

In addition to the ionic mechanisms of cell volume regulation (for review see [24]), some cell types, such as renal medulla cells and astrocytes specifically accumulate or release organic compounds, socalled organic osmolytes, in reponse to cell shrinkage or cell swelling, respectively (for review see [25-28]). Osmolytes need to be non-perturbing solutes that do not interfere with protein function even when occurring in high intracellular concentrations. Such a prerequisite explains why only a few classes of organic compounds, viz. polyols (e.g. myo-inositol, sorbitol), methylamines (e.g. betaine, α-glycerophosphorylcholine) and certain amino acids (e.g. taurine) have evolved as osmolytes. The osmolyte strategy (fig. 3) is used by renal medulla cells, astrocytes and lens epithelia. Whereas taurine is a major intracellular osmolyte in fish hepatocytes [29,30], little was known until recently about osmolytes in mammalian liver, except for a release of small quantities of myo-inositol [31] and taurine [32] from perfused rat liver following hypoosmotic cell swelling. More recently, betaine has been identified as an osmolyte in liver macrophages (Kupffer cells) [33] and mouse RAW 264.7 macrophages [34]. Upon hyperosmotic exposure these cells strongly induce the Na^+ and Cl^- dependent betaine transporter (fig. 4), which is encoded by the betaine-GABA-transporter (BGT1) gene and which functions to create intra/extracellular betaine concentration ratios of 500 and intracellular betaine concentrations of 10 mmol/l and more. It is likely that a hypertonic stress responsive element in the 5'-flanking region of the BGT1 gene, as found in studies on MDCK cells [35], is also involved in the induction of the transporter in Kupffer cells. Induction of betaine transport in response to hyperosmotic stress requires several hours and involves marked increases in BGT1 mRNA levels. Conversely, hypoosmotic exposure of Kupffer cells downregulates BGT1 mRNA levels and an almost instantaneous release of betaine from the cells [33] is probably due to an opening of volume-sensitive channels. Rat Kupffer cells also use taurine [36] and to a smaller extent myo-inositol (unpublished observation) as osmolytes. Betaine and taurine transport exhibit different osmosensitivities: whereas during hyperosmotic cell shrinkage betaine uptake is stronger induced than taurine uptake, hypoosmotic exposure leads to a stronger release of taurine than of betaine. Also sinusoidal endothelial cells exhibit an osmosensitive regulation of BGT1 mRNA levels and of the TAUT mRNA levels, which encodes for a Na^+-coupled taurine transporter. This strongly suggests that both betaine and taurine function as osmolytes in sinusoidal endothelial cells (U. Warskulat, F. Zhang and D. Häussinger, unpublished). Rat liver hepatocytes possess a Na^+-coupled taurine transporter in the plasma membrane. TAUT mRNA levels are upregulated in hyperosmolarity and decrease following hypoosmotic exposure, whereas BGT1 mRNA levels are not detectable in liver parenchymal cells and H4IIE hepatoma cells [37].

A **Organic osmolyte transporter mRNA levels in primary astrocytes**

255 305 355 | **Osmolarity (mosmol/l)**

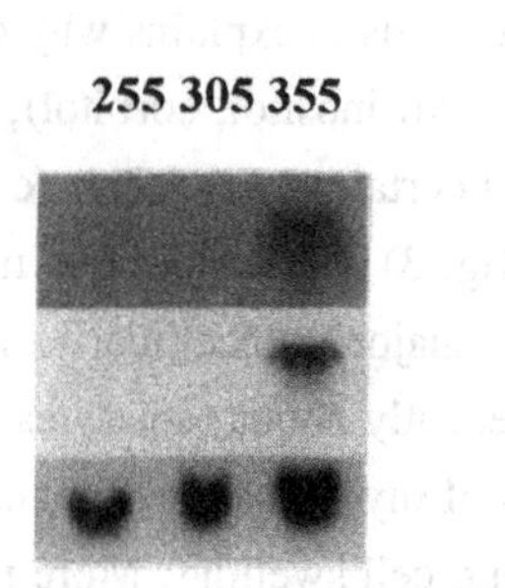

TAUT

SMIT

GAPDH

B **Organic osmolyte transporter mRNA levels in C6 glioma cells**

235 275 305 335 375 405 | **Osmolarity (mosmol/l)**

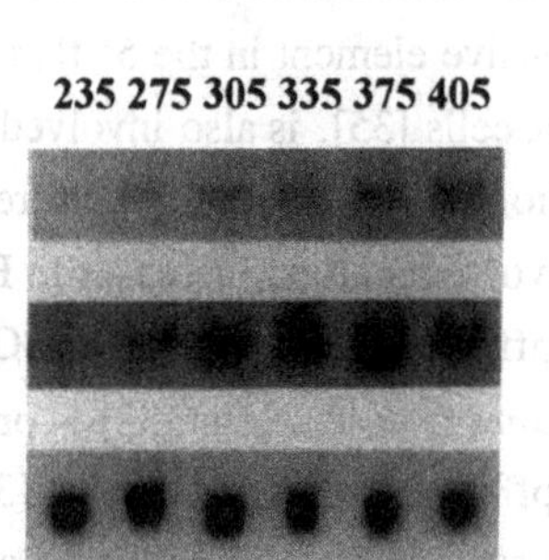

SMIT

TAUT

GAPDH

Fig. 5. ***Effect of hyperosmotic exposure on SMIT (myo-inositol transporter) and TAUT (taurine transporter) mRNA levels in cultivated rat astrocytes and C6 glioma cells.***

Cells were exposed for 12h to anisoosmolarity. Thereafter mRNA was extracted and subjected to Northern blot analysis. Glyceraldehyde phosphate dehydrogenase (GAPDH) mRNA levels are used as standards. In both cell types SMIT and TAUT mRNA levels are regulated by osmolarity with the basal mRNA levels under normoosmotic (305 mosmol/l) conditions being much higher in glioma cells than in primary astrocytes.

FUNCTIONAL SIGNIFICANCE OF THE OSMOLYTE STRATEGY IN LIVER MACROPHAGES

Whereas the functional significance of the osmolyte strategy employed by liver parenchymal cells, sinusoidal endothelial cells has not yet been established, recent data suggest that the osmolyte strategy in Kupffer cells is an important site of regulation of immune functions.

Recent studies have indicated that prostanoid formation by lipopolysaccharide-(LPS)-stimulated rat liver macrophages strongly depends upon ambient osmolarity. Increasing the osmolarity from 305 to 355 mosmol/l enhances prostaglandin E_2 formation almost 10-fold [38]. This is due to a strong induction and expression of cyclooxygenase-2, whereas hyperosmolarity does not affect the constitutively expressed cyclooxygenase-1 [38]. Hyperosmolarity-induced induction of cyclooxygenase-2 is abolished when betaine is present [33]. This finding may suggest that betaine is important for the formation of prostanoids in these cells. Phagocytosis of latex particles is accompanied by a release of betaine and taurine from Kupffer cells, which also occurs in response to hypoosmotic swelling of these cells [36,39]. Thus, one may speculate that these osmolytes play a role in the maintenance of Kupffer cell volume during ingestion of phagocytosable material. This may be important, because Kupffer cell swelling following phagocytosis might otherwise lead to sinusoidal obstruction. However, phagocytosis does not stimulate osmolyte efflux from RAW mouse macrophages.

Hypoosmotic exposure inhibits tumor necrosis factor-α production in LPS-stimulated Kupffer cells, whereas hyperosmotic cell shrinkage delayed the TNF response by these cells [40]. This latter effect of hyperosmolarity was counteracted by betaine [40]. However, nothing is known yet about the effects of cell volume on the formation of other cytokines.

OSMOLYTES AND THE PATHOGENESIS OF HEPATIC ENCEPHALOPATHY

Astrocytes use myo-inositol and taurine as osmolytes (fig. 5); the respective osmolyte transporters are upregulated (downregulated) following hyperosmotic (hypoosmotic) cell shrinkage (swelling) and astrocyte swelling leads to a rapid release of these osmolytes probably through an opening of unspecific channels in the plasma membrane [37,41-46]. Also betaine transporter BGT-1 mRNA is present in astrocytes and exhibits some osmosensitivity [37].

Astrocytes are the only cellular compartment in the brain capable of glutamine synthesis [47], which is the major pathway for cerebral ammonia detoxication. Brain edema in hepatic encephalopathy (HE) of acute liver failure is common and eventually determines the patients final outcome. Under these conditions astrocyte swelling due to an intracellular accumulation of glutamine is the most prominent neuropathological abnormality [48]. Although grade I-III portosystemic encephalopathy (PSE) in chronic liver disease was not considered in the past to involve cell swelling in the brain, recent *in vivo* evidence suggests that disturbances of astrocyte cell volume homeostasis (without clinically overt increase of intracranial pressure) may be an early event in HE in cirrhosis [49]. This suggestion is largely based on proton-magnetic resonance-(MR)-spectroscopic (^{1}H-MRS) studies.

^{1}H-MRS can be used to study metabolic abnormalities in the human brain *in vivo* and allows to pick up a myo-inositol signal, which was shown to be decreased in hepatic encephalopathy [50-52] and more recently identified to reflect an osmosensitive cerebral myo-inositol pool [49,53]. *In vitro* studies have shown that astrocytes contain high amounts of myo-inositol in contrast to neurons [54], suggesting that the myo-inositol signal in MRS-studies derived from whole brain is largely of glial origin.

There is a strong depletion of brain myo-inositol in humans with hepatic encephalopathy, as shown by *in vivo* ^{1}H-MR spectroscopy [49-52]. The loss of myo-inositol is accompanied by an increase of the glutamine/glutamate signal. Such alterations are also induced in the rat following portocaval shunting [52] and in humans following institution of a transjugular portosystemic intrahepatic stent shunt (TIPS) [49]. A high sensitivity and specificity of the myo-inositol signal for the diagnosis of hepatic encephalopathy in cirrhotics has been reported [56]. In fact, a decrease of the spectroscopic myo-inositol signal is already found in preclinical HE [49,56]. In view of the role of myo-inositol as an osmolyte in astrocytes, the MR-spectroscopic findings suggest that the markedly decreased myo-inositol signals in patients with HE reflect a disturbance of cell volume homeostasis in brain, which may occur already at preclinical stages of HE *in vivo*. This disturbance of brain cell volume homeostasis in HE may at least in part be attributed to an intracellular accumulation of glutamine in response to hyperammonemia, which tends to swell the cells. Indeed, cultured astrocytes swell under the influence of ammonia [57] and the ^{1}H-MR signal for glutamine is increased in parallel with the decrease of myo-inositol in both, latent and manifest HE, with the alterations being less pronounced in the latent stage. Apparently a volume-regulatory myo-inositol release occurs in response to ammonia-induced glutamine accumulation in astrocytes, indicating that astrocyte swelling may be an early event in HE in chronic liver disease. However, ammonia may not be the only mechanism by which astrocyte swelling is triggered in hepatic encephalopathy, because in vitro experiments indicate that astrocyte swelling also occurs under the influence of hyponatremia, some neurotransmitters [43], tumor necrosis factor-α [58] and benzodiazepines [59].

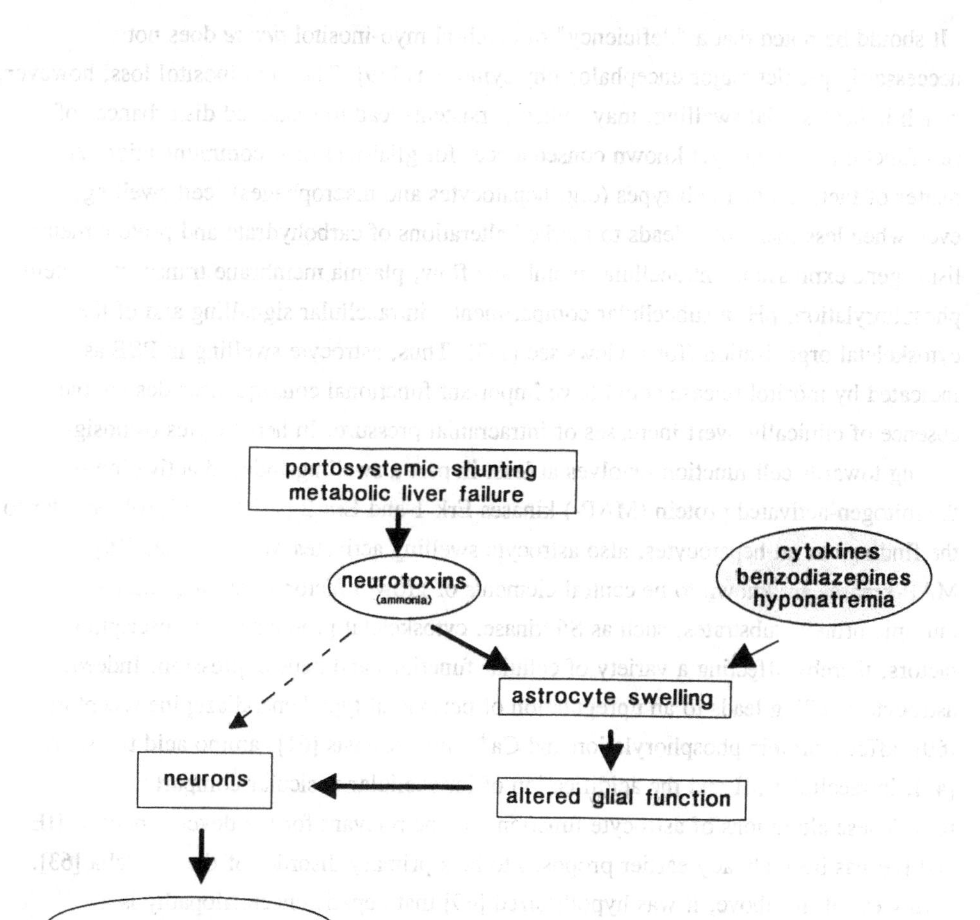

Fig. 6. *Hypothesis on glial swelling as a pathogenetic factor in hepatic encephalopathy.* Astrocyte swelling is induced by ammonia, tumor necrosis factor, benzodiazepines and hyponatremia. Glial swelling activates intracellular signalling pathways and produces alterations of glial function. This results in a disturbance of the glia-neuronal communication, triggering the clinical picture of HE.

It should be noted that a "deficiency" of cerebral myo-inositol *per se* does not neccessarily predict major encephalopathy symptoms [49]. The myo-inositol loss, however, which indicates glial swelling, may -when persistent- lead to sustained disturbances of cell function, with not yet known consequences for glial-neuronal communication. As a matter of fact, in other cell types (e.g. hepatocytes and macrophages), cell swelling, even when less than 10%, leads to marked alterations of carbohydrate and protein metabolism, gene expression, intracellular membrane flow, plasma membrane transport, protein phosphorylation, pH in subcellular compartments, intracellular signalling and of the cytoskeletal organization (for reviews see [1-3]. Thus, astrocyte swelling in PSE as indicated by inositol release could have important functional consequences despite the absence of clinically overt increases of intracranial pressure. In hepatocytes osmosignalling towards cell function involves at least in part a swelling-induced activation of the mitogen-activated protein (MAP-) kinases Erk-1 and Erk-2 [1,12,13,15,16]. Similar to the findings in rat hepatocytes, also astrocyte swelling activates MAP-kinases [19]. MAP-kinases are known to be central elements of growth factor signalling and have multiple protein substrates, such as S6 kinase, cytoskeletal proteins and transcription factors, thereby affecting a variety of cellular functions and gene expression. Indeed, astrocyte swelling leads to an upregulation of peripheral type benzodiazepine receptors [60], affects protein phosphorylation and Ca^{++} homeostasis [61], amino acid transport [43], intracellular pH and the acidification of intracellular vesicular compartments [62]. These alterations of astrocyte function may be relevant for the development of HE and HE has been already earlier proposed to be a primary disorder of the astroglia [63].

In view of the above, it was hypothesized [49] that hepatic encephalopathy is at least in part the result of astrocyte swelling with subsequent alterations of glial function and glioneuronal communication (fig. 6). This working model could explain why heterogenous factors can precipitate HE, because all these factors (e.g. ammonia, TNF, benzodiazepines, hyponatremia etc.) augment cell swelling and may thus act synergistically to trigger a common endpath, i.e. glia swelling with its functional consequences. Further, astrocyte swelling can trigger functional disturbances, which resemble several established phenomena in PSE, such as alterations of cerebral glucose metabolism, selective alterations of blood-brain permeability (which is equivalent to changes in astrocyte membrane transport), cytoskeletal changes and the upregulation of benzodiazepine receptors. However, further studies are required to establish the validity of this "swelling hypothesis".

PERSPECTIVE

The complex interplay between cell hydration and the cell function may have considerable impact on our understanding of organ function in health and disease. These interactions not only involve problems of cholestasis [13], protein turnover [64], hepatic encephalopathy [49] and viral replication [65], but also organ protection and preservation. Modulation of Kupffer and sinusoidal endothelial cell function by the hydration state, availability of osmolytes, such as betaine and taurine, and the expression of the respective osmolyte transporters may also have important consequences for the production of mediators of inflammation by these cells and could offer new potential sites for therapeutic intervention. It is hoped that this review will stimulate further research in this exciting area.

ACKNOWLEDGEMENTS

Our own work reported herein was supported by Deutsche Forschungsgemeinschaft, the Gottfried-Wilhelm-Leibniz-Prize and the Fonds der Chemischen Industrie.

REFERENCES

1 Häussinger D. & Lang, F. (1992) Cell volume and hormone action. Trends Pharmacol. Sci. 13, 371-373

2 Graf, J. & Häussinger, D. (1996) Ion transport in hepatocytes: mechanisms and correlations to cell volume, hormone actions and metabolism. J. Hepatol. 24, 53-77

3 Häussinger, D. (1996) The role of cell hydration in the regulation of cell function. Biochem. J. 313, 697-710

4 Minton, A.P., Colclasure, G.C. & Parker, J.C. (1992) Model for the role of macromolecular crowding in regulation of cellular volume. Proc. Nat. Acad. Sci. 89, 10504-10506

5 Parker, J.C. (1993) In defense of cell volume? Am. J. Physiol. 265, C1191-1200

6 Krapivinsky, G.B., Ackerman, M.J., Gordon, E.A., Krapivinsky, L.D. & Clapham, D.E. (1994) Molecular characterization of a swelling-induced chloride conductance regulatory protein $pICl_n$. Cell 76, 439-448

7 Sackin, H. (1994) Stretch-activated ion channels. In: Cellular and molecular physiology of cell volume regulation (Strange, K., ed.) pp. 215-240, CRC Press Boca Raton

8 Maeda, T., Wurgler-Murphy, S.M. & Saito, H. (1994) A two-component system that regulates an osmosensing MAP kinase cascade in yeast. Nature 369, 242-245

9 Nishida, E. & Gotoh, Y. (1993) The MAP kinase cascade is essential for diverse signal transduction pathways. Trends Biochem. Sci. 18,128-131

10 Waskiewicz, A.J. & Cooper, J.A. (1995) Mitogen and stress response pathways: MAP kinase cacades and phosphatase regulation in mammals and yeast. Curr. Op. Cell. Biol. 7, 798-805

11 Kyriakis, J.M., Banerjee, P., Nikolakaki, E., Dai, T., Rubie, E.A., Ahmad, M.F., Avruch, J. & Woodgett, J.R. (1994) The stress-activated protein kinase subfamily of c-Jun kinases. Nature 369, 156-160

12 Schliess, F., Schreiber, R., & Häussinger, D. (1995) Activation of of extracellular signal-regulated kinases Erk-1 and Erk-2 by cell swelling in H4IIE hepatoma cells. Biochem. J. 309, 13-17

13 Noé, B., Schliess, F., Wettstein, M., Heinrich, S. & Häussinger, D. (1996) Regulation of taurocholate excretion by a hypoosmolarity-activated signal transduction pathway in rat liver. Gastroenterology 110, 858-865

14 Finkenzeller, G., Newsome, W.P., Lang, F. & Häussinger, D. (1994) Increase of c-jun mRNA upon hypoosmotic cell swelling of rat hepatoma cells. FEBS Lett. 340, 163-166

15 Schreiber, R. & Häussinger, D. (1995) Characterization of the swelling-induced alkalinization of endocytotic vesicles in fluorescein isothiocyanate-dextran-loaded rat hepatocytes. Biochem. J. 309, 19-24

16 Busch, G.L., Schreiber, R., Dartsch, P.C., Völkl, H., vom Dahl, S., Häussinger, D. & Lang, F. (1994) Involvement of microtubules in the link between cell volume and pH of acidic cellular compartments in rat and human hepatocytes. Proc. Natl. Acad. Sci. USA 91, 9165-9169

17 vom Dahl, S., Stoll, B., Gerok, W. & Häussinger, D. (1995) Inhibition of proteolysis by cell swelling in the liver requires intact microtubular structures. Biochem. J. 308, 529-536

18 Häussinger, D., Saha, N., Hallbrucker, C., Lang, F. & Gerok W. (1993) Involvement of microtubules in the swelling-induced stimulation of transcellular taurocholate transport in perfused rat liver. Biochem. J. 291, 355-360

19 Schliess, F., Sinning, R., Fischer, R., Schmalenbach, C. & Häussinger, D. (1996) Calcium-dependent activation of Erk-1 and Erk-2 following hypoosmotic astrocyte swelling. Biochem. J. 320, 167-171

20 Sinning, R., Schliess, F., Kubitz, R. & Häussinger, D. (1996) Osmosignalling in C6 glioma cells. FEBS Lett. in press

21 O'Connor, E.R. & Kimelberg, H.K. (1993) Role of Ca^{++} in astrocyte volume regulation and the release of ions and amino acids. J. Neurosci. 13, 2638-2650

22 Bender, A.S., Mantelle, L.L. & Norenberg, M.D. (1994) Stimulation of calcium uptake in cultured astrocytes by hypoosmotic stress - effect of cyclic AMP. Brain Res. 645, 27-35

23 Fischer, R., Schliess, F. & Häussinger, D. (1996) Characterization of the hypoosmolarity-induced Ca^{++}-response in primary rat astrocytes. Glia, submitted

24 Lang, F. & Häussinger, D., eds. (1993) Interaction of cell volume and cell function. Springer Verlag Berlin.

25 Yancey, P.H., Clark, M.E., Hand, S.C., Bowlus, R.D. & Somero, G.N. (1982) Living with water stress: evolution of osmolyte systems. Science 217, 1214-1222

26 Burg, M.H. (1995) Molecular basis of osmotic regulation. Am. J. Physiol. 268, F983-F996

27 Chamberlin, M.E. & Strange, K. (1989) Anisosmotic cell volume regulation: a comparative view. Am. J. Physiol. 257, C159-C173

28 Kwon, H.M. & Handler, J.S. (1995) Cell volume regulated transporters of compatible osmolytes. Curr. Op. Cell. Biol. 7, 465-471

29 Ballatori, N., Simmons, T.W. & Boyer, J.L. (1994) A volume-activated taurine channel in skate hepatocytes: membrane polarity and role of intracellular ATP. Am. J. Physiol. 267, G285-G291

30 Ballatori, N. & Boyer, J.L. (1992) Taurine transport in skate hepatocytes. Am. J. Physiol. 262, G445-450 and G451-460

31 vom Dahl, S., Hallbrucker, C., Lang, F. & Häussinger, D. (1991) Role of eicosanoids, inositol phosphates and extracellular Ca^{++} in cell volume regulation of rat liver. Eur. J. Biochem. 198, 73-83

32 Brand, H.S., Meijer, A.J., Gustavson, L.A., Jörning, G.G.A., Leegwater, A.C.J., Maas, M.A.W. & Chamaleau, R.A.F.M. (1994) Cell swelling-induced taurine release from isolated perfused rat liver. Biochem. Cell. Biol. 72, 8-11

33 Zhang, F., Warskulat, U., Wettstein, M. & Häussinger, D. (1996) Identification of betaine as an osmolyte in rat liver macrophages. Gastroenterology 110, 1543-1552

34 Warskulat, U., Wettstein, M. & Häussinger, D. (1995) Betaine is an osmolyte in RAW 264.7 mouse macrophages. FEBS Lett. 377, 47-50

35 Takenaka, M., Preston, A.S., Kwon, H.M. & Handler, J.S. (1994) The tonicity-sensitive element that mediates increased transcription of the betaine transporter gene in response to hypertonic stress. J. Biol. Chem. 269, 29379-29381

36 Warskulat, U., Zhang, F. & Häussinger, D. (1996) Taurine is an osmolyte in rat liver macrophages (Kupffer cells). J. Hepatol. submitted

37 Warskulat, U., Wettstein, M. & Häussinger, D. (1996) Osmoregulated taurine transport in H4IIE hepatoma cells and perfused rat liver. Biochem. J. in press

38 Zhang, F., Wettstein, M., Warskulat, U., Schreiber, R., Henninger, P., Decker, K. & Häussinger D. (1995) Hyperosmolarity stimulates prostaglandin synthesis and cyclooxygenase-2 expression in activated rat Kupffer cells. Biochem. J. 312, 135-143

39 Warskulat, U., Zhang, F. & Häussinger, D. (1996) Modulation of phagocytosis by anisoosmolarity and betaine in rat liver macrophages (Kupffer cells) and RAW 264.7 mouse macrophages. FEBS Lett. 391, 287-292

40 Zhang, F., Warskulat, U. & Häussinger, D. (1996) Modulation of tumor necrosis factor-α release by anisoosmolarity and betaine in rat liver macrophages (Kupffer cells). FEBS Lett. 391, 293-296

41 Paredes, A., McManus, M., Kwon, H.M. & Strange, K. (1993) Osmoregulation of the Na^{+}- inositol cotransporter activity and mRNA levels in brain glial cells. Am. J. Physiol. 263, C1282-1288

42 Moran. J., Maar, T.E. & Pasantes-Morales, H. (1994) Impaired cell volume regulation in taurine-deficient cultured astrocytes. Neurochem. Res. 19, 415-420

43 Kimelberg, H.K., O'Connor, E.R. & Kettenmann, H. (1993) Effects of swelling on glial cell function. In: Interactions cell volume and cell function (Lang, F., Häussinger, D., eds,) pp. 158-186, Springer Verlag Heidelberg

44 Lien, Y.H.H., Shapiro, J.L. & Chan, L. (1990) Effects of hypernatremia on organic brain osmoles. J. Clin. Invest. 85,1427-1435

45 Murphy S. ed. (1993) Astrocytes - Pharmacology and function. Academic Press San Diego

46 Moats, R.A., Lien, Y.H.H., Filippi, D. & Ross, B.D. (1993) Decrease in cerebral inositols in rats and humans. Biochem. J. 295,15-18

47 Martinez-Hernandez, A., Bell, K.P. & Norenberg, M.D. (1977) Glutamine synthetase: glial localization in brain. Science 195, 1356-1358

48 Swain, M., Butterworth, R.F. & Blei, A.T. (1992) Ammonia and related amino acids in the pathogenesis of brain edema in acute ischemic liver failure in rats. Hepatology 15, 449-453

49 Häussinger, D., Laubenberger, J., vom Dahl, S., Ernst, T., Bayer, S., Langer, M. & Hennig, J. (1994) Proton magnetic resonance spectroscopic studies on human brain myo-inositol in hypoosmolarity and hepatic encephalopathy. Gastroenterology 107, 1475-1480

50 Kreis, R., Farrow, N.A. & Ross, B.D. (1990) Diagnosis of hepatic encephalopathy by proton magnetic resonance spectroscopy. Lancet 336,635-636

51 Kreis, R., Ross, B.D., Farrow, N.A. & Ackerman, Z. (1992) Metabolic disorders of the brain in chronic hepatic encephalopathy detected with H-1 MR spectroscopy. Radiology 182, 19-27

52 Moats, R.A., Lien, Y.H.H., Filippi, D. & Ross, B.D. (1993) Decrease in cerebral inositols in rats and humans. Biochem. J. 295, 15-18

53 Lee, J.H., Arcinue, E. & Ross, B.D. (1994) Organic osmolytes in the brain of an infant with hypernatremia. New Engl. J. Med. 331, 439-442

54 Brand, A. & Leibfritz, D. (1992) Metabolic markers in glial cells for differentiation of brain tissue. Abstr Commun 11th Ann. Meet. Soc. MR Med. 649

55 Kreis, R., Farrow, N.A. & Ross, B.D. (1990) Diagnosis of hepatic encephalopathy by proton magnetic resonance spectroscopy. Lancet 336, 635-636

56 Laubenberger, J., Häussinger, D., Bayer, S., Gufler, H., Hennig, J. & Langer, M. (1997) Demonstration of cerebral metabolic abnormalities in asymptomatic patients with liver cirrhosis by proton MR spectroscopy. Gastroenterology in press

57 Norenberg, M.D., Baker, L., Norenberg, L.O.B., Blicharska, J., Bruce-Gregorius, J.H. & Neary, J.T. (1991) Ammonia-induced astrocyte swelling in primary culture. Neurochem. Res. 16, 833-836

58 Bender, A.S., Rivera, I.V. & Norenberg, M.D. (1992) Tumor necrosis factor α induces astrocyte swelling. Trans. Amer. Soc. Neurochem. 23, 113

59 Norenberg, M.D. & Bender, A.S. (1994) Astrocyte swelling in liver failure: role of glutamine and benzodiazepines. In: Brain Edema IX (Ito, U., ed.), pp. 24-27 Springer Verlag Vienna

60 Itzhak, Y., Bender, A.S. & Norenberg, M.D. (1994) Effect of hypoosmotic stress on peripheral-type benzodiazepine receptors in cultured astrocytes. Brain Res. 644, 221-225

61 Bender, A.S., Neary, J.T. & Norenberg, M.D. (1992) Involvement of second messengers and protein phosphorylation in astrocyte swelling. Can. J. Physiol. Pharmacol. 70(Suppl):S362-366

62 Lang, F., Busch, G., Völkl, H. & Häussinger, D. (1994) Lysosomal pH- a link between cell volume and metabolism. Biochem. Soc. Trans. 22(2):504-507

63 Norenberg, M.D., Neary, J.T., Bender, A.S. and Dombro, R.S. (1992) Hepatic encephalopathy: a disorder in glial-neuronal communication. In: Progress in brain research (Yu, A.C.H., Hertz, L., Norenberg, M.D., Sykova, E. & Waxman, S.G., eds.) pp. 261-269, Elsevier Publ. Amsterdam

64 Häussinger, D., Roth, E., Lang, F. & Gerok, W. (1993) The cellular hydration state: an important determinant for protein catabolism in health and disease. Lancet 341, 1330-1332

65 Offensperger, W.B., Offensperger, S., Stoll, B., Gerok, W. & Häussinger, D. (1994) Effects of anisotonic exposure on duck hepatitis B virus replication. Hepatology 20, 1-7

EFFECTS OF ACID-BASE ALTERATIONS AND PROTEIN DEPLETION ON HEPATIC NITROGEN METABOLISM

Anton C. Schoolwerth[1] and Daniel J. O'Donovan[2]

[1]Division of Nephrology, Medical College of Virginia, Virginia Commonwealth University, USA

[2]Physiology Department, University College, Galway, Ireland

INTRODUCTION

An alteration in acid-base balance has wide-ranging effects on many systems in the body. It has long been recognized that acid-base regulation is linked to nitrogen metabolism. Ammonium (NH_4^+), which is a constituent of normal urine, is excreted in greater quantities in metabolic acidosis. Earlier work showed that the rise in NH_4^+ excretion in acidosis coincided with a decrease in the rate of urea excretion. When it was realized that the enzyme urease was lacking in mammalian tissues, it was concluded that urea is not a direct source of urinary NH_4^+. The discovery that the extraction of glutamine by the kidney contributed significantly to urinary NH_4^+ focused attention on the renal metabolism of glutamine. It is now well established that the extraction of glutamine by the kidney and the renal mitochondrial deamidation of glutamine are accelerated in chronic metabolic acidosis.

However, an increase in the renal utilization of glutamine in prolonged acidosis will ultimately place a drain on the nitrogenous resources of the body. A significant portion of the extra glutamine needed by the kidney in acidosis is supplied by muscle. NH_4^+ is utilized in the liver for the synthesis of both glutamine and urea. It is logical to assume that the hepatic synthesis of these two nitrogenous compounds would be influenced by the rate of conversion of glutamine to NH_4^+ in the kidney. Research in recent times has concentrated in trying to find the link between these two intriguing processes.

Large quantities of NH_4^+ and HCO_3^- are formed daily as end-products of neutral amino acid metabolism. HCO_3^- accumulation is prevented by hepatic urea synthesis, which also incorporates the excess NH_4^+. A reduction in urea formation in acidosis could spare HCO_3^- and thus reduce the severity of acidosis. It could also make NH_4^+ available for hepatic glutamine synthesis; this glutamine may be transported to the kidney, where it could be reconverted to

Advances in Cirrhosis, Hyperammonemia, and Hepatic Encephalopathy
Edited by Felipo and Grisolía, Plenum Press, New York, 1997

NH_4^+ by renal mitochondria. Most enzymes are pH sensitive, so that an alteration in acid-base balance may affect the enzymatic activity of many tissues. It has been demonstrated that lowering the pH decreases ureagenesis[1-3], thus making more NH_4^+ available for hepatic glutamine synthesis. An increased release of glutamine by the perfused rat liver in acidosis has also been observed[4]. However, an alteration in acid-base balance *in vivo* failed to alter urea formation when NH_4Cl was the acidifying agent used[5]. Factors other than enzymatic activity play a part in product availability. Thus NH_4^+ and HCO_3^- levels in the liver are dependent on the appropriate amino acids coming in contact with active sites on the enzymes. Prior to this the amino acids must be transported into the hepatocyte. Interestingly, the transport of glutamine across the plasma membrane is decreased at low pH[6].

Control of urea cycle activity is under complex short-term and long-term regulation[7]. The short-term flux through the cycle is modulated by the availability of substrate, N-acetyl-glutamate[8], which is an allosteric activator of carbamoylphosphate synthase (CPS)[9-11] and ornithine[12]. Decreased synthesis of N-acetylglutamate in acidosis could potentially explain the reduction of urea synthesis. There are several other steps which have been proposed as sites in which the main HCO_3^--utilizing process, the ornithine cycle, can be inhibited at low pH. These include protonation of NH_3, the true substrate for CPS, and inhibition of hepatic carbonic anhydrase. Urea synthesis can also be reduced at low pH by inhibition of hepatic glutamine degradation. Glutamine degradation is reduced at low pH, not only because of lower glutaminase activity, but also, as mentioned above, because glutamine transport across the plasma membrane is decreased at low pH[5]. An additional site at which urea synthesis may be inhibited at low pH is at the step of hepatic amino acid transport across the plasma membrane. This was suggested by *in vitro* studies performed by Boon and Meijer[7]. In contrast to the previously suggested sites, inhibition of amino acid uptake into the cell would not be expected to spare HCO_3^- in the liver and would imply that an important regulatory role for the ornithine cycle in acid-base homeostasis was unlikely.

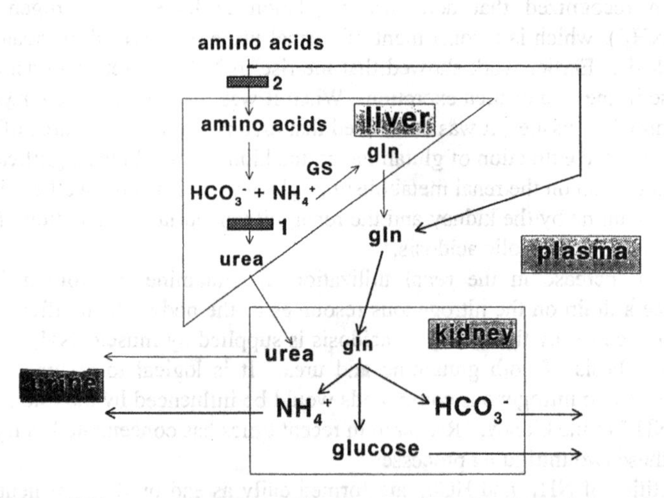

Fig. 1. Relationship of kidneys and liver in acid-base homeostasis. Traditional view of acid-base balance holds that HCO_3^- consumed by H^+ generated by diet and metabolism is resynthesized in kidneys from glutamine, a process closely linked to NH_4^+ formation and excretion. Also shown are potential sites of inhibition of urea formation in metabolic acidosis. *Site 1*, inhibition with the ornithine cycle; *site 2*, inhibition of amino acid transport across the hepatocyte plasma membrane. Thick arrows indicate pathways increased in acidosis, in the presence of inhibition at site 2. GS, glutamine synthetase. From Boon *et al*[18] with permission from the American Physiological Society.

Long-term regulation of urea cycle activity is mainly a function of the protein intake. The urea cycle enzyme activities reflect the level of dietary protein. The activities of the five hepatic enzymes increase when dietary protein is raised and decreased with a reduced protein intake[13-17]. The level of dietary protein has a profound effect on the disposition of NH_4^+ and amino acids within various tissues of the body. Change in the dietary protein, with and without ammonium chloride (NH_4Cl) ingestion, is an ideal model to determine the role of ureagenesis in acid-base regulation. Feeding a protein-free diet eliminates $HC0_3^-$ derived from ingested protein. Simultaneous administration of NH_4Cl produces metabolic acidosis and also provides NH_4^+ for hepatic urea synthesis. Under these circumstances, HCO_3^- should become the limiting factor in ureagenesis.

In the present manuscript, we review data assessing hepatic amino acid uptake in acute and chronic metabolic acidosis and $NaHCO_3$ feeding. We also review data from studies in which the effect of standard and protein-free diets, with and without NH_4Cl, on hepatic nitrogen metabolism and enzyme activities was evaluated. These data have been presented in separate form previously[18-20].

HEPATIC AMINO ACID UPTAKE IN ACUTE ACIDOSIS AND ALKALOSIS

Anesthetized rats received 1.8 mmol HCl or $NaHC0_3^-$ intravenously over a three hour period of time[18]. Thereafter, blood was obtained from the portal vein, hepatic vein, and aorta for amino acid analysis and liver tissue was obtained for amino acid determinations, protein, and DNA analysis. During the last hour of infusion, urine was collected for NH_4^+ and urea measurements[18]. After 3 hours of infusion of either HCl or $NaHC0_3$ mean blood pH was 7.1 and 7.7, respectively. Nitrogen excretion values are shown for this acute study in Table 1. Compared with alkalosis, NH_4^+ excretion was increased more than nine-fold and urea excretion was decreased 33% during acidosis. Total nitrogen excretion, estimated as the sum of NH_4^+ and urea excretion rates, was not significantly different in acute alkalosis and acidosis (703 $\pm$ 89 and 635 $\pm$ 48 µM N/h, respectively, $p > 0.05$). Plasma urea concentration was comparable during acute acidosis and alkalosis and averaged between 4 and 5 mM.

No differences were observed in hepatic vein-aortic plasma concentrations of amino acids, individually, or total in acidosis and alkalosis. However, substantial differences were noted in hepatic vein-portal vein concentration differences. These differences were reduced markedly for many amino acids in acidosis. Uptake of alanine, which is quantitatively the most important

Table 1. Urinary nitrogen excretion in acute acidosis and alkalosis

Urinary excretion	HCl Acidosis	$NaHCO_3$ Alkalosis	P
NH_4^+	201± 42	23± 9	<.01
Urea	434± 52	680± 94	<.01

Values are means ± SD for 6 rats in each group and are expressed as µmol N/h. NH_4^+, ammonium. Data from Boon *et al*[18].

amino acid for degradation in the liver, was strikingly reduced ($p < 0.01$) at low blood pH, as measured by hepatic vein-portal vein concentration differences. As shown in Table 2, total amino acid uptake, estimated from hepatic vein-portal vein concentration differences, decreased by 63% in acidosis compared with alkalosis. Hepatic vein amino acid concentrations, both individually and total, was approximately 45% higher in acidosis compared to alkalosis. Net hepatic NH_4^+ uptake, estimated from the concentration differences, was comparable during acute acidosis and alkalosis. However, NH_4^+ concentration in portal vein plasma was higher and remained elevated in hepatic vein plasma during acidosis compared with alkalosis ($p < 0.02$).

Table 2. Hepatic vein-portal vein differences in NH_4^+ and amino acid concentrations

Substance	HCl Acidosis	$NaHCO_3$ Alkalosis
NH_4^+	-116 ± 12	-102 ± 23
Alanine	-35 ± 16*	-129 ± 26
Glycine	-62 ± 12*	-93 ± 20
Glutamine	+40 ± 22	+55 ± 35
Threonine	-9.5 ± 5	-24 ± 8
Total amino acids	-188 ± 35*	-505 ± 71

Blood sample were obtained from portal vein and hepatic vein from rats after 3-h infusion with HCl (acidosis) and $NaHCO_3$ (alkalosis). NH_4^+ and amino acid concentrations are mean ± SE for 6 rats in each group, expressed in μM. A (-) indicates uptake, a (+) indicates release from the liver. *, $P < 0.05$ vs alkalosis. Data from Boon *et al* [18].

Extraction rates were estimated using the formula and flow rates reported by Welbourne *et al*[21]. By this calculation total amino acid extraction was approximately 55% lower in acidosis compared with alkalosis, consistent with the elevated concentrations of amino acids leaving the liver and the hepatic vein in this condition. For example, hepatic vein alanine increased from 120 ± 24 μM in alkalosis to 245 ± 17 μM in acidosis ($p < 0.01$; hepatic vein glycine was 114 ± 26 and 196 ± 13 μM in alkalosis and acidosis respectively ($p < 0.02$). Portal vein plasma amino acid concentrations were also increased in acidosis compared with alkalosis, although the differences were less marked than for the hepatic vein; for example, total amino acid concentration in portal vein plasma was 20% higher in acidosis than in alkalosis ($p < 0.02$).

Plasma concentration differences indicated a tendency for glutamine release from the liver but this difference was not significant. Moreover, release rates were not different in acidosis and alkalosis (Table 2). This is in contrast to the prediction from the intercellular glutamine cycle.[4]

The intracellular concentrations of alanine and serine were equal under both conditions, whereas the intracellular concentrations of glycine and threonine were decreased in the liver in alkalosis (data not shown). Intracellular glutamate and aspartate concentrations were lower in acidosis than alkalosis; intracellular NH_4^+ was also decreased in acidosis. Of these changes, the five-fold higher concentration of intracellular glutamate in alkalosis, probably due to increased amino acid influx followed by rapid transamination in this condition, was quantitatively the most important. Overall, the intracellular concentrations of readily transportable amino acids were not different in acidosis compared with alkalosis ($p > 0.05$).

Liver intracellular branched-chain amino acid concentrations were two-fold higher in acidosis compared to alkalosis although the differences were not significant. Since the branched-chain amino acids are not catabolized in rat liver, this finding suggested that an enhanced rate of proteolysis occurs during acidosis. Therefore, we determined the protein and DNA content in liver in both conditions. The protein-to-DNA ratio was 22% lower ($p < 0.05$) in acidosis than alkalosis. This finding, together with the suggested rise in intracellular branched-chain amino acid concentrations, is consistent with an accelerated rate of proteolysis in acute acidosis.

Overall these studies provide evidence *in vivo* confirming *in vitro* data published previously[7] indicating that amino acid uptake across the plasma membrane is reduced in acidosis. Since this occurs without a significant change in intracellular amino acid content, it is likely that the inhibition occurs at the level of amino acid transport across the plasma membrane. This effect of acidosis appears to be due entirely to a marked decrease in transport of Na^+-dependent amino acids (data not shown). However, the mechanism of acidosis induced inhibition of amino acid uptake and transport was not elucidated by these studies.

HEPATIC AMINO ACID CONSUMPTION IN CHRONIC METABOLIC ACIDOSIS

The mechanism responsible for the decline in urea synthesis was studied in chronic acidosis. Chronic metabolic acidosis and alkalosis were induced by feeding three groups of rats HCl, NH_4Cl, and $NaHC0_3$ (8 mmol/day) for seven days[19]; these substances were mixed with food which was provided to the animals daily in the evening. After seven days amino acids and NH_4^+ were measured in portal vein, hepatic vein, and aortic plasma, and arteriovenous differences were calculated. The rates of urinary NH_4^+ and urea excretion were also determined on the last day of the study.

Animals fed $NaHC0_3$ maintained weight (mean weight change + 2.8 $\pm$ 2.0 g, 1% body weight), whereas acidotic rats tended to lose weight. Mean weight change for HCl-fed rats was -5.3 $\pm$ 1.8 g (2.5% body weight, $p < 0.05$ vs. $NaHC0_3$), and for NH_4Cl-fed animals it was -1.7 $\pm$ 1.7 g (0.8% body weight, not significant vs. $NaHC0_3$). After seven days of feeding acid base parameters and urinary NH_4^+ and urea excretion were measured and are shown in Table 3. Mean blood pH and $HC0_3^-$ concentration were significantly lower in the groups given HCl and NH_4Cl than those given $NaHC0_3$. Urea excretion, which was similar in NH_4Cl and $NaHC0_3$-fed rats, was reduced by about 25% in rats given HCl ($p < 0.05$ vs $NaHC0_3$). Aortic plasma urea concentrations were approximately 6mM and not different in the three groups of rats, indicating that differences in excretion rates reflected altered urea production rates. Ammonium excretion during the last 24 hours was similar in both HCl and NH_4Cl groups and was about 96% lower in rats fed $NaHC0_3$ ($p < 0.05$)[19].

The effect of acidosis on the rate of urinary urea excretion was not consistent since estimation of the rate of urea excretion on the final day of chronic metabolic acidosis does not reveal the true picture. When rats were given 9 mmol HCl daily (mixed with food), the mean rate of urea excretion was significantly reduced for the 8 day period. However, when assayed on a daily

Table 3. Urinary nitrogen excretion in chronic acidosis and alkalosis

Urinary excretion	HCl	NH_4Cl	$NaHCO_3$
NH_4^+	3.98±0.22*	3.84±0.34*	0.14±0.05
Urea	7.54±0.36*	9.82±0.70	10.1±0.70

Values are as shown in Table 1 for HCl (n=6), NH_4Cl (n=4), and $NaHCO_3$ (n=4) fed rats. *, $P < 0.05$ vs $NaHCO_3$. Data from Boon *et al* [19].

basis it was seen that urea excretion decreased for the first four days and returned to control values by the eighth day (data not shown). A similar trend occurred with NH_4Cl feeding, except that in this case the mean rate of urea excretion was unchanged for the 7 day period (Lardner and O'Donovan, unpublished).

Plasma NH_4^+ and amino acid concentrations for rats fed HCl, NH_4Cl and $NaHC0_3$ were measured in these studies[19]. Compared to the $NaHC0_3$-fed group, aortic plasma threonine, serine, glutamine, glycine, and lysine were higher in HCl and NH_4Cl-fed animals ($p < 0.05$). Concentrations of several amino acids were higher in the hepatic vein, portal vein, and aorta in the acidotic groups than in the bicarbonate-fed animals. For example, several gluconeogenic amino acids (glycine, threonine, and serine) and arginine were significantly higher in the NH_4Cl

animals, with similar changes (arginine was not significantly higher) in the HCl group. With the notable exception of glycine, the concentrations of these amino acids were also higher in portal vein plasma in both acidotic groups compared with alkali-fed animals. The concentrations of branched-chain amino acids (valine, leucine, and isoleucine) were not affected by acidosis (data not shown).

Hepatic vein minus portal vein concentration differences (HV-PV) for NH_4^+ are shown in Table 4. Compared with the $NaHCO_3$ group, HV-PV for NH_4^+ was greater in HCl and was still greater in NH_4Cl (both $p < 0.05$). In contrast, HV-PV was less in acidosis than in the HCO_3^--fed group for alanine, glycine, methionine, and asparagine. Glutamine was the only amino acid released consistently from the liver; however, no difference in HV-PV and HV-A (not shown), was noted between acidosis and the alkali-fed animals. The difference in total amino acid concentrations in HV-PV in the two acidotic groups were less than one-half that seen in the HCO_3^- group; however, the differences did not reach statistical significance.

Table 4. Hepatic vein minus portal vein differences in NH_4^+ and amino acids: chronic study

Substance	HCl	NH_4Cl	$NaHCO_3$
NH_4^+	-187 ± 28*	-271 ± 60*	-57 ± 38
Asparagine	-66 ± 9.5*	-60 ± 13	-102 ± 14
Glutamine	+277 ± 47	+255 ± 95	+323 ± 123
Glycine	-159 ± 19*	-145 ± 27	-239 ± 31
Alanine	-118 ± 34	-83 ± 12	-199 ± 40
Methionine	-10 ± 2*	-7.3 ± 1.9	-23 ± 7.3
Total amino acids	-190 ± 173	-85 ± 119	-400 ± 224

Blood samples were obtained from portal vein and hepatic vein of rats after 7 days of HCl, NH_4Cl, or $NaHCO_3$ feeding. NH_4^+ and amino acid concentrations are means ± SE for 6 (HCl), 4 (NH_4Cl), and 4 ($NaHCO_3$) rats. Data are given in μM. *, $P < 0.05$ vs $NaHCO_3$. From Boon *et al* [19].

Intracellular NH_4^+ and amino acid contents and protein/DNA ratios were also measured in liver tissue in the chronic study (data not shown). Except for a 20-25% lower value of the NH_4^+ concentration in acidosis, and a 25-35% lower glutamine concentration in both HCl and NH_4Cl groups ($p < 0.05$) relative to the $NaHCO_3$ group, no consistent difference in hepatic amino acid concentrations were noted among the three groups, despite minor variations in several amino acids. Intracellular branched-chain amino acid concentrations (valine, leucine, and isoleucine) were also the same in chronic metabolic acidosis and in the $NHCO_3$ group. Liver protein/DNA ratios were not different for the animals fed the three different regimens.

Glutamine synthetase (GS) and CPS mRNA was quantitated in livers from animals fed the three dietary regimens (Table 5). Compared to liver from HCO_3^--fed rats, both GS and CPS mRNA abundance was greater in acidosis although this difference reached statistical significance only in the HCl-fed animals (p < 0,.05). In data not shown, no significant difference was seen in

Table 5. Relative abundance of GS and CPS mRNA in liver

mRNA	HCl	NH_4Cl	$NaHCO_3$
CPS	2.1 ± 0.23*	2.6 ± 0.44	1.15 ± 0.27
GS	3.48 ± 0.47*	3.16 ± 0.49	1.60 ± 0.16

The data are given as mean ± SD and expressed as μg per μg ribosomal RNA (measured using a 108 bp fragment of ribosomal RNA. *, $P < 0.05$ vs $NaHCO_3$. Data modified from Boon *et al* [20].

mRNA distribution as measured by in situ hybridization nor in enzyme protein as determined by immunohistochemistry.

The increase in urinary NH_4^+ excretion noted in chronic acidosis correlated with increased renal phosphoenolpyruvate carboxykinase (PEPCK) and phosphate-activated glutaminase (PAG) mRNA. No difference was noted in renal cortex glutamate dehydrogenase (GDH) mRNA content in acidosis compared to bicarbonate-fed animals (Table 6).

Table 6. Kidney mRNA content in acidosis and alkalosis

mRNA	HCl	NH_4Cl	$NaHCO_3$
PEPCK	2.4 ± 0.34*	1.97 ± 0.10*	0.94 ± 0.06
PAG	1.22 ± 0.15*	1.18 ± 0.19*	0.53 ± 0.07
GDH	1.65 ± 0.12	1.45 ± 0.13	1.29 ± 0.05
GS	0.76 ± 0.04	0.71 ± 0.05	0.71 ± 0.02

Results are mean ± SE for rats fed HCl (n=6), NH_4Cl (n=4), and $NaHCO_3$ (n=4). *, $P < 0.05$ vs $NaHCO_3$. Modified from Boon *et al* [20].

PROTEIN DEPLETION AND NITROGEN METABOLISM

The level of dietary protein has a profound effect on the disposition of NH_4^+ and amino acids within body tissues. The urea cycle in the liver is an effective mechanism for maintaining a low level of NH_4^+ in the blood. Glutamine synthetase in brain and skeletal muscle serves a similar role.

The data in Table 7 show the effects of feeding standard (17% protein) and protein-free diets, with and without NH_4Cl for ten days, on food and fluid intake of female Sprague-Dawley rats (Lardner and O'Donovan, unpublished observations). NH_4Cl groups were allowed free access to a 0.28 M NH_4Cl solution instead of tap water. Animals given the standard diet, with or without NH_4Cl had a constant food and fluid intake for the 10-day period. Food and fluid intake in the protein-free groups decreased throughout the 10-day period. Urine flow rates followed a similar pattern to fluid intake in all groups.

Table 7. Effects of NH_4Cl ingestion with a standard and protein-free diet on food and fluid intake on the 10th day

Diet	Food Intake (g)	Fluid Intake (ml)
Standard	25 ± 1.2	25 ± 1.1
Standard + NH_4Cl	23 ± 0.9	24 ± 0.9
Protein-free	12 ± 0.5	14 ± 0.4
Protein-free + NH_4Cl	12 ± 0.6	8 ± 0.4

Female rats were fed the indicated diets for 10 days. Results shown are for the final day. Standard (17% protein) and protein-free diets were offered *ad libitum* and the rats were allowed free access to 0.28 M NH_4Cl or tap water. From O'Donovan (unpublished observations).

The body weight and weights of the liver of the kidney were reduced following ingestion of a protein-free diet, with and without NH_4Cl. Table 8 demonstrates the activities of the hepatic urea cycle enzymes. The data were reported as units/g of liver, but the liver weight was reduced by 25% in the protein-free groups. The activities of CPS ornithine transcarbamylase (OTC) and argininosuccinate lyase (ASL) were reduced by 60% (units/g), while their total activities (units/liver) were decreased by 70% in the protein-free groups. The reduction in arginase

Table 8. Activities of urea cycle enzymes

Enzyme (Units/g liver)	Standard Diet	Standard Diet + NH_4Cl	Protein-free Diet	Protein-free Diet + NH_4Cl
CPS	18.4 ± 1.6	16.7 ± 0.8	6.0 ± 0.2	5.9 ± 0.4
OTC	300 ± 25	258 ± 17.4	118 ± 14.8	124.6 ± 5.6
ASL	4.6 ± 0.3	4.7 ± 0.3	1.8 ± 0.2	2.0 ± 0.1
Arginase	2018 ± 71	2012 ± 68	1664 ± 69	1647 ± 89

Effects of a protein-free diet ± NH_4Cl on urea cycle enzyme activities of rat liver. Enzymes were assayed at the end of a 10-day feeding period. From Lardner and O'Donovan, unpublished observations.

activity in the protein-free groups was only half that of the other three enzymes. Administration of NH_4Cl with the standard diet did not influence the activities of any of the four enzymes. Neither did it prevent the decrease in the activities of these enzymes with the protein-free diet.

The effects of a protein-free diet with and without NH_4Cl on the serum urea concentrations are shown in Table 9. It is obvious that the feeding of a protein-free diet drastically reduced the serum urea level. Administration of NH_4Cl to the standard and protein-free groups significantly increased the serum urea concentration.

Table 9. Serum urea concentration

Diet	Serum Urea (mM)
Standard	6.0 ± 0.3
Standard + NH_4Cl	8.4 ± 0.4
Protein-free	2.2 ± 0.1
Protein-free + NH_4Cl	3.8 ± 0.2

Effects of a protein-free diet, with and without the administration of NH_4Cl, on the serum urea concentration. From Lardner and O'Donovan (unpublished).

Ingestion of a protein-free diet produced a significant degree of metabolic acidosis. Administration of NH_4Cl to this group did not further augment the extent of acidosis. A reduction in plasma HCO_3^- concentration with the protein-free diet suggests that catabolism of dietary protein contributed significantly to the maintenance of acid-base balance. Surprisingly, ingestion of a protein-free diet did not influence the rate of urinary NH_4^+ excretion or the activity of renal phosphate-activated glutaminase (Table 8). However, both of these parameters were increased when NH_4Cl was administered the protein-free group. The increase in glutaminase activity resulting from NH_4Cl administration to the protein-free group is noteworthy, despite lack of dietary protein. This indirectly confirms increased protein turnover during metabolic acidosis. May *et al* [22] reported an acceleration of whole body turnover during metabolic acidosis in rats given a standard diet, reflected in a 70% increase in proteolysis, a 55% increase in protein synthesis, and a 145% increase in amino acid oxidation. Skeletal muscle would appear to be a major site of protein degradation during metabolic acidosis[22]. Muscle and liver branched-chain ketoacid dehydrogenase increases, while the activity of this enzyme decreases in the kidney in metabolic acidosis[23]. The data in Table 10 indicate that reincorporation of degraded body protein into phosphate-activated glutaminase was not affected by the lack of ingested protein.

Table 10. Renal phosphate-activated glutaminase (PAG) and urinary NH_4^+ excretion

Diet	PAG (Units/g kidney)	NH_4^+ excretion (mmol/day)
Standard	8.5 ± 1.0	0.47 ± 0.03
Standard + NH_4Cl	19.0 ± 1.4	2.3 ± 0.1
Protein-free	8.8 ± 1.1	0.45 ± 0.02
Protein-free + NH_4Cl	18.8 ± 1.9	4.6 ± 0.2

Urinary NH_4^+ excretion and renal phosphate-activated glutaminase (PAG) activity in rats consuming a standard or protein-free diet, with and without NH_4Cl ingestion, for 10 days. Data presented are for the 10th day. From Lardner and O'Donovan (In preparation).

DISCUSSION

The induction of both acute and chronic metabolic acidosis led to a significant reduction in urea excretion with an unchanged serum urea concentration. These findings indicate that urea synthesis is decreased in metabolic acidosis. However the data indicate strongly that the reduction in urea synthesis is due to a decreased uptake of amino acids across the hepatic plasma membrane rather than to an inhibitory effect somewhere in the ornithine cycle. Thus, the data suggest that in acute and chronic acidosis flux through the ornithine cycle is controlled by hepatic amino acid transport rather than by the activity of the ornithine cycle *per se*. These findings argue against a primary role for the ornithine cycle in the regulation of acid-base homeostasis. Rather, amino acids not taken up by the liver in acidosis are diverted to the kidney for enhanced glucose and NH_4^+ synthesis. Since glutamine is the major substrate for renal ammoniagenesis, it is likely, though not proven in these studies, that some amino acid conversions occur, resulting ultimately in enhanced delivery and extraction of glutamine by the kidney.

When animals were provided with a protein-free diet, urinary urea excretion was reduced compared to that of a standard diet. There was no further decrease upon feeding NH_4Cl to these animals. An increase in renal glutaminase and NH_4^+ excretion in protein-deprived rats consuming NH_4Cl indicates that the renal adaptation to metabolic acidosis is not compromised by a lack of dietary protein.

Taken together, these studies indicate that the liver plays a role in acid-base homeostasis. However, the regulatory steps reducing urea excretion in acidosis seem unlikely to occur in the urea cycle *per se*, but more likely occur at the level of amino acid entry into the hepatocyte. Moreover, depriving animals of protein in the diet did not have a significant effect on the ability of these animals to respond to an acidifying stimulus. The present *in vivo* experiments provide information clarifying the role of renal and hepatic metabolism during metabolic acidosis. The results do not support the hypothesis that ureagenesis is controlled in a fashion to regulate acid-base homeostasis directly. For this to be tenable, urea synthesis should be regulated within the ornithine cycle, or at least at a point beyond amino acid degradation and urea formation. Rather, it appears that the liver is important because hepatic amino acid transport is decreased in acidosis. As a result, amino acid availability for the kidneys is increased.

Acknowledgments

The studies summarized in this report were supported in part by the National Institute of Diabetes and Digestive and Kidney Diseases Grant DK-36922, a Fogarty International Fellowship TWO1711, the Netherlands Organization for Scientific Research, and an A.D. Williams Grant from Virginia Commonwealth University.

REFERENCES

1. D.E. Atkinson and M. Camien. The role of urea synthesis in the removal of metabolic bicarbonate and the regulation of blood pH. *Curr. Top. Cell. Regul.* 21:261-302 (1982).
2. D.E. Atkinson and E. Bourke. The role of ureagenesis in pH homeostasis. *Trends Biochem. Sci.* 7:297-300 (1984).
3. J. Oliver, A.M. Koelz, J. Costello, and E. Bourke. Acid-base alterations in glutamine metabolism and ureagenesis in perfused muscle and liver of the rat. *Eur. J. Clin. Invest.* 7:445-449 (1977).
4. D. Haussinger, H. Sies, and W. Gerok. Functional heterogeneity in ammonia metabolism. The intercellular glutamine cycle. *J. Hepatol.* 1:3-14 (1984).
5. M. L. Halperin, C.B. Chen, S. Cheema-Dhadli, M.L. West, and R.L. Jungas. Is urea formation regulated primarily by acid-base balance in vivo? *Am. J. Physiol.* 250 (*Renal Fluid Electrolyte Physiol.* 19):F605-F612 (1986).
6. C. Lenzen, S. Soboll, H. Sies, and D. Haussinger. pH control of hepatic glutamine degradation. Role of transport. *Eur. J. Biochem.* 166:483-488 (1987).
7. L. Boon and A.J. Meijer. Control by pH of urea synthesis in isolated hepatocytes. *Eur. J. Biochem.* 172:465-469, 1988.
8. B. Carey, C.W. Cheung, N.S. Cohen, S. Brusilow, and L. Raijman. Regulation of urea and citrulline synthesis under physiological conditions. *Biochem. J.* 292:241-247 (1993).
9. V. Felipo, M-D Minana, and S. Grisolia. Long-term ingestion of ammonium increases acetyl glutamate and urea levels without affecting the amount of carbamoyl-phosphate synthase. *Eur. J Biochem.* 176:567-571 (1988).
10. H.E.S.J. Hensgens, A.J. Verhoeven, and A.J. Meijer. The relationship between intra-mitochondrial n-acetylglutamine activity and carbamoyl phosphate synthetase (ammonia). *Eur. J. Biochem.* 107:197-205 (1980).
11. K. Shigesada, K. Aoyagi, and M. Tatibana. Role of n-acetylglutamate in ureotelism. Variations in acetylglutamate level and its possible significance in control of urea synthesis in mammalian liver. *Eur. J. Biochem.* 85:385-391 (1978).
12. N.S. Cohen, S.W. Cheung, and L. Raijman. The effects of ornithine on mitochondrial carbamoyl phosphate synthesis. *J. Biol. Chem.* 255:10248-10255 (1980).
13. V. Felipo, M-D Minana, and S. Grisolia. Control of urea synthesis and ammonia utilization in protein deprivation and refeeding. *Arch. Biochem. Biophys.* 285:351-356 (1991).
14. T. Saheki, M. Tsuda, T. Tanaka, and N. Katunuma. Analysis of regulatory factors for urea synthesis by isolated perfused rat liver. *J. Biochem.* 77:671-678 (1975).
15. T. Saheki, T. Katsunuma, and M. Sase. Regulation of urea synthesis in rat liver. Changes in ornithine and n-acetylglutamate concentration in the livers of rats subjected to dietary transitions. *J. Biol. Chem.* 237:459-468 (1977).
16. R.T. Schimke. Differential effects of fasting and protein-free diets on levels of urea cycle enzymes in rat liver. J. Biol. Chem. 237:1921-1924 (1962)
17. R. Zaragosa, J. Renu-Piqueras, M. Portoles, J. Hernandez-Yago, A. Jorda, and S. Grisolia. Rats fed prolonged high protein diets show an increase in nitrogen metabolism and liver megamitochondria. *Arch. Biochem. Biophys.* 258:426-435 (1987).
18. L. Boon, P.J.E. Blommaart, A.J. Meijer, W.H. Lamers, and A.C. Schoolwerth. Acute acidosis inhibits amino acid transport: no primary role for the urea cycle in acid-base balance. *Am. J. Physiol.* 267 (*Renal Fluid Electrolyte Physiol.* 36):F1015-F1020 (1994).
19. L. Boon, P.J.E. Blommaart, A.J. Meijer, W.H. Lamers, and A.C. Schoolwerth. Response of hepatic amino acid consumption to chronic metabolic acidosis. *Am. J. Physiol.* 271 (*Renal Fluid Electrolyte Physiol.* 40):F198-F202 (1996).

20. L. Boon, P.J.E. Blommaart, A.J. Meijer, W.H. Lamers, and A.C. Schoolwerth. Effect of chronic acidosis on hepatic amino acid uptake and gene regulation: implications for control of acid-base balance. *Contr. Nephrol.* 110:138-143 (1994).
21. T.C.Welbourne, D. Childress, and G. Givens. Renal regulation of interorgan glutamine flow in metabolic acidosis. *Am. J. Physiol.* 251 (*Regulatory Integrative Comp. Physiol.* 20):R858-R866 (1986).
22. R.C. May, R.A. Kelly, and W.E. Mitch. Metabolic acidosis stimulates protein degradation in rat muscle by a glucocorticoid dependent mechanism. *J. Clin. Invest.* 77:614-621 (1986).
23. R.C. May, T. Masud, B. Logue, J. Bailey, and B.K. England. Metabolic acidosis accelerates whole body protein degradation and leucine oxidation by a glucocorticoid dependent mechanism. *Miner. Electrolyte Metab.* 18:245-249 (1992).

GLUCOSE AND INSULIN METABOLISM IN CIRRHOSIS

Christopher O. Record

Liver Unit, Royal Victoria Infirmary and
University of Newcastle upon Tyne
NE1 4LP, UK

Abnormalities in Carbohydrate metabolism in cirrhosis have been known for very many years and the term hepatogenous diabetes was coined by Naunyn in 1906 to describe those patients with cirrhosis where diabetes was also present. Overt diabetes is now recognised in about 30% of cirrhotics whereas abnormalities of glucose tolerance occur in excess of 50% [1].

It is not surprising that diabetes occurs in cirrhosis since the liver maintains a tight control of nutrient supply to the tissues, glucose being taken up during feeding for glycogen synthesis and being released during fasting by glycogenolysis or gluconeogenesis. The liver is also responsible for fatty acid and triglyceride synthesis during feeding and beta oxidation of fat and the formation of ketone bodies during fasting. Since the advent of insulin assay in the 1960s, it has been recognised that the diabetes of cirrhosis is paradoxically characterised by high insulin concentrations and insulin resistance. Other metabolic abnormalities recognised in cirrhosis are a decrease in insulin growth factor (IGF1), an increase in glucagon and growth hormone concentrations, increases in non esterified fatty acids (NEFA) and increases in lactate pyruvate and glycerol. The branch chain amino acids, valine, leucine and isoleucine however are characteristically decreased [1].

Hyperinsulinaemia is almost universal in cirrhosis but cirrhotic patients with impaired glucose tolerance or overt diabetes have lower levels of insulin than those with normal glucose tolerance [1]. This suggests the late development of pancreatic beta cell dysfunction. There has been much controversy as to the mechanism of the hyperinsulinaemia in cirrhosis prior to the development of overt diabetes and an increase in pancreatic islet cell secretion or a decrease in hepatic degradation of insulin have been suggested. A decrease in hepatic degradation is suggested by the finding that the liver extracts about 40–60% of insulin secreted by the pancreas [2] and that basal portal insulin concentrations are similar in cirrhotics to controls [3,6] By infusing insulin into the portal vein Nygnen et al [6] showed that the fractional hepatic insulin extraction was only 13% compared to 51% in controls. Portal insulin stimulated by glucose or arginine is lower in cirrhotics than controls [3,5], while C peptide concentrations which are not degraded by the liver are normal after oral glucose in cirrhotics suggesting normal insulin secretion [7]. Other workers however have found that both basal and stimulated C peptide concentrations are increased in cirrhotics suggesting increased insulin secretion [8,9,10,11]. Furthermore, C peptide levels suppressed only 54% in cirrhotics compared to 100% in controls in response to an insulin infusion despite similar insulin levels, once again suggesting an increase in pancreatic insulin secretion [12].

Advances in Cirrhosis, Hyperammonemia, and Hepatic Encephalopathy
Edited by Felipo and Grisolía, Plenum Press, New York, 1997

The shunting of portal blood into the systemic circulation in cirrhosis effectively bypassing the liver may also influence peripheral insulin concentrations but Holdsworth et al [13] found no change in glucose tolerance or insulin concentrations following the creation of a surgical portacaval shunt. This may have been due to the spontaneous portal systemic shunting present prior to the creation of the surgical shunt. In patients with normal liver function but portal vein thrombosis, peripheral C peptide and insulin concentrations are similar to controls [14]. Such patients can have very considerable portasystemic shunting but the extraction of insulin from the hepatic arterial supply by the normal liver may compensate for the shunting of portal blood. Conversely the arterial–hepatic venous insulin extraction in cirrhotic patients with side to side portacaval shunts was similar to controls (51% versus 48%; [15]). This finding suggests normal hepatic degradation of insulin in cirrhosis implying shunting as the main cause of peripheral hyperinsulinaemia. An important role for portal systemic shunting of insulin is also suggested by the finding that basal peripheral insulin concentrations in cirrhotics with portal hypertension are greater than hepatic venous insulin levels. In controls however basal peripheral insulin concentrations are less than hepatic venous levels [16].

In practice, the likely sequence of events is:

1. A decrease in hepatic insulin degradation and/or portasystemic shunting leads to peripheral hyperinsulinaemia and the development of peripheral insulin resistance.

2. The development of peripheral insulin resistance leads to impaired peripheral glucose uptake and high peripheral glucose concentrations stimulate further insulin secretion. Chronic hyperglycaemia and hyperinsulinaemia ultimately leads to beta cell exhaustion and the development of overt diabetes.

Insulin Resistance

Resistance to the action of insulin may be due to a decrease in sensitivity when more insulin is required to achieve a normal maximal response or a decrease in responsiveness when the maximal response which can be achieved by insulin is diminished. It is thought that a maximal insulin response is achieved when only 10% of insulin receptors are occupied and thus a greater than 90% loss of receptors would be required to lead to a decrease in responsiveness. A receptor defect is thus likely to lead to a decrease in insulin sensitivity and a post receptor defect a decrease in sensitivity and responsiveness. Some authors have found a decrease in adipose tissue receptor function in cirrhotics [11,17] while others [18] have found that they are normal. Adipose tissue and muscle however (the principle site of peripheral insulin resistance) may behave differently. Whole body leucine turnover in cirrhotics [19] is normal in patients with cirrhosis, even in those with impaired glucose tolerance [20] and this finding suggests a post receptor defect for glucose intolerance since the same insulin receptor is thought to be responsible for the modulation of both glucose and protein metabolism. Insulin sensitivity is affected by exercise, a high carbohydrate diet, the development of obesity, starvation and pregnancy and we have suggested that post receptor insulin sensitivity may be regulated by intracellular diacylglycerol concentrations and protein kinase signalling [21].

Glucose Uptake

Glucose intolerance in cirrhosis may be due to a decrease in peripheral glucose uptake, a decrease in splanchnic glucose uptake or a decrease in suppression of hepatic glucose output. These may be due to a decrease in receptor/post receptor function, altered substrate competition between glucose and fatty acids (Randle Cycle) or due to abnormalities of counter regulatory hormones. Various studies have been undertaken to try and characterise the importance of each of these individual factors. Several have shown that hepatic glucose production is normal in cirrhosis and suppresses normally during euglycaemic hyperinsulinaemic clamps [11,22,20]. In our early studies of the uptake of oral glucose in cirrhotics, we found that forearm glucose uptake was normal when compared to controls [23]. However the normal forearm uptake of glucose was only achieved by having high circulating glucose and insulin

Table 1. Hyperglycaemic clamp studies [26]

	Cirrhotics [10]	Controls [6]	p
Forearm glucose uptake mg/100 ml/min	0.39±0.06	1.24±0.26	0.001
Basal hepatic glucose production ($6-^3H$ glucose infusion)	1.84±0.12	1.92±0.12	NS
Net splanchnic glucose uptake (hepatic vein catheter) mg/kg/min	1.59±0.14	1.27±1.7	NS
Whole body glucose uptake ('M' value) mg/kg/min	3.7±0.3	8.7±1.8	0.004

Blood sugar maintained at 10 mmol/l by a variable glucose infusion

levels implying insulin resistance in the periphery. We subsequently undertook euglycaemic hyperinsulinaemia clamp studies in cirrhotics when blood glucose concentrations were maintained at basal levels by constant glucose infusion during the course of an insulin infusion. Under these circumstances the uptake of glucose in the forearm was decreased ten fold in cirrhotics compared to controls [24]. This finding was subsequently confirmed by Petrides et al [20] when hepatic glucose output was also shown to suppress normally and furthermore, it was shown that glucose oxidation assessed by indirect calorimetry was normal. This suggested impaired muscle glycogen synthesis in glucose intolerant cirrhotics and indeed a decrease in glycogen deposition in muscle biopsies in cirrhotics was noted by Kruszynska et al [25]. In hyperglycaemia clamp studies (blood sugar maintained at 10 mmol/l by variable glucose infusion), we also showed gross impairment of peripheral glucose uptake (Table 1; [26]). When hyperglycaemia was combined with a somatostatin infusion to block hormone secretion, free fatty acid concentrations were exceedingly high but when non esterified fatty acid concentrations were suppressed with acipimox, there was no alteration in whole body glucose uptake (Table 2) suggesting that the operation of the Randle cycle does not have any influence upon the development of impaired glucose uptake in cirrhotics [26].

Effect of Growth Hormone and IgF1

Growth hormone concentrations have been recognised as being increased in cirrhotics for many years and there is a paradoxical rise after glucose administration [1]. An elevation in growth hormone concentration is associated with the development of insulin resistance in acromegaly, starvation and pregnancy. Growth hormone infusions lead to a 30–60% decrease in forearm glucose uptake [27,28]. In euglycaemic hyperinsulinaemic clamp studies [29] we assessed the effect of growth hormone suppression with somatostatin on forearm and whole body glucose uptake. During these studies insulin and

Table 2. Effect of nefa suppression with acipimox on glucose uptake [26]

	Cirrhotics [6]	Controls [5]	p
Whole body glucose uptake Somatostatin ('M' value) mg/kg/min	2.49±0.10	2.09±0.06	NS
Whole body glucose uptake Somatostatin + Acipimox ('M' value) mg/kg/min	2.42±0.12	1.97±0.57	NS

Hyperglycaemic clamp at 10 mmol/l
Somatostatin infusion to block hormone secretion

Table 5. Insulin-like growth factor binding protein 1 (igf-1) levels-links with insulin resistance [30]

	Controls [6]	Cirrhotics [6]	p
Growth Hormone mu/l	0.5±0.4	6.1±0.4	<0.01
IGF-1 nmol/l	36±9	16±4	<0.05
IGFBP-3 mg/l	3.67±0.36	1.16±0.22	<0.001
IGF-1/IGFBP-3 molar ratio	0.3±0.1	0.4±0.1	NS
IGFBP-1 ug/l	3.2±0.2	26.8±8.4	<0.001

Values during euglycaemic hyperinsulinaemic clamp

Table 6. Insulin-like growth factor binding protein 1 (igf-1)-effect of growth hormone [30]

	Controls [6]	Cirrhotics [6]	p
Growth hormone mU/l	2.1±1.0	1.8±0.6	NS
IGF-1* nmol/l	75±12	46±14	NS
IGFBP-3*	6.1±0.6	4.1±0.9	NS
IGFBP-1	2.1±0.4	10.6±3.7	<0.05

Values during euglycaemic hyperinsulinaemic clamp after five days of growth hormone
In cirrhotics change in IGFBP-1 with growth hormone correlated with change in insulin sensitivity
$r = 0.84$; $p<0.05$

patients with cirrhosis it was possible to decrease endogenous growth hormone concentrations to a similar value to that in controls and this resulted in an increase in IGF1 and IGFBP3 concentrations similar to the control group. IGFBP1 levels however, although decreased by growth hormone administration, were still significantly elevated (Table 6). In cirrhotics the change in IGFBP1 concentrations correlated with the change in insulin sensitivity during the clamp ($R=0.84$) ($p<0.05$). This suggests an important role for IGF1 and IGFBP1 in the determination of insulin sensitivity in cirrhosis [30]. In conclusion, high IGFBP1 levels in cirrhosis diminish bioactivity of IGF1 and lead to apparent insulin resistance. IGFBP1 may be the signal from the liver to the periphery indicating an increased hepatic demand for available substrates.

References

1. Shmueli E, Record CO & Alberti K G M M. Liver diseases, carbohydrate metabolism and diabetes. Clin Endocrinol and Metabol 1992; 6: 719–743.
2. Ferrannini E, Wahren J, Faber OK et al. Splanchnic and renal metabolism of insulin in human subjects: A dose response study. Am J Physiology 1983; 244: E517–E527.
3. Greco AV, Crucitti F, Ghirlanda G et al. Insulin and glucagon concentrations in portal and peripheral veins in patients with hepatic cirrhosis. Diabetologia 1979; 17: 23–28.
4. Pelkonen R, Kallio H, Suranta H, Karonen SL. Plasma insulin, C-peptide and blood glucose in portal, hepatic and peripheral veins in liver cirrhosis. Effect of intravenous tolbutamide. Acta Endocrinologica 1981; 97: 496–502.
5. Ohnishi K, Mishima A, Takashi Me et al. Effects of intra and extra hepatic portal systemic shunts on insulin metabolism. Digestive Diseases and Sciences 1983; 28: 201–206.
6. Nygren A, Adner N, Sunblad L, Wiechel K. Insulin uptake by the human alcoholic cirrhotic liver. Metabolism 1985; 34: 48–52.

7. Johnston DG, Alberti KGMM, Faber OK, Binder C, Wright R. Hyperinsulinism of hepatic cirrhosis: Diminished degradation or hypersecretion. Lancet 1977; i: 10–12.
8. Riggio O, Merli M, Cangiano C et al. Glucose intolerance in liver cirrhosis. Metabolism 1982; 31: 627–634.
9. Shankar TP, Solomon SS, Duckworth WC et al. Studies of glucose intolerance in cirrhosis of the liver. J Lab and Clin Med 1983; 102: 459–469.
10. Proietto J, Dudley FJ, Aitken P, Alford FP. Hyperinsulinaemia and insulin resistance of cirrhosis: The importance of insulin hypersecretion. Clin Endocrinology 1984; 21: 657–665.
11. Cavallo-Perin P, Cassader M, Bozzo C et al. Mechanism of insulin resistance in human liver cirrhosis. Evidence of a combined receptor and post receptor defect. J Clin Invest 1985; 75: 1659–1665.
12. Cavallo-Perin P, Bruno A, Nuccio P et al. Feedback inhibition of insulin secretion is altered in cirrhosis. J Clin Endocrinology & Metabolism 1986; 63: 1023–1027.
13. Holdsworth CD, Nye L & King E. The effect of portacaval anastomosis on oral carbohydrate tolerance and on plasma insulin levels. Gut 1972; 13: 58–63.
14. Smith-Laing G, Sherlock S, Faber OK. Effects of spontaneous portal-systemic shunting on insulin metabolism. Gastroenterology 1979; 76: 685–690.
15. Sherwin RS, Fisher M, Bessoff J et al. Hyperglucagonemia in cirrhosis: Altered secretion and sensitivity to glucagon. Gastroenterology 1978; 74: 1224–1228.
16. Bosch J, Gomis R, Kravetz D et al. Role of spontaneous portal-systemic shunting in hyperinsulinism of cirrhosis. Am J Physiology 1984; 247: G206–G212.
17. Taylor R, Heine RJ, Collins J, James OFW, Alberti KGMM. Insulin action in cirrhosis. Hepatology 1985; 5: 64–71.
18. Harewood MS, Proietto J, Dudley F, Alford FP. Insulin action and cirrhosis: Insulin binding and lipogenesis in isolated adipocytes. Metabolism 1982; 31: 1241–1246.
19. Mullen KD, Denne SC, McCullough AJ et al. Leucine metabolism in stable cirrhosis. Hepatology 1986; 6: 622–630.
20. Petrides AS, Groop LC, Riely CA, DeFronzo RA. Effect of physiological hyperinsulinaemia on glucose and lipid metabolism in cirrhosis. J Clin Invest 1991b; 88: 561–570.
21. Shmueli E, Alberti KGMM, Record CO. Diacylglycerol/protein kinase C signalling: a mechanism for insulin resistance?. J Int Med 1993; 234: 397–400.
22. Proietto J, Alford FP, Dudley FJ. The mechanism of the carbohydrate intolerance of cirrhosis. J Endocrinology & Metabolism 1980; 51: 1030–1036.
23. Leatherdale BA, Chase RA, Rogers J et al. Forearm glucose uptake in cirrhosis and its relationship to glucose tolerance. Clinical Science 1980; 59: 191–198.
24. Butler PC, Thompson CJ, Alberti KGMM, Record CO. The contribution of skeletal muscle to insulin resistance in hepatic cirrhosis. J Hepatology 1987; 56: 515.
25. Kruszynska Y, Williams N, Perry M, Home PD. The relationship between insulin sensitivity and skeletal muscle enzyme activities in hepatic cirrhosis. Hepatology 1988; 8: 1615–1619.
26. Shmueli E, Walker M, Alberti G, Record CO. Normal splanchnic but impaired peripheral insulin-stimulated glucose uptake in cirrhosis. Hepatology 1993; 18: 86–95.
27. Moller N, Butler PC, Antsiferov MA, Alberti KGMM. Effects of growth hormone on insulin sensitivity and forearm metabolism in man. Diabetologia 1989; 32: 105–110.
28. Moller N, Jorgensen JOL, Schmitz O et al. Effects of a growth hormone pulse on total and forearm substrate fluxes in humans. Am J Physiology 1990; 258: E86–E91.
29. Shmueli E, Stewart M, Alberti KGMM, Record CO. Growth hormone, insulin-like growth factor-1 and insulin resistance in cirrhosis. Hepatology 1994; 18: 322–328.
30. Shmueli E, Miell JP, Stewart M, Alberti KGMM, Record CO. High insulin-like growth factor binding protein 1 levels in cirrhosis: Link with insulin resistance. Hepatology 1996; 24: 127–133.

AN AMMONIA HYPOTHESIS OF ALZHEIMER DISEASE

Nikolaus Seiler

Groupe de Recherche en Thérapeutique Anticancéreuse, URA, CNRS 1529
Institut de Recherche Contre le Cancer, Faculté de Médecine, Université de Rennes 1, 2 av. du Pr. Léon Bernard, F-35043 RENNES, Cedex, France

1. INTRODUCTION

"All this has been said before,
but since nobody listened, it must be said again."
André Gide

There is little doubt that dementia of the Alzheimer type (DAT) is a multifactorial disease. The existence of a major gene for DAT is equivocal, however, a genetic predisposition is considered to be likely from the high concordance of DAT in monozygotic and dizygotic twins (1), and an increased frequency of the disease in relatives of affected patients (2). The long arm of chromosome 21 is the locus of predisposition (3). The expression of a number of genes encoding for various neuronal and non-neuronal proteins is also changed in DAT brains (4).

In Table 1 suggestions regarding pathogenetic events and factors which may contribute to the etiology or progression of DAT are summarized. The list is still growing, and it is more and more difficult to decide which factors are important. Among the numerous hypotheses the formation of neurotoxic amyloid depositions due to abnormal processing of the precursor protein of β-amyloid (βAPP) has attracted by far the greatest interest, because plaques and fibrillary tangles are hallmarks of DAT. The fact that certain mutations in the gene encoding βAPP are known to lead to familial forms of DAT (5) is the most convincing argument in favor of the β-amyloid hypothesis, although it has repeatedly been shown that plaque formation is not correlated with the severity of cognitive impairments in aged (6-8).

It has been hypothesised that risk factors in DAT increase with age (9). If this is true, one has to consider consequences of general age-related changes in organ functions as con-

Advances in Cirrhosis, Hyperammonemia, and Hepatic Encephalopathy
Edited by Felipo and Grisolía, Plenum Press, New York, 1997

tributing factors. Among these the impairment of the blood-brain barrier function (10) is of especial importance. In agreement with this idea pathogenetic effects of environmental factors, such as aluminum, and infection with spirochetes (11) have been considered as a consequence of the dysfunction of the blood-brain barrier.

Enhanced exposure of the organism to oxygen free radicals, e.g. due to reduced catalase and superoxide dismutase activities, may be another general noxious event, although direct evidence for the validity of this idea with respect to DAT is scarce. But oxygen free radicals have nevertheless been implicated as etiological agents in the process of aging (12), and in several neurodegenerative disorders, including DAT (13,14).

Table 1. Potential pathogenetic events and factors of Alzheimer disease

Event / factor	Reference
Genetic predisposition	(1, 2,)
Formation of neurotoxic β-amyloid depositions	(5, 38, 39)
Neurofibrillary degeneration (abnormal phosphorylation of Tau protein)	(15)
Impairment of neuronal functions	
Degeneration of selected neurons (cholinergic, serotoninergic, noradrenergic, somatostatinergic)	(16 - 21)
Changes in receptor density and function (serotonin, dopamine, glutamate etc.)	(22 - 26)
Impairment of glial functions	
Astroglia	(27)
Microglia	(28)
Lack of trophic factors	(29)
Neurotoxins	
Cytokines	(30)
Aluminum	(31 - 34)
Radicals	(13, 14, 35)
Glutamate	(36, 37)
Colchicin-like factor	(40)
Ammonia	(41)
Infections	
Treponema pallidum	(11)
Viral agents	(42)

Ammonia is the most important endogenous neurotoxic agent. It is a normal metabolite in all tissues, but it is also taken up from the gastrointestinal tract. In Fig. 1 ammonia movements in the vertebrate organism are shown. In the following ammonia and ammonium (salt) will be used synonymously, keeping in mind that at pH 7.4 1.7 % of ammonia is present in the vertebrate organism in non-protonated form (NH_3), while 98.3 % are protonated (NH_4^+) (43). Most tissues take up ammonia from the arterial blood and release corresponding amounts of glutamine. Detoxification occurs in liver by urea formation. Since NH_3 easily passes cell membranes, the blood-brain barrier can be passed by diffusion.

Our present knowledge of ammonia in humans is mainly based on observations of patients with impaired liver function (fulminant hepatic failure, liver cirrhosis, etc.), and of children with hereditary deficiencies of urea cycle enzymes. It is evident from the course of these diseases that DAT is not a direct consequence of hyperammonemia. However, hepatic encephalopathy and DAT have common features (see below). Therefore, it seems conceivable that chronic elevation of brain ammonia, together with other factors, may affect, or determine the severity and progression of DAT.

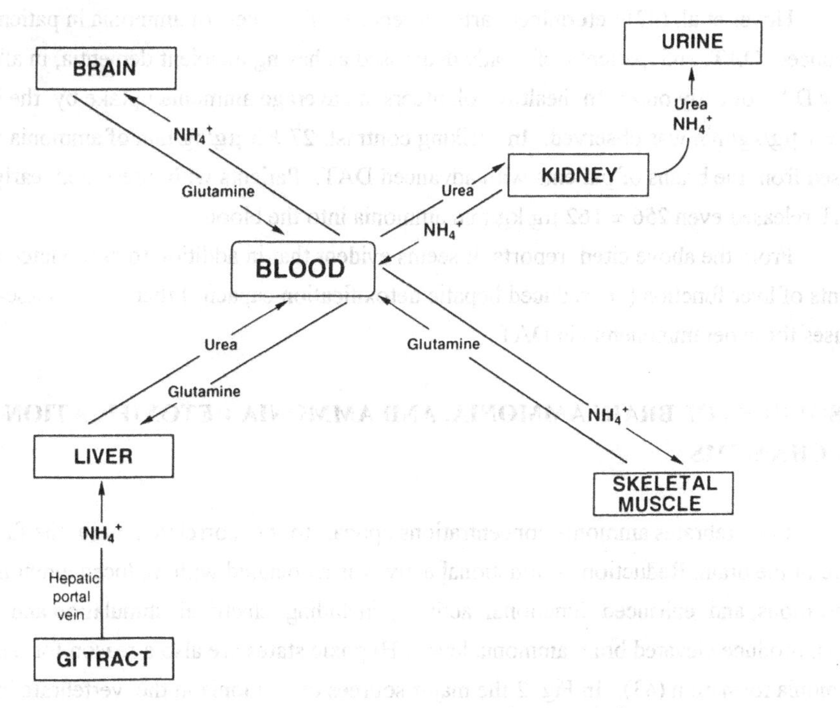

Fig. 1. Ammonia movements in the vertebrate organism

2. EVIDENCE FOR ELEVATED AMMONIA CONCENTRATIONS IN BLOOD AND BRAIN IN DAT

Owing to technical difficulties data on ammonia concentrations in blood and CSF show considerable variation (Table 2). The human brain values have been extrapolated from animal studies, since ammonia concentrations increase rapidly after death.

Table 2. Ammonia in human brain and body fluids

Brain	100 - 300 nmol/g
Cerebrospinal fluid (CSF)	20 - 100 nmol/ml
Arterial blood/plasma	70 - 113 nmol/ml
Venous blood/plasma	20 - 100 nmol/ml

Data from ref. 43.

Ammonia has not attracted attention as a pathogenetic factor of DAT. Therefore, no systematic investigations have been carried out, and direct evidence is scarce. Fisman et al. (44,45) demonstrated in two reports that postprandial blood ammonia levels were significantly higher in DAT patients than in matched control subjects. Some DAT patients had tri-phasic waves on EEG, a wave form suggestive for metabolic encephalopathy. In subjects with DAT, which were free of liver diseases and urinary tract infections, Branconnier et al. (46) found 122 ± 80 nmol ammonia per ml of plasma. The normal range in this study was 12 - 55 nmol/ml; 83 % of the patients had blood ammonia levels above the normal limit.

Hoyer et al. (47) determined arterio-venous differences of ammonia in patients with advanced DAT, and patients clinically diagnosed as having incipient dementia, in all probability DAT of early onset. In healthy volunteers an average ammonia uptake by the brain of 72 ± 7 μg/kg/min was observed. In striking contrast, 27 ± 3 μg/kg/min of ammonia was released from the brains of patients with advanced DAT. Patients with presumed early onset DAT released even 256 ± 162 μg/kg/min ammonia into the blood.

From the above cited reports it seems evident that in addition to age-related impairments of liver function (i.e. reduced hepatic detoxification capacity) there are disease-related causes for hyperammonemia in DAT.

3. SOURCES OF BRAIN AMMONIA, AND AMMONIA DETOXIFICATION MECHANISMS

In vertebrates ammonia concentrations appear to be correlated with the functional state of the brain. Reduction in functional activity is associated with reduced ammonia concentrations, and enhanced functional activity, including electrical stimulation and convulsions, produce elevated brain ammonia levels. Hypoxic states are also a reason for enhanced ammonia formation (43). In Fig. 2 the major sources of ammonia in the vertebrate brain are summarized. A considerable proportion of the ammonia of the vertebrate organism originates from the gastrointestinal tract. Deficient hepatic detoxification causes hyperammonemia, and since ammonia easily passes the blood-brain barrier, elevated ammonia accumulates in brain above normal concentrations. In hepatic encephalopathy resulting from acute or chronic liver disease, ammonia of gastrointestinal origin is a key pathogenetic factor (48,49). Bacterial infections of the urinary tract is another potential cause of hyperammonemic encephalopathy (43). Proteins, nucleic acids and hexosamines have long been suggested as sources of cerebral ammonia (50). Hydrolysis of glutamine and asparagine, oxidative deaminations of primary amines, glycine catabolism via the glycine cleavage system, deaminations of purines, pyrimidines and glucosamine-6-phosphate, among others, are well known ammonia generating reactions, which may contribute to the steady-state level of brain ammonia (51).

Glutamate dehydrogenase links the tricarboxylic acid cycle with ammonia. The direction of the glutamate dehydrogenase-catalysed reaction appears to be regulated by the intracellular $NAD(P)^+/NAD(P)H$-ratio. In the absence of glucose, when this ratio is high, glutamate is oxidatively deaminated. In the presence of glucose, when 2-oxoglutarate is not rate limiting, reductive amination of 2-oxoglutarate to glutamate is favored. Paradoxically, in hyperammonemic states the synaptic (in contrast with non-synaptic) mitochondrial glutamate dehydrogenase is stimulated in direction of glutamate oxidation (52). This reaction counteracts presumably the hyperammonemia-induced decrease of cerebral 2-oxoglutarate formation in other metabolic pathways, and thus supports energy production via the tricarboxylic acid cycle.

Hepatic urea formation is the most important ammonia detoxifying reaction of the mammalian organism. In brain the urea cycle is not functional. The ATP-dependent formation of glutamine in astrocytes, and its release into the bloodstream is nearly exclusively responsible for the limitation of brain ammonia concentrations (43, 51).

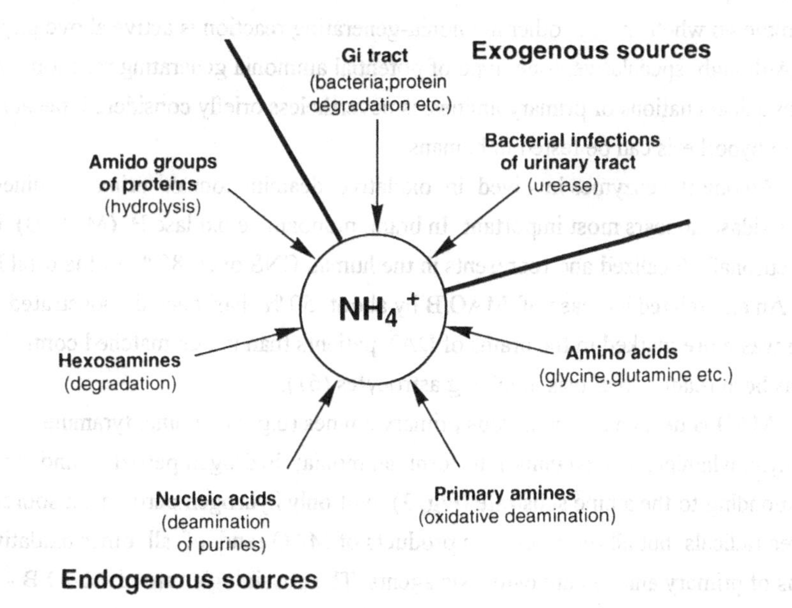

Fig. 2. Ammonia sources of the vertebrate brain.
Endogenous sources denote ammonia forming reactions within the organism. Most ammonia generating reactions are, however, also active within the CNS.

4. BRAIN AMMONIA METABOLISM IN DAT

In mammals the enhancement of brain ammonia concentration with age is presumably a general phenomenon. The release of ammonia from the brain in DAT patients (47) suggests the pathologic enhancement of ammonia formation, or deficient detoxification mechanism, or both.

Age-related gradual reduction of astroglial glutamine synthetase activity has been reported, with significantly lower activities of this enzyme in the brains of DAT patients (53, 54). In contrast, the phosphate-activated glutaminase, the enzyme responsible for the intraneuronal liberation of glutamate from glutamine, is unchanged in DAT patients (55). It is well established that ammonia is involved in the regulation of the (phosphate-activated) glutaminase. Its activity is reduced in the presence of ammonia. In aged animals glutamine hydrolysis was found to be significantly less sensitive to inhibition by ammonia than the enzyme in the brains of young rats (56). Thus it appears that the reduction of glial glutamine formation, and the derangement of the intraneuronal control of ammonia release are important aberrations of ammonia detoxification mechanisms in the aged brain.

A major reason for the loss of glutamine synthetase during aging is presumably the sensitivity of this enzyme to damage by oxygen free radicals. This is suggested by its greatly reduced activity in the brains of aged gerbils (57) and the rapid loss of glutamine synthetase during ischemia/reperfusion-induced brain injury (58).

Whether the imbalance between glutamine formation and its hydrolytic cleavage is a sufficient explanation for an ammonia excess in the brain of DAT patients is not known. It is also unknown whether any other ammonia-generating reaction is active above physiological level. Although speculative, one type of potential ammonia generating reaction, namely the oxidative deaminations of primary amines, is nevertheless briefly considered, because the underlying hypothesis can be tested in humans.

Among the enzymes involved in oxidative deaminations of primary amines, monoamine oxidase appears most important. In brain, monoamine oxidase B (MAO B) is mostly extraneuronally localized and represents in the human CNS over 80 % of the total MAO activity. An age-related increase of MAO B by about 50 % has been demonstrated. This increase was more marked in the brains of DAT patients than in age-matched controls (59,60), and has been related to gliosis involving astrocytes (61).

MAO B deaminates numerous primary amines (e.g. dopamine, tyramine, tryptamine, β-phenylethylamine, benzylamine) to form ammonia; hydrogen peroxide and an aldehyde corresponding to the amine substrate (Fig. 3). Not only hydrogen peroxide, a source of oxygen free radicals, but all three reaction products of MAO (and of all other oxidative deaminations of primary amines) are cytotoxic agents. The physiologic rate of MAO B - catalysed reactions in brain, and rates of related oxidases is not known. The impaired blood-brain barrier of DAT patients (10) may allow the enhanced intrusion of substrates of the oxidases from the blood into the brain, and consequently oxidative deaminations may occur at a rate considerably above physiological rates. It appears likely that the improvement of the cognitive functions of DAT patients during treatment with an inhibitor of MAO B (62) is in part due to the reduced formation of noxious metabolites of this enzyme. But other explanations may be as relevant (63).

$$R\text{-}CH_2\text{-}CH_2\text{-}NH_2 + H_2O + O_2 \xrightarrow[\text{Monoamine oxidase}]{} R\text{-}CHO + NH_3 + H_2O_2$$

$$H_2O_2 + Fe^{2+} \longrightarrow {}^{-}OH + {}^{\circ}OH + Fe^{3+}$$

Fig. 3. Oxidative deamination of a primary amines and radical formation from hydrogen peroxide.

5. TOXIC EFFECTS OF AMMONIA AND ALZHEIMER PATHOLOGY

In experimental animals key toxic manifestations of enhanced brain ammonia concentrations are independent of the genesis of the state of hyperammonemia, i.e. the symptoms are much the same after impairment of liver function (e.g. by portacaval shunting), hyperammonemia produced by urease injections, or by inactivation of glutamine synthetase, using methionine sulfoximine (64-66). They resemble pathophysiological observations in the brains of patients with hepatic encephalopathy and hereditary defects of urea cycle enzymes (48). Based on these facts, it may not surprise that the following features of hyperammonemic states are also observed in patients with DAT:

Impaired cognitive functions and behavioral abnormalities
Impaired blood-brain barrier
Astrocytosis
Impaired glucose utilization and energy metabolism
Reduced glutamine synthetase activity
Enhanced extracellular glutamate
Loss of NMDA-type glutamate receptors
Enhanced MAO B activity
Impaired lysosomal processing of proteins

5.1. Ammonia intoxication and synaptic transmission

Based on experimental results it was calculated that a 2 - 5-fold increase of ammonia in brain is sufficient to disturb the major excitatory (glutamate), and inhibitory neuronal systems (GABA, glycine), and to produce widespread enhanced neuronal excitability, and to initiate the encephalopathy related to acute ammonia intoxication (67). In view of the possibility that chronic exposure to ammonia may produce long-term changes in the activity of large populations of neurons, it seems likely that gradually progressing pathogenetic mechanisms are initiated even at brain ammonia levels only slightly above physiological concentrations.

5.2. Reduced glucose utilization

The reduced utilization of glucose with concomitantly decreased rates of energy metabolism is one of the most conspicuous findings in experimental and disease-related hyperammonemic states (66,68). Analogous observations have been made in DAT: In PET studies cerebral glucose utilization was predominantly reduced in the parietal cortex, in agreement with morphological abnormalities (69-71). Overall cerebral glucose utilization was diminished by about 50 %, with normal oxygen consumption in early onset (72), but reduced oxygen consumption in late onset DAT (73). The impairment of brain energy metabolism in DAT, and of enzymes involved in energy metabolism was the topic of several investigations (e.g. see ref. 74-76).

5.3. Impairment of astroglia function and excitotoxicity

Astrocytic alterations, characterised as "Alzheimer type II gliosis", are invariable characteristic histopathological consequence of sustained hyperammonemia, both in experimental animals (77), and in patients with hepatic encephalopathy (78). Frederickson (27) summarised observations supporting the idea that reactive astrocytosis may mediate neuropathologic events of DAT, including the facilitation of extracellular depositions of β-AP.

Astrocytic damage by ammonia is followed by a decrease of glutamate synthetase activity, as was evidenced from the reduction of the activity of this enzyme by 15 % in rats with portacaval shunts (79). However, this decrease in synthetase activity may cause further damage to astrocytes. It is well established that glutamine synthetase is critically involved in the regulation of intracellular ammonia and acid-base balance. Any derangement of the function of this enzyme will be followed by the amplification of ammonia toxicity. Therefore, it is not surprising that an increased intracellular pH, and swelling of astrocytes was observed in hyperammonemic rats (80).

Presumably the most conspicuous difference between the amino acid patterns of cirrhotic (48) and DAT patients (57) is the several-fold increase of glutamine in all brain regions of cirrhotics, but unchanged concentrations of this amino acid in the brains of DAT patients. Likewise, no increase of glutamine was detected in the CSF of patients with DAT (81), whereas the level of this amino acid was elevated in the CSF of rats with portal-systemic encephalopathy (82). These finding suggest the inability of the brains of DAT patients to enhance glutamine formation above a certain level. They may be taken as an indication for the sensitivity of DAT brains even to a small increase in the rate of ammonia formation.

Due to the loss of glutamatergic neurons the concentrations of glutamate in the brains of DAT patients are lower than in age-matched controls (57), but CSF levels of glutamate are elevated, both in DAT (81) and in portal systemic encephalopathy (82). The elevation of extracellular glutamate has been demonstrated in shunted rats by microdialysis experiments (83). It is a major effect of ammonia-induced astrocytosis, and most probably due to the impairment of glutamate uptake by the functionally compromised astrocytes. In view of its excitotoxic properties, neuronal degeneration is the logical consequence of chronically enhanced extracellular glutamic acid concentrations. Based on other considerations several authors suggested glutamate-induced excitotoxicity as potenetial pathogenetic mechanism in DAT (27,36,37). Excitotoxic mechanisms in the pathogenesis of DAT are attractive, since they are able to explain symptoms of cortical disconnection (e.g. aphasia) and memory dysfunction.

From the key observations reported in the preceeding sections the scenario schematized in Fig. 4 appears evident. Damage of glutamine synthetase (and of other proteins) e.g. by oxygen free radicals, or the impairment of astroglia function by toxins would provoke the reduction of the capacity of the brain to detoxify ammonia. This, in turn initiates positive feed-back mechanisms wich result in progressive astrocytosis and accumulation of ammonia, impairment of energy metabolism and disturbance of synaptic functions. Impairment of astrocyte function favors the accumulation of extracellular glutamate, which may initiate neuronal damage mediated by glutamate receptors.

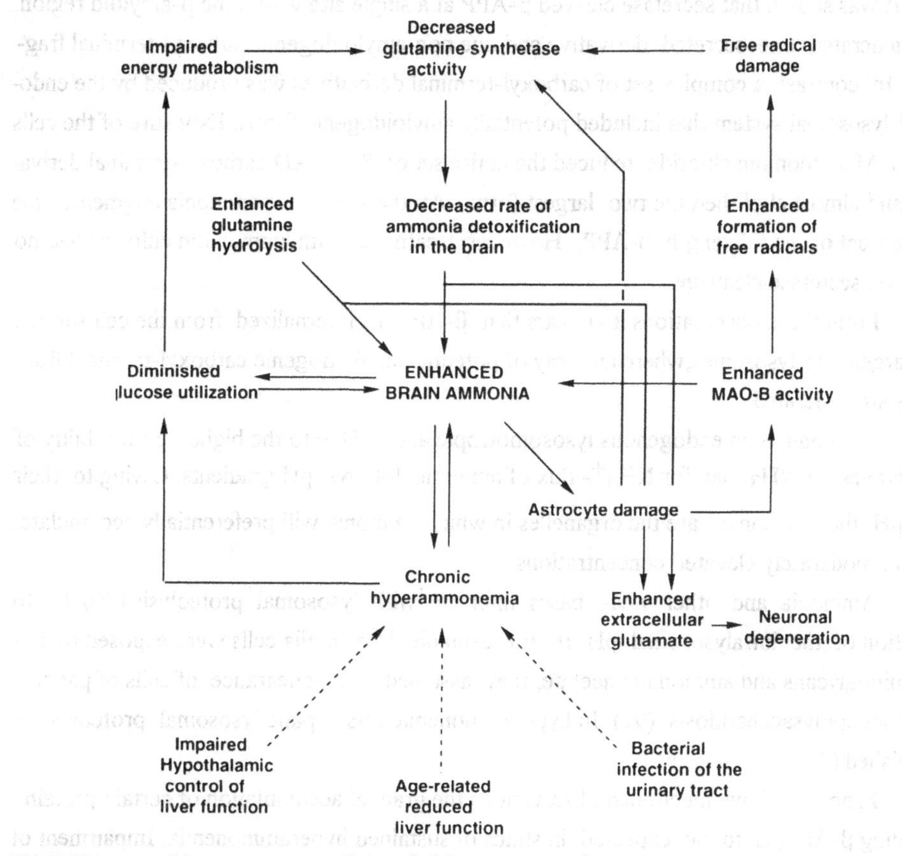

Fig. 4. Some possible consequences of chronic hyperammonemia.
Positive feedback regulatory cycles are induced in states of enhanced brain ammonia concentrations, which may lead to progressive functional impairment of astroglia function and to neuronal damage by excitotoxic mechanisms.

Reduction of glucose utilization is a possible primary event in DAT (72). The decrease in brain energy supply is assumed to initiate analogous vicious circles, as have been suggested to be consequential to the impairment of ammonia detoxification (Fig. 4)

5.4 Lysosomes, β-amyloid precursor protein, and ammonia

The opinion concerning the importance of lysosomes in the processing of βAPP has repeatedly changed in the past; nevertheless, several lines of evidence are in favor of a role of the endosomal - lysosomal system in the pathogenesis of DAT:

(a) β-APP was localized in lysosomes (84-86).

(b) Lysosomal proteinase antigens are prominently localized with senile plaques (87).

(c) The degradation but not the secretion of β-APP by PC12 cells was impaired by inhibitors of lysosomal function (e.g. by ammonium chloride and chloroquine) (85,88).

(d) Golde et al. (89) generated deletion mutants of CEP4b cells which produced the normal set of carboxyl-terminal derivatives of β-APP, and shortened secreted derivatives were studied. It was shown that secretase cleaved β-APP at a single site within the β-amyloid region, and generated one secreted derivative and one non-amyloidogenic carboxyl-terminal fragment. In contrast, a complex set of carboxyl-terminal derivatives was produced by the endosomal-lysosomal system that included potentially amyloidogenic forms. Exposure of the cells to 50 mM ammonium chloride reduced the entire set of 8 - 12 kD carboxyl-terminal derivatives and almost abolished the two largest forms. At the same time ammonia augmented the cell content of the full length β-APP. However, treatment with ammonium chloride had no effect on secretase cleavage.

From these observations it appears that β-APP is internalized from the cell surface and targeted to lysosomes,where an array of potential amyloidogenic carboxyl-terminal fragments are generated.

Ammonia is an endogenous lysosomotropic agent. Due to the higher permeability of membranes for NH_3 than for NH_4^+- flux of ammonia follows pH gradients. Owing to their low pH the lysosomes are the organelles in which ammonia will preferentially accumulate, even at moderately elevated concentrations.

Ammonia and other weak bases interfere with lysosomal proteolysis (90) due to elevation of the intralysosomal pH. If, for example, human glia cells were exposed to glycosaminoglycans and ammonium acetate, they assumed the appearance of cells of patients with mucopolysaccharidosis (91). In hyperammonemic rats hepatic lysosomal proteolysis is diminished (92).

From the above mentioned observations the gradual accumulation of certain proteins, including β-APP, is to be expected in states of sustained hyperammonemia. Impairment of lysosomal proteolysis does not imply that hydrolysis of all proteins is equally affected since both, activation and inhibition of lysosomal hydrolases may occur due to ammonia-induced changes of their environment.

The invasion of microglia into cortical and other brain areas with prevailing normal neuronal degeneration is a potential source of lysosomal components of senile plaques (93). The enhancement of the activity of a lysosomal enzyme in those areas of DAT brains which exhibited pre-mortem reduced glucose utilization has been demonstrated by post-mortem determination of β-glucuronidase (69). In this connection it is also worth mentioning that the proteolysis of MAP-2, a protein controlling together with Tau protein the polymerization of microtubules, was enhanced in rats with severe hyperammonemia (94).

Ammonia, is known to release lysosomal enzymes from cells (95,96). In DAT brains different classes of lysosomal enzymes have been localized in extra-lysosomal compartments (e.g. in the perikarya and proximal dendrites of many cortical neurons, and in senile plaques) (97-99). It was recently shown (100,101) that in the presence of ammonia, microglia cell lines reduce their phagocytic capacity. This may contribute to the accumulation of incompletely degraded cell constituents. In addition, the cytokine production of astroglioma and immortalized microglia cells was affected by ammonia in a complex manner. Among other observations the enhanced release of the inflammatory and chemotactic interleukin-8 (IL-8) was found (101). Since IL-8 is known to cause the release of lysosomal enzymes (102), its effect on cytokine production may be an important mechanism of the lysosomotropic effect of ammonia. Inflammatory proteins have been found in the brains of DAT patients (103) and anti-inflammatory agents have been envisaged several years ago as a potential therapeutic approach to Alzheimer disease (104).

6. POTENTIAL CONSEQUENCES OF ENHANCED BRAIN TRYPTOPHAN METABOLISM

The enhanced uptake and turnover of tryptophan in hepatic failure (105) was considered as a pathogenetic factor in hepatic encephalopathy (106). But hyperammonemia in the absence of any derangement of liver function also causes the enhancement of tryptophan up-take by the brain (107). The reports concerning the rate of tryptophan and serotonin metabolism in DAT are controversial. The following considerations may nevertheless be valid in view of the data which support a role of hyperammonemia in the pathogenesis of DAT.

Kynurenine is a toxic metabolite of tryptrophan. It is formed by oxidative cleavage of the pyrrole ring to N-formyl kynurenine, and enzymatic removal of the formyl residue. Quinolinic acid is formed from kynurenine. It is excitotoxic, similar to glutamate and kainic acid (108). Enhanced kynurenine concentrations in plasma, CSF and brains of hyperammonemic patients (with liver cirrhosis) have been recognized as a consequence of enhanced tryptophan levels (109). Increased quinolinic acid formation in brain seems not to be a direct consequence of enhanced kynurenine formation in brain. However, quinolinic acid concentrations were found to be elevated in the brains of aged rats (110). Therefore, they may be a consequence of enhanced quinolinic acid formation in liver, and increased uptake by the brain due to the age-related impairment of the blood-brain barrier (10).

Based on these informations, it is not difficult to imagine a scenario for aged subjects with chronic hyperammonemia, as is depicted in Fig. 4. In addition to excitotoxic damage generated by quinolinic acid and kynurenine, the impairment of lysosomal proteolysis by both, tryptophan and kynurenine (111) is a likely consequence of chronically elevated brain ammonia concentrations.

7. CONCLUSIONS

It has not been generally recognised that there is considerable evidence in favor of the idea that hyperammonemia may be a common feature of DAT. Although age-related reduction of liver function could contribute, the derangement of the physiological ammonia detoxification mechanisms in the brain, and the enhanced formation of ammonia in certain parts of the CNS are more likely causes of hyperammonemia in DAT.

Hepatogenic hyperammonemias differ considerably from DAT with respect to disease progression and symptoms. However, the derangement of astrocyte metabolism and astrocytosis, the decreased glucose utilization and energy metabolism, the enhanced formation and release of excitotoxic amino acids, and the presumptive derangement of neurotransmission of GABAergic, glycinergic and glutamatergic neurons, together with symptoms of cognitive impairment and memory defects are common to both diseases, and may hint at a common source: *ammonia.*

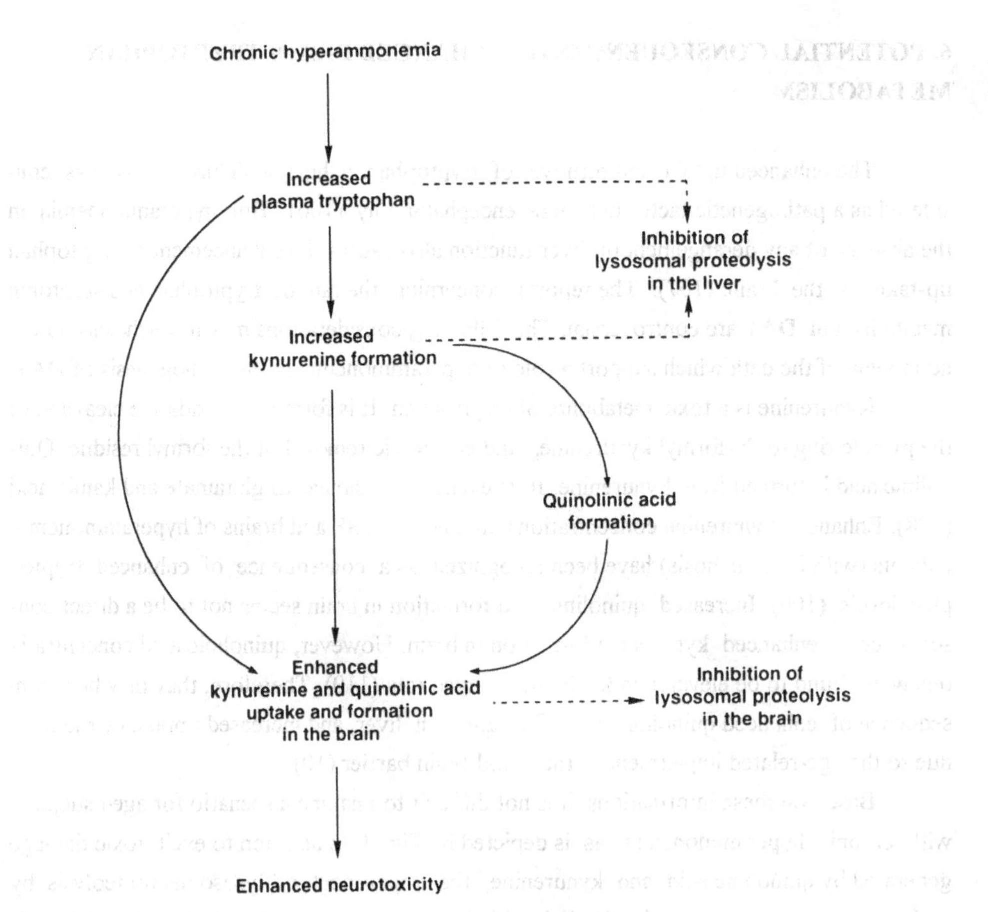

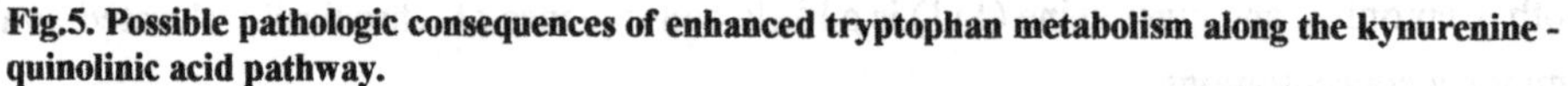

Fig.5. Possible pathologic consequences of enhanced tryptophan metabolism along the kynurenine - quinolinic acid pathway.

A major difference between brain-born hyperammonemia, as is suggested for DAT, and hyperammonemia generated by liver dysfunction, are differences in regional affection of the brain. Brain-born hyperammonemias are expected to be localized, although ammonia presumably spreads out from the foci of its excessive generation. Ammonia accumulating in brain from peripheral sources is expected to spread more or less over the entire brain according to vascularisation and physicochemical parameters which influence its distribution in the brain. Another difference is that in hyperammonemias generated by liver dysfunction, not only ammonia, but aliphatic amines, mercaptans and other toxins, which are generated in the gastrointestinal tract, enter the brain an contribute to the pathophysiology of the disease (49, 112).

Most probably ammonia is not a primary cause of DAT. However, the consequences of elevated brain ammonia concentrations have obvious implications in several of the major current hypotheses concerning the etiology of DAT: β-amyloid formation, excitotoxic neuronal damage, astrocyte dysfunction, and impairment of glucose utilization. Moreover, effects of ammonia on microglia function and lysosomal enzymes may contribute to the pathologic accumulation of abnormal materials. Therefore, it seems likely that ammonia is a cause of manifestations and progression of DAT.

Considerable efforts are presently put on the identification of targets which may allow the development of symptomatic and preventive therapies. In the light of the arguments presented in this overview, the amelioration or prevention of hyperammonemia seems a worth-while target. Inhibition of ornithine aminotransferase has been shown to enhance ammonia detoxification in experimental animals with acute or chronic hyperammonemias. A suitable non-toxic inactivator of ornithine aminotransferase, (S,S)-5-(fluoromethyl)ornithine, is at our disposal (113); it awaits clinical testing.

In order to avoid overinterpretation of the scarce data available at present on hyperammonemic states in DAT, no attempt was made in this review to connect hyperammonemia to selective vulnerability of cholinergic or other neurons, or to cognitive or behavioral abnormalities in DAT. If the role of ammonia in the pathophysiologic manifestations of DAT will have attracted more general attention, it can be expected that refined and specifically designed experiments will soon provide answers to those open quenstion that are needed to allow one to draw a more detailed and more precise picture of the role that ammonia appears to play in the etilogy of DAT.

8. REFERENCES

1. Jarvik,L.F., Ruth,V. and Matsuyama,S.S. 1980, Organic brain syndrome and aging. A 6 year follow-up of surviving twins. Arch. Gen. Psychiatry **37**: 280-286.
2. Heston,L.L. and White,J. 1980, A family study of Alzheimer disease and senile dementia; an interim report. In *Psychopathology in the Aged* (Cole,J.O and Barrett,J.E. Eds.) Raven Press, New York, pp 63-72
3. St. George-Hyslop,P.H., Tanzi,R.E., Polinski,R.J., Haines,J.L., Nee,L., Watkins,P.C., Myers,R.H., Feldman,R.G., Pollen,D., Drachman,D., Growdon,J., Bruni,A., Foncin,J.F., Salmon,D., Frommet,P., Amaducci,L., Sorbi,S., Piacentini,S., Stewart,G.D., Hobbs,W.J., Coneally,P.M. and Gusella,J.F. 1987, The genetic defect causing familial Alzheimer's disease maps on chromosome 21. Science **235**: 885-890.
4. Boyes,B.E., Walker,D.G., McGeer,P.L., and McGeer,E.G. 1992, Identification and characterization of a large human brain gene whose expression is increased in Alzheimer disease. Mol. Brain Res. **12**: 47-57.

5. Selkoe,D.J. 1991, The molecular pathology of Alzheimer's disease. Neuron **6**: 487-498.
6. Delaere,P., Duyckaerts,C., Brion,J.T., Poulain,V. and Hauw,J.J. 1989, Tau, paired helical filaments and amyloid in the neocortex: A morphometric study of 15 cases with graded intellectual status in aging and senile dementia of Alzheimer type. Acta Neuropathol. **77**: 645-653.
7. Terry,R.D., Masliah,E., Salmon,D.P., Butters,N., De Theresa,R., Hill,R., Hausen, L.A. and Katzman,R. 1991, Physical basis of cognitive alterations in Alzheimer's disease: synaptic loss is the major correlate of cognitive impairment. Ann. Neurol. **30**: 572-580.
8. Lassmann,H., Fischer,P. and Jellinger,K. 1993, Synaptic pathology of Alzheimer's disease. In *Amyloid Precursor Proteins, Signal Transduction and Neural Transplantation*. Proc. 7th Meeting of the Intern. Study Group on the Pharmacology of Memory Disorders Associated with Aging, pp 41-47.
9. Henderson,A.S. 1988, The risk factors of Alzheimer's disease: a review and an hypothesis. Acta Psychiatr. Scand. **78**: 257-275.
10. Alafuzoff,I., Adolfsson,R., Grundke-Iqbal,I. and Winblad,B. 1987, Blood-brain barrier in Alzheimer's dementia and in non-demented elderly. An immunocytochemical study. Acta Neuropathol. **73**: 160-166.
11. Miklossy,J. 1993, Alzheimer's disease, a spirochetosis? Neuro Report **4**: 841-848.
12. Harman,D. 1984, Free radical theory of aging: The "free radical" diseases. Age **7**: 111-131.
13. Jeandel,C., Nicolas,M.B., Dubois,F., Nabet-Belleville,F., Penin,F. and Cuny,G. 1989, Lipid peroxidation and free-radical scavengers in Alzheimer's disease. Gerontology **35**: 275-282.
14. Volicer,L. and Crino,P.B. 1990, Involvement of free radicals in dementia of the Alzheimer type: an hypothesis. Neurobiol. Aging **11**: 567-571.
15. Crowther,R.A. 1993, Tau protein and paired helical filaments of Alzheimer's disease. Current Opinion Struct. Biol. **3**: 202-206.
16. Fowler,C.J., Cowburn,R.F. and O'Neill,C. 1992, Brain signal transduction distrubances in neurodegenerative disorders. Cell. Signal. **4**: 1-9.
17. Christensen,H., Maltby,N., Jorm,A.F., Creasey,H. and Broe,G.A. 1992, Cholinergic "blockade" as a model of the cognitive deficits in Alzheimer's disease. Brain **115**: 1681-1699.
18. Davies,P. and Maloney,A.J.R. 1976, Selective loss of central cholinergic neurons in Alzheimer's disease. Lancet ii 1403.
19. Benton,J.S., Bowen,D.M., Allen,S.J., Haan,E.A., Davison,A.N., Neary,D., Murphy,R.P. and Snowden,J.S. 1982, Alzheimer's disease as a disorder of isodendritic care. Lancet ii 456.

20. McGeer,P.L., McGeer,E.G., Suzuki,J., Dolman,C.E. and Nagai,T. 1984, Aging, Alzheimer disease and the cholinergic system of the basal forebrain. Neurology **34**: 741-745.

21. Palmer,A.M. and Dekosky,S.T. 1993, Monoamine neurons in aging and Alzheimer disease. J. Neural Transm. **91**: 135-139.

22. Giacobini,E. 1991, Nicotinic cholinergic receptors in human brain: effects of aging and Alzheimer. Adv. Exp. Med. Biol. **296**: 303-315.

23. De Keyser,J. 1992, Loss of high-affinity agonist receptor binding in Alzheimer's disease. Ann. Neurol. 31: 231-232.

24. Greenamyre,J.T. and Maragos,W.G. 1993, Neurotransmitter receptors in Alzheimer disease. Cerebrovasc. Brain Metab. Rev. **5**: 61-94.

25. Blin,J., Baron,J.C., Dubois,B., Crouzel,C., Fiorelli,M., Attar-Levy,D., Pillon,B., Fournier,D., Vidailhet,M. and Agid,Y. 1993, Loss of brain 5HT-2 receptors in Alzheimer's disease. Brain **11**: 497-510.

26. Joyce,J.N., Kaeger,C.,Ryoo,H. and Goldsmith,S. 1993, Dopamine D2 receptors in the hippocampus and amygdala in Alzheimer's disease. Neurosci. Lett. **154**: 171-174.

27. Frederickson,R.C.A. 1992, Astroglia in Alzheimer's disease Neurobiol. Aging **13**: 239-253.

28. McGeer,P.L., Kawamata,T., Walker,D.G., Akiyama,H., Tooyama,I. and McGeer,E.G. 1993, Microglia in degenerative and neurological disease. Canad. Sci. Neurol. **16**: 511-515.

29. Hefti,F. and Schneider,L.S. 1991, Nerve growth factor in Alzheimer's disease. Clin. Neuropharmacol. **14**, Suppl. 1, S62-S76.

30. Vandenbeele,P. and Fiers,W. 1991, Is amyloidogenesis during Alzheimer's disease due to IL-1/Il-6 - mediated acute phase response in the brain? Immunol. Today **12**: 217-219.

31. Markesbury,W.R., Ehmann,W.D., Hossain,T.I.M., Alauddin,M. and Goodin,D.T. 1981, Instrumental neutron activation analysis of brain aluminum in Alzheimer disease and aging. Ann. Neurol. **10**: 511-516.

32. Thompson,C.M., Markesbery,W.R., Ehmann,W.D., Mao,Y.X. and Vance,D.E. 1988, Regional brain trace element studies in Alzheimer's disease. Neurotoxicology **9**: 1-8.

33. Deloncle,R. and Guillard,O. 1990, Mechanism of Alzheimer's disease: Arguments for a neurotransmitter-aluminium complex implication. Neurochem. Res. **15**: 1239-1245.

34. Good,P.F., Perl,D.P., Bierer,L.M. and Schmeidler,J. 1992, Selective accumulation ofaluminum and iron in the neurofibrillary tangles of Alzheimer's disease: a laser microprobe (LAMMA) study. Ann. Neurol. **31**: 286-292.

35. Evans,P.H., Klinowski,J., Yano,E. and Urano,N. 1989, Alzheimer's disease: a pathogenetic role for aluminium silicate-induced phagocytic free radicals. Free Rad. Res. Commun. **6**: 317-321.

36. Maragos,W.F., Greenamyre,T., Penney,Jr. J.B. and Young,A.B. 1987, Glutamate dysfunction in Alzheimer's disease, an hypothesis. TINS **10**: 65-68.

37. Lawlor,B.A. and Davis,K.L. 1992, Does modulation of glutamatergic function represent a viable therapeutic strategy in Alzheimer's disease? Biol. Psychiatry **31**: 337-350.

38. Hardy,J. and Allsop,D. 1991, Amyloid deposition as the central event in the aetiology of Alzheimer's disease. TIPS **12**: 383-388.

39. Pike,C.J., Burdick,D., Walencewicz,A.J., Glabe,C.G. and Cotman,C.W. 1993, Neurodegeneration induced by β-amyloid peptides in vitro: The role of peptide assembly state. J. Neurosci. **13**: 1676-1687.

40. Gorenstein,C. 1987, A hypothesis concerning the role of endogenous colchicin-like factors in the etiology of Alzheimer's disease. Med. Hypotheses **23**: 371-374.

41. Seiler,N. 1993, Is ammonia a pathogenetic factor in Alzheimer's disease? Neurochem. Res. **18**: 235-245.

42. Prusiner,S.D. 1984, Some speculations about prions, amyloid and Alzheimer's disease. N. Engl. J. Med. **310**: 661-663.

43. Cooper,A.J.L. and Plum, F. (1987) Biochemistry and physiology of brain ammonia. Physiol. Rev. **67**: 440-519.

44. Fisman,M., Ball,M. and Blume,W. 1989, Hyperammonemia and Alzheimer's disease. J. Am. Ger. Soc. **37**: 1102.

45. Fisman,M., Gordon,B., Felcki,V., Helmes,E., Appell,J. and Rabhern,K. 1985, Hyperammonemia in Alzheimer's disease. Am. J. Psychiatry **142**: 71-73.

46. Branconnier,R.J., Dessain,E.C., McNiff,M.E. and Cole,J.O. 1986, Blood ammonia and Alzheimer disease. Am. J. Psychiatry **143**: 1313.

47. Hoyer,S., Nitsch,R. and Oesterreich,K. 1990, Ammonia is endogenously generated in the brain in the presence of presumed and verified dementia of Alzheimer type. Neurosci. Lett. **117**: 358-368.

48. Butterworth,R.F., Giguere,J.F., Michaud,J., Lavoie,J. and Pomier-Layrargues,G. 1987, Ammonia: Key factor in the pathogenesis of hepatic encephalopathy. Neurochem. Pathol. **6**: 1-12.

49. Zieve,L. 1987, Pathogenesis of hepatic encephalopathy. Metabolic Brain Dis. **2**: 147-165.

50. Weil-Malherbe,H. and Drysdale,A.C. 1957, Ammonia formation in brain. III. Role of protein amide groups and of hexosamines. J. Neurochem. **1**: 250-257.

51. Kvamme,E. 1983, Ammonia metabolism in the CNS. Progr. Neurobiol. **20**: 109-132.

52. Faff-Michalak,L. and Albrecht,J. 1993, Hyperammonemia and hepatic encephalopathy stimulate rat cerebral synaptic mitochondrial glutamate dehydrogenase activity specifically in the direction of glutamate oxidation. Brain Res. **618**: 299-302.
53. Smith,C.D., Carney,J.M., Starke-Reed,P.E., Oliver,C.N., Stadtman,E.R., Floyd,R.A. and Markesbery,W.R. 1991, Excess brain protein oxidation and enzyme dysfunction in normal aging and in Alzheimer disease. Proc. Natl. Acad. Sci. USA **88**: 10540-10543.
54. Le Prince,G., Delaere,P., Fages,C., Lefrancois,T., Touret,M. and Tardy,M. 1995, Glutamine synthetase (GS) expression is reduced in senile dementia of the Alzheimer Type. Neurochem. Res. **20**: 859-862.
55. Procter,A.W., Palmer,A.M., Francis,T.D., Low,S.L., Neary,D., Murphey,E., Doshi, R. and Bowen,D.M. 1988, Evidence of glutamatergic denervation and possible abnormal metabolism in Alzheimer's disease. J. Neurochem. **50**: 790-802.
56. Wallace,D.R. and Dawson,Jr. R. 1992, Ammonia regulation of phosphate-activated glutaminase displays regional variation and impairment in the brain af aged rats. Neurochem. Res. **17**: 1113-1122
57. Carney,J.M., Starke-Reed,P.E., Oliver,C.N., Landeem,R.W., Cheng,M.S., Wu,J.F. and Floyd,R.A. 1991, Reversal of age-related increase in brain protein oxidation, decrease in enzyme activity, and loss in temporal and spatial memory by chronic administration of the spin-trapping compound N-tert.butyl-α-phenylnitrone. Proc. Natl. Acad. Sci. USA 88: 3633-3636..
58. Oliver,C.N., Starke-Reed,P.E., Stadtman,E.R., Liu,G.J., Carney,J.M. and Floyd,R.A. 1990, Oxidative damage to brain proteins, loss of glutamine synthetase activity and production of free radicals during ischemia/reperfusion-induced injury to gerbil brain. Proc. Natl. Acad. Sci. USA **87**: 5144-5147.
59. Adolfsson,R., Gottfries,C.G., Oreland,L. and Winblad,B. 1980, Increased activity of brain and platelet monoamine oxidase in dementia of Alzheimer type. Life Sci. **27**: 1029-1034.
60. Rainikainen,K.J., Paljärvi,L., Halonen,T., Malminen,O., Kosma,V.M., Laakso,M. and Riekkinen,P.J. 1988, Dopaminergic system and monoamine oxidase B activity in Alzheimer's disease. Neurobiol. Aging **9**: 245-252.
61. Nakamura,S., Kawamata,T., Akiguchi,I., Kamayama,M., Nakamura,N. and Kimura, H. 1990, Expression of monoamine oxidase B activity in astrocytes of senile plaques. Acta Neuropathol. **80**: 419-425.
62. Mangoni,A., Grassi,M.P., Frattola,L., Piolti,R., Bassi,S., Motta,A., Marcone,A. and Smirne,C. 1991, Effect of an MAO B inhibitor in the treatment of Alzheimer disease. Eur. Neurol. **31**: 100-107.
63. Li,X.M., Juorio,A.V. and Boulton,A.A. 1995, Some new mechanisms underlying the actions of (-)deprenyl: possible relevance to neurodegeneration. Progr. Brain Res. **106**: 99-112.

64. Raabe, W.A. and Onstad,G.A. 1982, Ammonia and methionine sulfoximine intoxication. Brain Res. **242**: 291-298.

65. Yamamoto,T., Iwasaki,K., Sato,Y., Yamamoto,H. and Konno,H. 1989, Astrocytic pathology of methionine sulfoximine-induced encephalopathy. Acta Neuropathol. **77**, 357-368.

66. Jessy,J., Mans,A.M., De Joseph,R.M., and Hawkins,A. 1990, Hyperammonemia causes many of the changes found after portacaval shunting. Biochem. J. **272**, 311-317.

67. Raabe,W.A. 1987, Synaptic transmission in ammonia intoxication. Neurochem. Pathol. **6**: 145-166.

68. Lockwood,A.H., Yap,E.W.G. and Wong,W.H. 1991, Cerebral ammonia metabolism in patients with severe liver disease and minimal hepatic encephalopathy. J. Cerebral Blood Flow Metab. **11**: 337-341.

69. McGeer,E.G., McGeer,P.L., Akiyama,H. and Harrop,R. 1989, Cortical glutaminase and glucose utilization in Alzheimer's disease. J. Canad. Sci. Neurol. **16**: 511-515.

70. Foster,N.L., Chase,T.N., Mansi,L., Brooks,R., Fedio,P., Patronas,N.J. and Dichiro, G. 1984, Cortical abnormalities in Alzheimer's disease. Ann. Neurol. **16**: 649-654.

71. Fukuyama,H. Harada,K., Yamauchi,H.,Miyoshi,T., Yamagushi,S., Kimura,J., Kameyama,M., Senda,M., Yonekura,Y. and Konishi,J. 1991, Coronal reconstruction images of glucose metabolism in Alzheimer's disease. J. Neurol. Sci. **106**: 128-134.

72. Hoyer,S. 1991, Abnormalities of glucose metabolism in Alzheimer's disease. Ann. N.Y. Acad. Sci. **640**: 53-58.

73. Frackowiak,R.S., Possili,C., Legg,N.J., Du Boulay,G.H., Marshall,J., Lenzi,G.L. and Jones,T. 1981, Regional cerebral oxygen supply and utilization in dementia. A clinical and physiological study with oxygen-15 and positron tomography. Brain **104**: 753-778.

74. Heiss,W.D., Szelies,B., Kessler,J. and Herholz,K. 1991, Abnormalities of energy metabolism in Alzheimer's disease studied with PET. Ann. N.Y. Acad. Sci. **640**: 65-71.

75. Parker,Jr.W.D., 1991, Cytochrome oxidase deficiency in Alzheimer's disease. Ann. N.Y. Acad. Sci. USA **640**: 59-64.

76. Liguri,G., Taddei,N.,Nassi,P., Matorraca,S., Nediani,C. and Sorbi,S. 1990, Changes in Na^{+},K^{+}-ATPase, Ca^{2+}-ATPase and some soluble enzymes related to energy metabolism in brains of patients with Alzheimer's disease. Neurosci. Lett. **112**: 338-342.

77. Gibson,G.E., Zimber,A., Krook,L., Richardson,E.P. and Visek,W.J. 1974, Brain histology and behavior of mice injected with urease. J. Neuropathol. Exp. Neurol. **33**: 201-211.

78. Martin,H., Voss,K., Hufnagl,P., Wack,R. and Wassilew,G. 1987, Morphometric and densitometric investigations of protoplasmic astrocytes and neurons in hepatic encephalopathy. Exp. Pathol. **32**: 198-237.

79. Butterworth,R.F., Girard,G. and Giguère,J.F. 1988, Regional differences in the capacity for ammonia removal by brain following portacaval anastomosis. J. Neurochem. **51**: 486-490.

80. Swain,M.S., Blei,A.T., Butterwortth,R.F. and Kraig,R.P. 1991, Intracellular pH rises and astrocytes swell after portacaval anastomosis in rats. Am; J. Physiol. **261** R1491-R1496.:

81. Pomara,N., Singh,R., Deptula,D., Chou,J.C.Y., Banay-Schwartz,M. and Le Witt, P.A. (1992) Glutamate and other CSF amino acids in Alzheimer's disease. Am. J. Psychiatry **149**: 251-254.

82. Therrien,G. and Butterworth,R.F. 1991, Cerebrospinal amino acids in relation to neurological status in experimental portal-systemic encephalopathy. Metabolic Brain Dis. **6**: 65-74.

83. Tossman,U., Delin,A., Eriksson,L.S. and Ungerstedt,U. 1987, Brain cortical amino acids measured by intracerebral dialysis in portacaval shunted rats. Neurochem. Res. **12**: 265-269.

84. Benowitz,L.I., Rodriguez,W., Paskevich,P., Mufson,E.J., Schenk,D. and Neve,R.L. 1989, The amyloid precursor protein is concentrated in neuronal lysosomes in normal and Alzheimer disease subjects. Exp. Neurol. **106**: 237-250.

85. Cole,G.M., Huynh,T.V. and Saitoh,T. 1989, Evidence for lysosomal processing of amyloid beta-protein precursor in cultured cells. Neurochem. Res. **14**: 933-939.

86. Kawai,M., Cras,P., Richey,P., Tabaton,M., Lowery,D.E., Gonzalez-deWitt,P.A., Greenberg,B.G., Gambetty,P. and Perry,G. 1992, Subcellular localization of amyloid precursor protein in senile plaques of Alzheimer's disease. Am. J. Pathol. **140**; 947-958.

87. Cataldo,A.M., Thayer,C.Y., Bird,E.D., Wheelock,T.R. and Nixon,R.A. 1990, Lysosomal proteinase antigens are prominently localized within senile plaues of Alzheimer's disease: evidence for a neuronal origin. Brain Res. **513**: 181-192.

88. Caporaso,G.L., Gandy,S.E., Buxbaum,J.D. and Greengard,P. 1992, Chloroquine inhibits intracellular degradation but not secretion of Alzheimer β–A4 amyloid precursor protein. Proc. Natl. Acad. Sci. USA **89**: 2252-2256.

89. Golde,T.E., Estus,S., Younkin,L.H., Selkoe,D.J. and Younkin,S.G. 1992, Processing of the amyloid precursor protein to potentially amyloidogenic derivatives. Science **255**: 728-730.

90. Segelen,P.O. 1983, Inhibitors of lysosomal function. Meth. Enzymol. **96**: 737-765.

91. Glimelius,B., Westermark,B. and Wasteson,A. 1977, Ammonium ion interferes with the lysosomal degradation of glycosaminoglycans in cultures of human glial cells. Exp. Cell Res. **107**: 201-217.

92. Felipo,V., Minana,M.D., Wallacer,R. and Grisolia,S. 1988, Long-term ingestion of ammonium inhibits lysosomal proteolysis in rat liver. FEBS Lett. **234**: 213-214.

93. Dickson,D.W., Farlo,J., Davies,P., Crystal,H., Fuld,P. and Yen,S.H. 1988, Alzhei-

mer's disease: a double-labeling immunohistochemical study of senile plaques. Am. J. Pathol. **132**: 86-101.

94. Felipo,V., Grau,E., Minana,M.D. and Grisolia,S. 1993, Ammonium injection induces N-methyl-D-aspartate receptor - mediated proteolysis of the microtubule-associated protein MAP-2. J. Neurochem. **60**: 1626-1630.

95. Tsuboi,M., Harasawa,K., Izawa,T., Komabayashi,T., Fujinami,H. and Suda,K. 1993, Intralysosomal pH and release of lysosomal enzymes in the rat liver after exhaustive exercise. J. Appl. Physiol. **74**: 1628-1634.

96. Leoni,P. and Dean,R.T. 1983, Mechanism of lysosomal enzyme secretion by human monocytes. Biochim. Biophys. Acta **762**: 378-389.

97. Cataldo,A.M. and Nixon,R.A. 1990, Enzymatically active lysosomal proteases are associated with amyloid deposits in Alzheimer brain. Proc. Natl. Acad. Sci. USA **87**: 3861-3865.

98. Cataldo,A.M., Paskevich,P.E., Kominami,E. and Nixon,R.A. 1991, Lysosomal hydrolases of different classes are abnormally distributed in brains of patients with Alzheimer disease. Proc. Natl. Acad. Sci. USA **88**: 10998-11002.

99. Nakamura,Y, Takeda,M., Suzuki,H., Hattori,H., Tada,K., Hariguchi,S., Hashimoto, S. and Nishimura,T. 1991, Abnormal distribution of cathepsins in the brain of patients with Alzheimer's disease. Neurosci. Lett. **130**: 195-198.

100. Atanassov,C.L., Muller,C.D., Sarhan,S., Knödgen,B., Rebel,G. and Seiler,N. 1994, Effect of ammonia on endocytosis, cytokine production and lysosomal enzyme activity of a microglial cell line. Res. Immunol. **145**: 277-288.

101. Atanassov,C.L., Muller,C.D., Dumont,S., Rebel,G., Poindron,P. and Seiler,N. 1995, Effect of ammonia on endocytosis and cytokine production by immortalized human microglia and astroglia cells. Neurochem Int. **27**: 417-424.

102. Mukaida,N., Harada,A., Yasumoto,K. and Matsushima,K. 1992, Properties of pro-inflammatory cell type-specific leukocyte chemotactic cyokines, interleukin-8 (IL-8) and monocyte chemotactic and activating factor (MCAF). Microbiol. Immunol. **36**: 773-789.

103. Berkenbosch,F., Biewenga,J., Brouns,M., Rozemuller,J.M., Strijbos,P. and Van Dam,A.M. 1992, Cytokines and inflammatory proteins in Alzheimer's disease. Res. Immunol. **143**: 657-663.

104. McGeer,P.L. and Rogers,J. 1992, Anti-inflammatory agents as a therapeutic approach to Alzheimer's disease. Neurology **42**: 447-448.

105. Curzon,G., Kantamaneni,B.D., Winch,J., Rochas-Bueno,A., Murray-Lyon,I.M. and Williams,R. 1973, Plasma and brain tryptophan changes in experimental acute hepatic failure. J. Neurochem. **21**: 137-145.

106. Record,C.O. 1991, Neurochemistry of hepatic encephalopathy. Gut **32**: 1261-1263.

107. Bachmann,C. and Colombo,J.P. 1983, Increased tryptophan uptake into the brain in hyperammonemia. Life Sci. **33**: 2417-2424.

108. Foster,A.C. and Schwarcz,R. 1989, Neurotoxic effects of quinolinic acid in the mammalian central nervous system. In *Quinolinic Acid and Kynurenines* (Stone, W. Ed.) CRC Press, Boca Raton, pp 173-192.

109. Kornhüber,J., Wichart,I., Riederer,P., Kleinberger,G. and Jellinger,K. 1989, Kynurenine in hepatic encephalopathy. *In Quinolinic acid and Kynurenines* (Stone,T.W. Ed.) CRC Press, Boca Raton, pp 275-281.

110. Moroni,F., Lombardi,G. and Carla,V. 1989, The measurement of quinolinic acid in the mammalian brain: Neuropharmacological and physiopathological studies. In *Quinolinic Acid and Kynurenines* (Stone,T.W. Ed.) CRC Press, Boca Raton, pp 53-62.

111. Grinde,B. 1989, Kynurenine and lysosomal proteolysis. In *Quinolinic Acid and Kynurenines* (Stone,T.W. Ed.) CRC Press, Boca Raton, pp 91-97.

112. Uribe,M. 1989, Nutrition, diet and hepatic encephalopathy. In *Hepatic Encephalopathy: Pathophysiology and Treatment* (Butterworth,R.F. and Pomier Layrargues, Eds.) Humana Press, Clifton, pp. 529-547.

113. Seiler,N. 1997, Ornithine aminotransferase as a therapeutic target in hyperammonemias. This volume.

LIVING RELATED LIVER TRANSPLANTATION

James B. Piper

Westchester County Medical Center
Macy Pavilion
Valhalla, New York 10595

Since 1988, there has been a rapid increase in both the number of centers performing liver transplantation and the number of patients being transplanted, with more than 2000 recipients receiving livers in 120 centers last year in the United States.[1] This dramatic increase is in large part due to the improving results seen following liver transplantation, and has resulted in a tripling of the number of patients on the waiting list. Despite this increase in demand, the number of cadaveric donors has remained stagnant over a similar time period.[2] Consequently, there has been an increasing organ donor shortage with an alarming increase in the number of patients dying while awaiting transplantation. Unfortunately no adequate solutions have been identified which could potentially eliminate this severe shortage of donor organs.

The pediatric population has historically been the most disadvantaged in competing for the limited number of organs available. This is because of the disparity between the epidemiology of liver disease and the conditions causing brain death in children. According to national health statistics data, 55% of the children born with liver disease will die before their second birthday if not transplanted.[3] Full size liver transplants can only be used in recipients who are within 20–30% of the donor's weight and unfortunately the pediatric population produces very few organ donors. These factors historically have resulted in higher pre–transplant mortality rates in children than were seen in adult patients (Table 1).[4] This shortage prompted many surgeons to develop mechanisms by which small children could be transplanted utilizing organs from larger livers.

The surgical reduction of cadaveric grafts for use in children was first reported in 1984 by Bismuth and Broelsch.[5,6] This technique rapidly proliferated throughout the world and resulted in a dramatic decrease in the pre–transplant mortality rate for children, compared with centers not utilizing this technique (Table 1).[4] Critics of this procedure argued that graft reduction simply redistributed organs that would otherwise be utilized in larger individuals, suggesting that this would lead to a further increase in the organ donor shortage for adults. Reduced size liver transplants were also considered to be 'experimental' and less effective than full size grafts. This assumption was later proven inaccurate, as children less than one year of age have been shown to

Table 1. Waiting list mortality rates

Center	Year	Mortality
Pittsburgh	1981–1984	55/216 (25%)
Hannover	1982–1984	25/85 (30%)
Los Angeles	1984–1987	9/45 (20%)
Colorado	1981–1987	9/33 (27%)
Pittsburgh	1987–1989	16/113 (14%)
Los Angeles	1984–1989	18/84 (17%)
Chicago	1986–1989	2/164 (2%)

have improved survivals using reduced size techniques compared to children receiving full sized organs and older children's survivals appear to be similar whether a reduced size or full size graft is used.[7] With increased experience in this technique, reduced size liver transplantation has now become the standard of care at most major pediatric liver transplant centers world wide.[8,12]

Split liver transplant, the surgical division of a cadaveric graft with the transplantation of both sides, was first performed by Pichlmeyer in Germany and Bismuth in Paris in 1988.[13,14] The first large series of split liver transplants was reported by Broelsch at The University of Chicago in 1989 and then again by Emond in 1990.[15] Split liver transplantation was exciting, as this was the first operation ever performed that created new organs that otherwise would not have been available for transplantation. If successful, split liver transplantation could help alleviate the increasing organ donor shortage. Unfortunately, our experience at The University of Chicago, encompassing forty–two cases, concluded that graft and patient survivals were lower than similar control groups receiving full and reduced size grafts. Of great concenr was that these decreased survivals appeared to be persistent throughout the entire series and did not improve with technical advances.[16] Split liver transplantation did serve a crucial role however, in proving that two livers could be obtained from a single organ, thus paving the way for living donor liver transplantation.

The technical feasibility of living donor liver transplantation was first described by Smith in 1969,[17] but it was not for almost another twenty years until the first attempt at human transplantation was reported by Raia in Brazil.[18] Although both of the recipients died from apparent medical complications, further supporting the technical feasibility of this exciting new procedure. Strong in Australia was the first to report a successful transplant using the left lobe of the child's mother.[19] Broelsch, at The University of Chicago, was the first to report a full series of living donor liver transplants, where 22 grafts were transplanted into 20 recipients.[20] The overall patient and graft survivals of this first series, 80% and 70%, were similar to that of other pediatric cadaveric series. In a follow–up study from The University of Chicago, the techniques of living donor liver transplantation had been refined and a 94% one year patient survival was reported.[21] In Japan, cadaveric transplantation is nonexistant because of Japan's lack of brain death laws. Due to Japan's unique needs, Tanaka established a program at Kyoto University which has now become the largest living donor transplant experience in the world, with survival statistics similar to that seen in the recent University of Chicago series.[22]

Donor Evaluation

The donor pool consists of healthy adults over the age of 18 years who are ABO compatible with the recipient. In the initial 20 cases only first degree relatives were considered to be suitable donors. Once living donor liver transplantation was accepted by our institution as the standard of care, distant relatives and even unrelated individuals have been evaluated and utilized as living donors. After a potentially suitable donor is identified, a thorough medical evaluation is performed by an independent physician who ensures that the potential donor has no medical illnesses or liver disease that would increase the surgical risk, or produce a sub optimal graft. All patients undergo blood testing which includes serum chemistries and serologic testing to ensure the absence of any transmittable viral illnesses. Evaluation of the cardiovascular system and a psychosocial assessment are obtained. In the initial twenty cases, the protocol mandated all potential donors to undergo a psychiatric evaluation. A two week consent process was also required initially to ensure that the potential donor, and their families, fully comprehended the risks and benefits of the surgical procedure, and were aware of all alternative treatment options. Following the completion of the first twenty transplants, the evaluation process was modified, the two week consent process was eliminated which allowed even those children who were in urgent need of liver transplantation to benefit from this exciting new procedure. The mandatory psychiatric evaluation was also eliminated, but was offered to any potential donor whom the independent physician, social worker, patient or patient's family felt it may benefit.

After the successful completion of the medical and psychosocial evaluation, an assessment of the graft is performed. Computed tomographic evaluation of the abdomen is obtained in order to rule out any lesions of the hepatic parenchyma which might produce a sub-optimal graft or place the potential donor at undue risk. Steatosis, a condition that would yield an unacceptable graft, can often be diagnosed by the computed tomography scan. A volumetric analysis of the segments to be removed was performed in our early series in order to judge the appropriateness of the graft size to the recipient's needs. We no longer require volumetric analysis, as it rarely supplied information that would result in the elimination of a potential donor. Small grafts have been shown to rapidly regenerate[23] and larger grafts undergo apoptosis[24] to achieve the correct size requirements of the recipient. Apoptosis takes days to weeks, so the recipients of larger grafts often can not be primarily closed because the deleterious effects of increased intra abdominal pressure on the perfusion of the new graft and on peak airway pressures. The University of Chicago has recently published the use of temporary PTFE abdominal wall patches in order to normalize intra abdominal pressure during this time of apoptosis of the transplanted graft.[25]

Hepatic arteriography continues to be required in our center, as well as many other centers which perform living donor liver transplant. Angiography is used to identify the blood supply to the liver segments to be removed and to ensure that no vascular anomalies exist that would place the child at a higher risk of post transplant arterial complications. Some authors have suggested that with the use of current microsurgical techniques, angiography is no longer required since all anomalous vasculature can be adequately reconstructed.[26] Although we concur that most anomalies can be reconstructed with the use of the microscope, we continue to perform arteriography in all donors and use it to guide the dissection of the arterial trunks in the donor operation.

Liver biopsy remains a controversial test in the donor evaluation process. The University of Chicago currently requires that potential male donors with abnormal liver function studies and all women undergo liver biopsy. The rationale for requiring all women to undergo liver biopsy is that this is the population where steatosis is most commonly identified. There have been at least four patients in two centers (unpublished data) where patients have been found to have unacceptable grafts secondary to steatosis only after the donor operation was initiated. Retrospective review of the CT scans failed to show any evidence of steatosis, raising concern about the accuracy of CT scans in identifing this condition. Cholangiography is not routinely necessaryin all donors. In selective cases, where the recipient has Alagiels syndrome, we will require a potential donor who is a first degree relative to undergo cholangiography to insure that a sub clinical form of the disease is not present within the graft.

Surgical Technique

The surgical technique has been described thoroughly in several publications.[20,27] The procedure has had only minor revisions since its inception, and we will briefly describe the current technique which is shown in Figure 1.

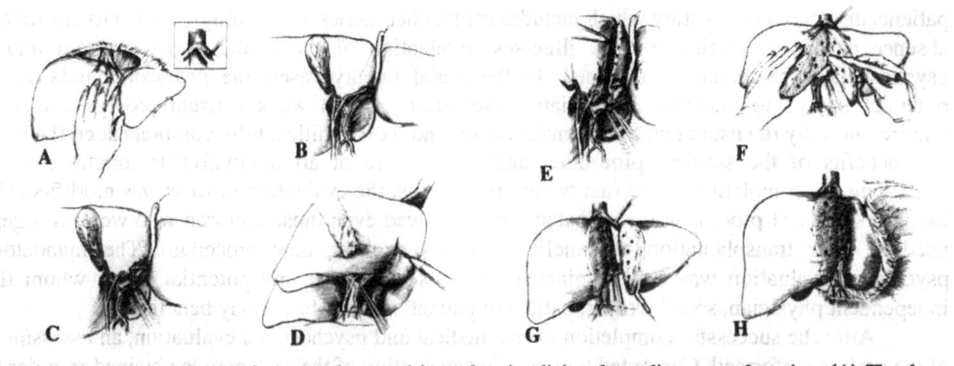

Figure 1. **Overview of the surgical procedure used in performing living donor liver transplantation. (A) The donor liver is mobilized revealing the left hepatic vein, which is encircled. (B) The hilum is exposed and (C) the left hepatic artery and the left branch of the portal vein are mobilized. The bile duct is divided. (D) The capsule over the umbilical fissure is opened and (E) is extended to the line of division to the right of the falciform ligament. (F) The parenchymal division is continued, achieving homeostasis with suture ligatures. (G) The vascular pedicles are clamped and the graft is removed. (H) The vascular pedicles are repaired and final homeostasis is achieved.**

A subcostal incision with a midline extension is used to expose the liver. The falciform and left triangular ligaments are taken down exposing the left and middle hepatic veins. The vein(s) feeding the segments to be removed is encircled with a vessel loop (Figure 1A). The peritoneum surrounding the porta hepatis is opened exposing the left hepatic artery (Figure 1B). Just posterior to this, the portal vein is identified and all small branches leading to the caudate lobe are individually ligated. The bile duct is divided close to the common bile duct bifurcation so that a single bile duct anastomosis is likely in the recipient (Figure 1C). If a left lateral segment graft is to be obtained, the round ligament is retracted to the left and all the vascular and biliary structures entering segment 4 are individually divided. If a full left lobe graft is required, these structures are left intact. The left lateral segment is retracted medially and the capsule overlying the umbilical fissure is opened to the level of the left hepatic vein (Figure 1D). If a full left lobe graft is to be performed, intraoperative ultrasound is used to identify the course of the middle hepatic vein, which is included within the graft. For a left lateral segment graft, the parenchymal dissection proceeds just to the right of the falciform ligament achieving hemostasis utilizing ligature and mattress sutures (Figure 1E, 1F). After completion of the parenchymal dissection, the vessels are clamped and divided (Figure 1G). The graft is removed and immediately flushed with the heparinized preservation solution on the back table, first via the portal vein and finally via the hepatic artery. The vascular pedicles of the donor are then repaired, ensuring that no stenosis are created in the vasculature that remains in the donor (Figure 1H). A segment of saphenous vein is harvested from the thigh in all cases, it can be used as a vascular extension graft if this is required in the recipient.

Donor Complications

The development of reduced size liver transplantation has greatly reduced the organ donor shortage for small children by redistributing organs from larger cadaveric donors. Because of this reduction in pretransplant mortality, some have questioned whether it is ethical to place a healthy adult at risk in order to supply a graft for transplantation. Living donor liver transplantation has consistently produced results that are equal, or superior, to cadaveric grafts.[20,22] Living donors also create new grafts that would otherwise be unavailable for transplantation, helping to alleviate the organ donor shortage. It has been the position of The University of Chicago that living donor liver transplantation should be utilized routinely as long as donors are not placed in an unacceptably

Table 2. Major complications

Splenectomy
3 bile leaks
Bile duct injury
Brachial plexus injury
Bleeding gastric ulcer
Hepatic artery thrombosis
Gastric outlet obstruction

high risk. Internationally, there have been more than five hundred living donor hepatectomies performed, with only one reported death.[28]

Removing the left lateral segment along with its vascular pedicles places both segments 1 and 4 at a theoretical risk of ischemia. Some authors still recommend removing these segments at the completion of the procedure to prevent abscess formation.[27] Most of the patients in our series had evidence of ischemia of segment 1, but none of these patients developed complications that could be attributed to necrosis of this segment. Segment 4 rarely looks ischemic at the completion of the procedure, and we do not believe that segment 4 ischemia has significantly contributed to any of the complications we have seen.

The first three donors at our institution all underwent full left lobectomies that were then surgically reduced to left lateral segmentectomies prior to implantation, because of the concern for the blood supply to segment 4. All of these donors had complications which were considered major. The first patient required a splenectomy for a retractor injury and the next two patients both developed bile leaks, one of which required a reoperation. In the subsequent donors left lateral segmentectomies were performed, unless more parenchyma was needed to meet the recipients' needs. After the revision of the procedure, only 7% of the patients developed complications that were considered major and 7% developed complications that were considered minor. The complications are summarized in Tables 2 and 3. Bile leaks that required reoperation were considered major, and those requiring percutaneous drainage were considered minor. All bile leaks were from the cut edge of the liver, none were from injuries of the common or right hepatic ducts. The only bile duct injury in our series was recognized at the time of donor hepatectomy and was repaired with a Roux-en-Y choledochojejunostomy. One patient developed an hepatic artery thrombosis after dual arteries to the left lateral segment were removed on a common patch and the arteriotomy was repaired primarily. Thrombectomy and vein patch angioplasty was used to reestablish arterial flow to the right lobe. A patient with a gastric ulcer had been using high doses of non-steroidal anti-inflammatory drugs, and required a Graham patch to repair anterior gastric perforation. The only donor to have a lasting disability suffered a brachial plexus injury from positioning the arm at the time of surgery.

Five donors developed either transient or near complete gastric outlet obstructions. Four of these donors had left hepatic arteries arising from left gastric arteries, suggesting that in the process of dissecting this common arterial variant, a partial vagotomy may result. It should be noted that not everyone with replaced left hepatic arteries developed gastric outlet obstruction, as this arterial anomoly was found in 19 of the 100 donors.

Table 3. Minor complications

2 Bile leaks
Seroma
Lymphocele
4 transient gastric outlet obstructions

Table 4. Indications for liver transplantation in children

	University of Chicago	National
Biliary Atresia	61%	55%
Metabolic	9%	13%
Fulminant	7%	11%
Other Cirrhosis	5%	7%
Bylers disease	3%	-
Cholestatic	2%	2%
Malignancy	1%	2%
Other	13%	10%

Recipients

Biliary atresia remains the most common indication for liver transplantation at our institution, as well as the nation. Because of our interest in primary familial intrahepatic cholestasis (Byler's disease), we have transplanted a surprising large population with this rare disorder. Table 4 lists the indications for primary liver transplant at our institution and the nation.

Recipient Procedure

The recipient operation is similar to the implantation of a reduced size cadaveric liver. The vena cava is preserved and the right hepatic and all short hepatic veins are oversewn. The confluence of the middle and left hepatic vein are opened and this is extended down the vena cava in order to make a large triangulated opening for the anastomosis (Figure 2). The hepatic vein of the graft is then cut down the segment 3 branch to create a similar triangulated opening for the anastomosis. The hepatic vein anastomosis is then created insuring that the inferior–most aspect of the vena cava is anastomosed through the inferior most aspect of the cut going down the segment 3 hepatic vein branch. This rotates the graft to the right to insure that there will be adequate outflow from the graft. The portal vein anastomosis is then performed. In the early series, portal vein conduits were used, which will be discussed in a later section. Our current technique is that of opening the confluence of the right or left hepatic vein and doing a direct portal vein anastomosis to the graft (Figure 3). The graft is reperfused, prior to the arterial anastamosis. Whenever possible, a direct anastomosis to the recipient hepatic artery is performed in an end–to–end fashion using the aid of a surgical microscope. If the recipient hepatic artery is deemed unsuitable for an

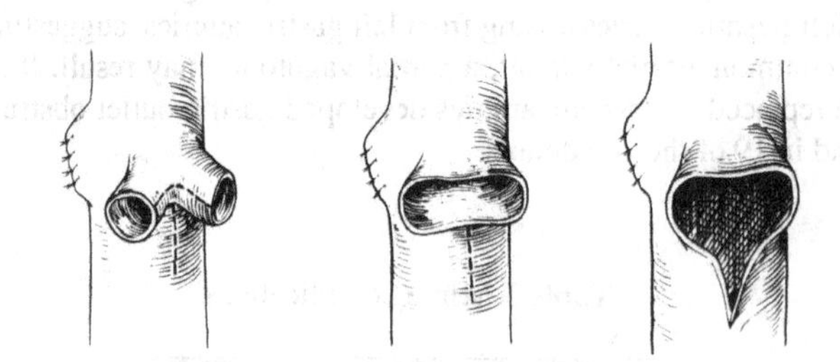

Figure 2. The recipient vena cava is left intact. The right hepatic vein is oversewn and the confluence of the left and middle hepatic veins are opened. The new orifice is spatulated inferiorly to create a large triangulated orifice for the hepatic vein anastamosis.

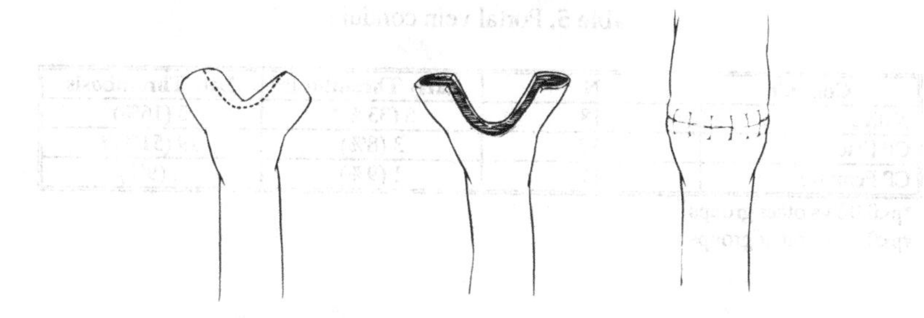

Figure 3. The recipient portal vein is opened between the right and left branches, which leads to extra length and a large anastomosis free of strictures

anastomosis, then the previously procured donor saphenous vein is used as a conduit to the supraceliac aorta. The biliary anastomosis is performed to a Roux-en-Y jejunal conduit. By transecting the donor's left hepatic bile duct farther to the right in the donor operation, a single biliary anastomosis can now usually be performed.

Portal Vein Conduits

Living donor liver transplantation, as initially described by Broelsch, resulted in the graft rotating approximately 45 degrees into the right upper quadrant. This required an extension of the portal vein of the recipient in order to allow for this rotation. There are no easily accessible vessels that can be obtained from the donor which would be a good size match for the recipient's portal vein. In order to accomplish this vein extension, the inferior mesenteric vein or saphenous vein was procured and reconstructed as shown in Figure 4A.

This resulted in a conduit that had twice the diameter and half the length. This group of patients had a 33% early thrombosis rate which was significantly greater than a matched series of cadaveric grafts. In order to provide a better conduit, iliac veins were procured from cadaveric donors and cryopreserved. When the cryopreserved veins were utilized, the early thrombosis rate decreased to 8%. Iliac veins from adult donors were not good size matches for pediatric recipients, so these veins often required down-sizing as shown in Figure 4B. Femoral veins from adult donors are a much better size match for a pediatric recipient, so the next series utilized cryopreserved femoral veins. After we had converted to cryopreserved femoral vein conduits, we noticed a concerning finding in the cryopreserved iliac vein population. The late incidence of portal vein stenosis or thrombosis in this group was 51%, much higher than our cadaveric population. This raised a concern about whether the cryopreservation process resulted in a propensity for late strictures and resulting thrombosis. We stopped utilizing portal extension conduits unless

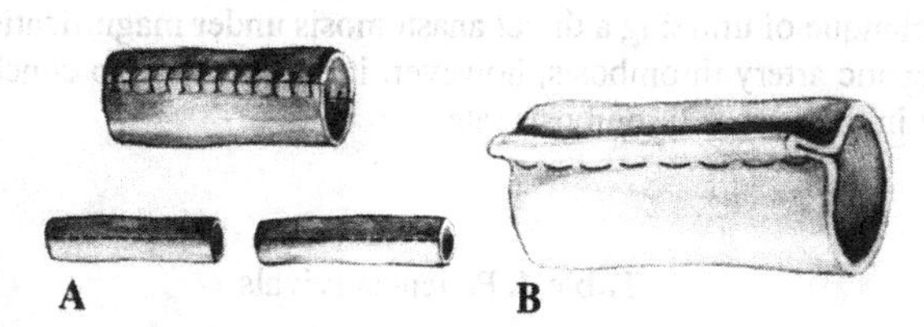

Figure 4. Portal vein conduits. (A) Saphenous or inferior mesenteric vein which are opened and sewn together to create a conduit of larger diameter. (B) A cryopreserved iliac vein which has required downsizing to create an appropriate sized conduit.

Table 5. Portal vein conduits

Conduit	N	Early Thrombosis	Late Thrombosis
Native	18	6 (33%)*	3 (16%)
CP Iliac	37	3 (8%)	19 (51%)#
CP Femoral	11	1 (9%)	1 (9%)

*p<0.02 vs other groups
#p<0.02 vs other groups

absolutely necessary, and in the population where it was deemed necessary, recipient internal jugular vein was obtained and utilized for the conduit. With further follow–up it became clear that the cryopreserved femoral veins did not have the same problem with late portal vein stenosis that was seen in the cryopreserved iliac vein population, suggesting that it was not the cryopreservation that resulted in the late strictures. Table 5 summarizes our data from The University of Chicago. It is our current recommendation that, when ever possible, no conduit should be utilized. If a conduit is necessary, recipient internal jugular vein or cryopreserved femoral vein should be used.

Table 6. Rejection episodes

	Cadaver	LRD
Number	59	40
Survival	73%	90%
Rejection	41 (69%)	28 (70%)
Resistant	21 (36%)	5 (13%)*
Rejection	–	–

*P<0.05

Arterial Thrombosis

Since the initial series published at The University of Chicago, arterial thrombosis has been the leading cause of graft loss in our living donor transplant series. Historically, we had always reconstructed the hepatic artery utilizing saphenous vein conduits so that an anastomosis could be made to the recipient hepatic artery at the level of the gastroduodenal artery, or taken to the supraceliac aorta. Utilizing this technique, we have seen arterial thrombosis rates of 16%, a rate not statistically different from our overall pediatric population. The Kyoto group has reported excellent results using a direct microsurgical anastomosis between the graft hepatic artery and the recipient hepatic artery, which has led to an overall risk of arterial thrombosis of only 2.5%.[26,27] We have now adopted the technique of utilizing a direct anastomosis under magnification for our last twelve cases without an hepatic artery thrombosis, however, it is premature to conclude this represents a significant decrease in the arterial thrombosis rate.

Table 7. Patient survivals

	Patient	No. Cases
University of Chicago	86%	100
Kyoto	85%	70
Nebraska	93%	14
Hamburg	78%	23
UCLA	90%	–

Rejection Episodes

We had initially hoped that there would be an immunologic benefit in transplanting liver allografts from closely related individuals, even though this phenomenon had never been demonstrated in retrospective cadaveric series. Despite our early optimism, we showed that if there was a benefit of genetic matching, it played only a minimal role in outcomes following liver transplantation. A group a living donor liver transplant recipients were compared to a group of cadaveric recipients from the same time period at The University of Chicag and the incidence of rejection was similar in both groups. We did show that the severity of the rejection episodes, as measured by steroid resistance, was less in the living donor group. [29] The initial twenty living donor transplants, during the period living donor liver transplants were considered experimental, were excluded from this study, and all patients had a minimum of a one year follow up. The results are summarized in Table 6.

Patient and Graft Survival

As discussed previously, there has been an evolution of the living donor transplantation procedure, culminating in the current operation which is similar in most institutions. Because of the benefit gained from the technical descriptions described in the first series published by Broelsch, most recent series show patient survivals of greater than the 85%. The current survival rates at The University of Chicago show a patient survival of 86%, and a graft survival of 72% at one year. Table 7 summarizes an overview of the published experience.

Living Donor Transplant in Older Recipients

Most living donor liver transplants have been performed in a pediatric population where small children receive left lateral segment grafts. Larger children, and even adults, have been successfully transplanted by obtaining more hepatic parenchyma from the donor, utilizing either a left hepatic lobe or a right hepatic lobe grafts. If living donor transplantation can be safely expanded so that large children and adults could be transplanted utilizing this modality, this could have a major impact on the organ donor shortage. When we look at our own series, 16 patients five years of age or older have been transplanted using living donor left lobe grafts, with a graft and patient survival of 75% and 43%. The graft losses were seen early after transplantation from vascular thromboses. It is too early to speculate on the etiology of this increase in graft loss, but it causes enough concern to mandate caution whenever larger children are to be transplanted. As mentioned previously, another alternative which could supply increased amounts of liver parenchyma, is transplantation of the right lobe. This has been reported by two separate centers with mixed results. Because of the implications living donor liver transplantation could have on the adult population, further study is warranted, but only by groups that have extensive experience in pediatric living donor transplantation.

References

1. UNOS Update, May/June, 1996.
2. United Network for Organ Sharing 1993 annual report of the US Scientific Registry of Transplant Recipients and the organ procurement and transplantation network--transplant date: 1988–1991. Bethesda, MD, Division of Organ Transplantation, Bureau of Health Resources Development, Health Resources and Services Administration, U.S. Department of Health and Human Services, 1993.
3. National Health Statistics, 1988.
4. Piper J, Whitington PF, Woodle ES, et al: Pediatric liver transplantation at the University of Chicago Hospitals. Terasaki P (ed.), Clinical Transplants 1992. Los Angeles, CA: UCLA Tissue Typing Laboratory.
5. Bismuth H, Houssin C: Reduced size orthotopic liver graft in hepatic transplantation in children. Surgery 95:367–370, 1984.
6. Broelsch CE, Neuhas P, Burdelski M, et al: Orthotopic transplantation of hepatic segments in infants with biliary aytresia. In: Kosloski L, (ed.), Chirurgisches Forum '84f. Experim u. Klinische Forschung Hrsg. Berlin/Heidelberg, Springer, 1984.

7. So SKS, Concepcion W, Cox K, et al: Factors affecting survival after orthotopic liver transplantation (OLT) in infants. Presented at the American Society of Transplant Physicians 14th Annual Meeting, Chicago, IL, 1995.
8. Ryckman FC, Flake AW, Fisher RA, et al: Segmental orthotopic hepatic transplantation as a means to improve patient survival and diminish waiting-list mortality. J Pediatr Surg 26:422–428, 1991.
9. Otte JB, de Ville de Goyet J, Sokal E, et al: Size reduction of the donor liver is a safe way to alleviate the shortage of size-matched organs in pediatric liver transplantation. Ann Surg 211:146–157, 1990.
10. Houssin D, Couinaud C, Boillot O, et al: Controlled hepatic bipartition for transplantation in children. Br J Surg 78:75–80, 1991.
11. Kalayouglu M, D'Alessandro AM, Sollinger HW, et al: Experience with reduced-size liver transplantation. Surg Gynecol Obstet 171:139–147, 1990.
12. Cox K, Nakazato P, Berquist W, et al: Liver transplantation in infants weighing less than 10 kilograms. Transplant Proc 23:1579–1580, 1991.
13. Pichlmayr R, Ringe B, Gubernatis G, et al: Transplantation einer Spenderleber auf Zwei Empfanger (Split liver transplantation): Eine neue Methode in der Weiterentwicklung der Lebersegmenttransplantatione. Langenbecks Arch Chir 373:127–130, 1989.
14. Bismuth H, Morino M, Castaing D, et al: Emergency orthotopic liver transplantation in two patients using one donor liver. Br J Surg 76:722–724, 1989.
15. Emond JC, Whitington PF, Thistlethwaite JR, et al: Transplantation of two patients with one liver: Analysis of a preliminary experience with 'split liver' grafting. Ann Surg 212:14–22, 1990.
16. Emond JC, Heffron TG, Thistlethwaite JR Jr, et al: Innovative approaches to donor scarcity: A critical comparison between split liver and living related liver transplantation. Hepatology 14:92A, 1991.
17. Smith B: Segmental liver transplantation from a living donor. J Pediatr Surg 4:126–132, 1969.
18. Raia S, Nery JR, Mies S: Liver transplantation from liver donors. Lancet ii:497, 1988.
19. Strong RW, Lynch SV, Ong TN, et al: Successful liver transplantation from a living donor to her son. N Engl J Med 322:1505–1507, 1990.
20. Broelsch CE, Whitington PF, Emond JC, et al: Liver transplantation in children from living related donors. Ann Surg 214:428–439, 1992.
21. Emond JC, Heffron TG, Kortz EO, et al: Improved results of living-related liver transplantation with routine application in a pediatric program. Transplantation 55:835–840, 1993.
22. Tokunaga Y, Tanaka K, Uemoto S, et al: Risk factors and complications in living related liver transplantation. Transplant Proc 30:140–144, 1994.
23. Emond JC, Xia RC: Reduced-size liver transplants (RLT) provide evidence of host regulation of hepatic regeneration. Gastroenterology 100:A739, 1991.
24. Oberhammer F, Bursch W, Tiefenbacher R, et al: Apoptosis is induced by transforming growth factor-b1 within 5 hours in regressing liver without significant fragmentation of the DNA. Hepatology 18:1238–1247, 1993.
25. Seaman DS, Newell KA, Piper JB, et al: Use of polytetrafluoroethylene patch for temporary wound closure after pediatric liver transplantation. Transplantation 62:7, 1996.
26. Tanaka K, Uemoto S, Tokunaga Y, et al: Surgical techniques and innovations in living related liver transplantation. Ann Surg217:82–91, 1993.
27. Ozawa K: The Operative Process. In Ozawa, ed. Living Related DonorLiver Transplantation, Krager, 1994
28. Rogiers X, Schroeder T, Tuttlewski K, Broelsch CE: First report of the international living donor liver registry. Presented at the XVIth International Congress of the Transplantation Society meeting, Barcelona, Spain, 1996.
29. Alonso A, Piper J, Echols G, et al: Allograft rejection in pediatric recipients of living related liver transplants. Hepatology 23(1):40–44, 1996.

CONTRIBUTORS

APELQVIST, G.
Department of Clinical Pharmacology
Lund University Hoospital
S-221 85 Lund
Sweden

BASILE, A. S.
Laboratory of Neuroscience
NIDDK, National Institutes of Health
Bethesda, MD 20892
U.S.A.

BENDER, A. S.
Laboratory of Neuropathology
Department of Pathology
University of Miami
School of Medicine
P.O. Box 016960
Miami, FL 33101
U.S.A.

BENGTSSON, F.
Department of Clinical Pharmacology
Lund University Hoospital
S-221 85 Lund
Sweden

BERGQVIST, P. B. F.
Department of Clinical Pharmacology
Lund University Hoospital
S-221 85 Lund
Sweden

BLUML, S.
Magnetic Resonance Spectroscopy
Laboratory
Hungtington Medical Research Institute
Pasadena, CA 91105
U.S.A.

BUTTERWORTH, R. F.
Neuroscience Research Unit
André-Viallet Clinical Research Center
Hôpital Saint-Luc
Montreal, Quebec
H2X 3J4 Canada

CARLA, V.
Dipartimento di Farmacologia
Preclinica e Clinica
Universita di Firenze
50134 Firenze
Italia

CARPENEDO, R.
Dipartimento di Farmacologia
Preclinica e Clinica
Universita di Firenze
50134 Firenze
Italia

CHAMULEAU, R. A.
J. van Gool Laboratory of
Experimental Internal Medicine
Academic Medical Centre
1105 AZ Amsterdam
The Netherlands

CHIARUGI, A.
Dipartimento di Farmacologia
Preclinica e Clinica
Universita di Firenze
50134 Firenze
Italia

CUCARELLA, C.
Instituto de Investigaciones Citologicas
Fund. Valenciana Investig.Biomédicas
46010 Valencia
Spain

FELIPO, V.
Instituto de Investigaciones Citologicas
Fundación Valenciana de
Investigaciones Biomédicas
46010 Valencia
Spain

GALLI, A.
Dipartimento di Farmacologia
Preclinica e Clinica
Universita di Firenze
50134 Firenze
Italia

GRISOLIA, S.
Fundación Valenciana de
Estudios Avanzados
Valencia
Spain

HA, J. H.
Department of Pharmacology
Yeungnam University
School of Medicine
Taegu
Korea

HÄUSSINGER, D.
Abteilung Gastroenterologie
und Infectiologie
Heinrich Heine Universitat
40225 Düsseldorf
Germany

HERMENEGILDO, C.
Instituto de Investigaciones Citologicas
Fundación Valenciana de
Investigaciones Biomédicas
46010 Valencia
Spain

HORIUCHI, M.
Department of Biochemistry
Faculty of Medicine
Kagoshima University
Sakuragaoka 8-35-1
890 Kagoshima
Japan

IMAMURA, Y.
Department of Biochemistry
Faculty of Medicine
Kagoshima University
890 Kagoshima
Japan

ITZHAK, Y.
Laboratory of Neuropathology
Department of Pathology
University of Miami
School of Medicine
Miami, FL 33101
U.S.A.

JONES, E. A.
Department of Gastrointestinal and
Liver Diseases
Academic Medical Center
1105 AZ Amsterdam ZO
Netherlands

KANAMORI, K.
Magnetic Resonance Spectroscopy
Laboratory
Hungtington Medical Research Institute
Pasadena, CA 91105
U.S.A.

KNAUER, S.
Department of Anesthesiology
Johns Hopkins University
School of Medicine
Baltimore, MD.
U.S.A.

KNECHT, K.
Neuroscience Research Unit
André-Viallet Clinical Research Center
Hôpital Saint-Luc
Montreal, Quebec
H2X 3J4 Canada

KOBAYASHI, K.
Department of Biochemistry
Faculty of Medicine
Kagoshima University
890 Kagoshima
Japan

LLANSOLA, M.
Instituto de Investigaciones Citologicas
Fundación Valenciana de
Investigaciones Biomédicas
46010 Valencia
Spain

MANNAIONI, G.
Dipartimento di Farmacologia
Preclinica e Clinica
Universita di Firenze
50134 Firenze
Italia

MICHALAK, A.
Neuroscience Research Unit
André-Viallet Clinical Research Center
Hôpital Saint-Luc
Montreal, Quebec
H2X 3J4 Canada

MIÑANA, M. D.
Instituto de Investigaciones Citologicas
Fundación Valenciana de
Investigaciones Biomédicas
46010 Valencia
Spain

MONTOLIU, C.
Instituto de Investigaciones Citologicas
Fundación Valenciana de
Investigaciones Biomédicas
46010 Valencia
Spain

MOODY, E.
Department of Anesthesiology
Johns Hopkins University
School of Medicine
Baltimore, MD.
U.S.A.

MORONI, F.
Dipartimento di Farmacologia
Preclinica e Clinica
Universita di Firenze
50134 Firenze
Italia

MUSA, D. A. A.
Department of Biochemistry
Faculty of Medicine
Kagoshima University
Sakuragaoka 8-35-1
890 Kagoshima
Japan

NORENBERG, M.
Laboratory of Neuropathology
Department of Pathology
University of Miami
School of Medicine
P.O. Box 016960
Miami, FL 33101
U.S.A.

O'DONOVAN, D. J.
Department of Physiology
University College
Galway
Ireland

PIPER, J.
University of Chigago
School of Medicine
Section of Transplantation
Department of Surgery(MC5027)
5841 South Maryland Avenue
Chicago, IL 60637
U.S.A.

QURESHI, I. A.
Division of Medical Genetics
Centre de Recherche
Hôpital Sainte-Justine
Université de Montreal
Montreal, Quebec
H3T 1C5 Canada

RAO, K. V. R.
Division of Medical Genetics
Centre de Recherche
Hôpital Sainte-Justine
Université de Montreal
Montreal, Quebec
H3T 1C5 Canada

RECORD, C.O.
Liver Unit
Royal Victoria Infirmary
University of Newcastle
Newcastle upon Tyne
NE1 4LP
United Kingdom

ROSS, B. D.
Magnetic Resonance Spectroscopy
Laboratory
Hungtington Medical Research Institute
Pasadena, CA 91105
U.S.A.

SAHEKI, T.
Department of Biochemistry
Faculty of Medicine
Kagoshima University
Sakuragaoka 8-35-1
890 Kagoshima
Japan

SCHLIESS, F.
Abteilung Gastroenterologie
und Infectiologie
Heinrich Heine Universitat
Moorenstrasse 5
40225 Düsseldorf
Germany

SCHOOLWERTH, A. C.
Division of Nephrology
Medical College of Virginia
POB 980160
Richmond, VA 23298
U.S.A.

SEILER, N.
Groupe de Recherche en
Therapeutique Anticancereuse
Laboratoire de Biologie Cellulaire
URA CNRS 1529
Faculté de Medicine
Université de Rennes 1
F-35043 Rennes Cedex
France

TOMOMURA, A.
Department of Biochemistry
Faculty of Medicine
Kagoshima University
890 Kagoshima
Japan

TOMOMURA, A.
Department of Biochemistry
Faculty of Medicine
Kagoshima University
890 Kagoshima
Japan

VOGELS, B. A. P. M.
J. van Gool Laboratory of
Experimental Internal Medicine
Academic Medical Centre
1105 AZ Amsterdam
The Netherlands

WARSKULAT, U.
Abteilung Gastroenterologie
und Infectiologie
Heinrich Heine Universitat
40225 Düsseldorf
Germany

INDEX

9780306455988